PSYCHIATRY

by T

PSYCHIATRY

by Ten Teachers

Edited By

Nisha Dogra BM DCH FRCPsych MA PhD
Senior Lecturer in Child and Adolescent Psychiatry,
The Greenwood Institute of Child Health,
University of Leicester

Brian Lunn MB ChB FRCPsych
Honorary Clinical Senior Lecturer,
Newcastle University

Stephen Cooper MD FRCPI FRCPsych
Professor of Psychiatry,
Queen's University Belfast

CRC Press
Taylor & Francis Group
Boca Raton London New York

CRC Press is an imprint of the
Taylor & Francis Group, an **informa** business

CRC Press
Taylor & Francis Group
6000 Broken Sound Parkway NW, Suite 300
Boca Raton, FL 33487-2742

© 2011 by Taylor & Francis Group, LLC
CRC Press is an imprint of Taylor & Francis Group, an Informa business

No claim to original U.S. Government works

Visit the Taylor & Francis Web site at
http://www.taylorandfrancis.com

and the CRC Press Web site at
http://www.crcpress.com

Contents

The Ten Teachers

Simon Budd *MBChB MMedSc FHEA*

Honorary Senior Lecturer in Psychiatry, University of Leeds

Ian Collings *MB BS DPM MRCPsych PGDME*

Specialist Registrar, Rehabilitation Psychiatry, Whitchurch Hospital, Cardiff Honorary Clinical Tutor, Cardiff University

Richard Day *MBChB BSc(MedSci) MRCPsych*

Clinical Senior Lecturer and Honorary Consultant Psychiatrist, Ninewells Hospital, University of Dundee

Nisha Dogra *BM DCH FRCPsych MA PhD*

Senior Lecturer in Child and Adolescent Psychiatry, The Greenwood Institute of Child Health, University of Leicester

Stephen Cooper *MD FRCPI FRCPsych*

Professor of Psychiatry, Queen's University Belfast

Ilana Crome *MA MPhil MB ChB MD FRCPsych*

Professor of Addiction Psychiatry and Academic Director of Psychiatry, Keele University and Consultant Addiction Psychiatrist, North Staffordshire Combined Healthcare NHS Trust, Stoke-on-Trent

John Eagles *MB ChB MPhil FRCPsych*

Consultant Psychiatrist, Royal Cornhill Hospital, Aberdeen

Brian Lunn *MB ChB FRCPsych*

Honorary Clinical Senior Lecturer, Newcastle University

Ciaran Mulholland *MB BCh BAO DMH MRCPsych MD*

Senior Lecturer and Consultant Psychiatrist, Queen's University Belfast

Howard Ring *BSc MBBS MD FRCPsych*

Lecturer, Department of Experimental Psychology, University of Cambridge

Preface

Most of those students reading this textbook will not become psychiatrists. However, as doctors, all of you, whether in your Foundation posts or later, will encounter patients with significant mental health problems and symptoms of psychiatric illnesses. In order to carry out your role as a doctor effectively you will require the necessary knowledge and skills. This book has been written to try to address the needs of all students, whatever their career intentions.

The book is largely based around the Core Curriculum devised as part of the editors' work for the Royal College of Psychiatrists' Scoping Group on Undergraduate Education. The 'core curriculum' arose from a consensus around this work.

In each subject we have tried to be explicit about why the area covered is relevant to you as a medical student and each chapter gives clinical examples to illustrate the points made. We have sought to avoid overloading you with details but have instead focused on essential information to help you meet the mental health needs of all patients.

In some chapters, for example 1, 3 and 4, you are asked to reflect on your own perspectives as we consider that many societal and professional attitudes towards those with mental illness need to be challenged. We hope you find that this book helps you to get as much as possible from your clinical placements and by the end feel confident that you could recognise and manage mental health problems when you qualify.

It is worth emphasising that no clinical placement will be successful unless you practice your skills and no book can substitute for spending time with patients. However, it is helpful to have a framework around which to organise your experience. Whilst this textbook is focused on the needs of all medical students, we would be delighted if using it during your placements makes you consider becoming a psychiatrist. We would be happy to receive any feedback and sincerely hope the book works as it is intended to.

Nisha Dogra
Brian Lunn
Stephen Cooper

Acknowledgements

We would like to thank all those that helped produce this text. Nisha would like to thank the following colleagues and medical students who reviewed various drafts at different stages:

Nick Brindle
Guy Brookes
Dr Melanie Hobbs
Akshay Kansagra
Dr Khalid Karim
Ruby Lekwauwa
Professor James Lindesay
Dr Pablo Ronzoni
Dr Daniel Smith
Dr Mark Steels
Professor Scott Weich

Thanks also to Jo Welch for her administrative support.

Abbreviations

BSE	Bovine spongiform encephalopathy
CAMHS	Child and Adolescent Mental Health Services
CPN	Community psychiatric nurse
CSF	Cerebrospinal fluid
CVD	Cardiovascular disease
EEG	Electroencephalography
FSH	Follicle-stimulating hormone
GABA-BDZ	Gamma-aminobutyric acid/ benzodiazepine
LH	Luteinizing hormone
MMN	Mismatch negativity
MRI	Magnetic resonance imaging
NMDA	N-Methyl-D-aspartic acid
OCD	Obsessive–compulsive disorder
PCP	Phencyclidine
PET	Positron emission tomography
PRN	*Pro re nata* – as needed
SPET	Single photon emission computed tomography

CHAPTER 1

DEFINING MENTAL HEALTH AND MENTAL ILLNESS

Nisha Dogra and Stephen Cooper

KEY CHAPTER FEATURES

- Discussion of the terminology around mental health, mental health problems and mental illness
- Outline of the scale of individual suffering from mental health problems and a public health dimension of the scale of the problems
- Define stigma, how it is perpetuated and its consequences on individuals and practice
- The evidence regarding which interventions may reduce stigma
- The steps you may need to take to reflect on your views and their impact on your practice

Introduction

In this chapter we define mental health, mental health problems and mental illness. This is important because, although it sounds fairly straightforward, our discussion will demonstrate the difficulties that abound with the terminology. The scale of the problem and access to services at a public health level are outlined. We then discuss stigma generally, explore the reasons for it and possible sequelae. We also review the interventions to reduce stigma before asking you to reflect on your own perspective and their potential impact on your future practice.

Defining mental health, mental illness and mental health problems

It is important to state at the outset that there is no widely agreed consensus on the meaning of these terms and their use. Many outside the health arena challenge the terms, and mental illness as a concept is widely challenged by the anti-psychiatry movement (which does include doctors). However, the reality

Exercise

On your own or with some peers answer the following questions? (You will get more from the exercise if you answer as honestly as you can.)

What is your own understanding of mental health, mental illness and mental health problems?

What sorts of problems do people experience that could be described as mental health problems or mental illness?

How can you tell if someone is experiencing mental health problems or mental illness?

How often do you use words that reflect on patients with mental health in a less than complimentary way?

How do you think you have formed your views on mental illness and what part might your cultural background have played in forming these views?

remains that if an individual experiences difficulties which impact on their emotional and inner worlds, their functioning can be affected. Mental health and mental illness can be viewed as two separate, yet related, issues.

Mental health

The World Health Organization (WHO) definition of health is: 'A state of complete physical, mental and social well-being, and not merely the absence of disease.' (www.who.int/topics/mental_health/en/) This is supported by the Royal College of Psychiatrists, who have argued that there is no health without mental health. The WHO adds:

Mental health is not just the absence of mental disorder. It is defined as a state of well-being in which every individual realizes his or her own potential, can cope with the normal stresses of life, can work productively and fruitfully, and is able to make a contribution to her or his community.

Another way of looking at this is that mental health includes how people look at themselves, their lives and the other people in their lives; how they feel about these different components, evaluate their challenges and problems; and how they explore choices. This includes handling stress, relating to other people and making decisions. However, even a cursory glance at the definition raises important questions as the concept is clearly rooted in societal norms and expectations. The way that the normal stresses of life are defined will vary from society to society and within subgroups. The contribution to the community is also societal and culturally based. Perhaps a useful way of viewing the definition in practice is that someone is considered as having mental health when they manage day-to-day living without too much difficulty in a way that satisfies them and fulfils familial and societal expectations of them without causing them undue stress. Immediately this alerts you to consider the plight of those who do not meet familial or societal expectations as they conflict with individual perspectives and the significant impact this can have on mental health (for example, consider being gay in countries in which homosexuality is illegal, or forced marriages). Culture and its influence on how mental health is understood are discussed later in this chapter.

Definitions of mental health relating specifically to children have been provided by several bodies and emphasize the expectations of a healthy child. So, a mentally healthy child is one who can for example:

- develop emotionally, creatively, intellectually and spiritually;
- initiate, develop and sustain mutually satisfying personal relationships;
- face problems, resolve them and learn from them.

This could easily apply to adults and in some ways is developmentally rather than culturally contextual, as these functions apply in whichever society the young person is living.

Mental health problems

The term 'mental health problems' is one that encompasses a range of experiences and situations. Mental health might usefully be viewed as a continuum of experience, from mental well-being through to a severe and enduring mental illness. Mental health problems cover a wide range of problems which affect someone's ability to get on with their daily life. Mental health problems can affect anyone, of any age and background, as well as having an impact on the people around them such as their family, friends and carers. Mental health problems result from a complex interaction of biological, social and psychological factors. Major life events such as bereavement, relationship break-up or serious illness can impact significantly on how we feel about ourselves and subsequently on our mental state and health. A minority of people may experience mental health problems to such a degree that they may be diagnosed as having a mental illness. Common mental health problems include anxiety (including phobias), obsessive compulsive disorders, adjustment disorders and milder mood problems.

Mental illness

A mental illness is an illness that causes disturbances in thinking, perception and behaviour beyond those that might be experienced even in an acutely distressed state. They can be severe, seriously interfering with a person's life, significantly impairing a person's ability to cope with life's ordinary demands and routines, and even causing a person to become disabled. The majority of people will not experience mental illness, but will undoubtedly experience mental health problems at different times in their lives.

Another common term is mental disorder, and this is often used in the sense that a person who is mentally ill is suffering from a mental disorder – the use is usually in the context of legislation. In practice most clinicians tend to use mental health problems for less serious disorders and mental illness for more severe disorders. A complicating factor is that subjective components are also relevant. A clinician may feel that the anxiety symptoms their patient has are fairly mild but for the patient the impact on their life may be significant. Some patients who are seriously mentally ill (for example someone who is manic or acutely psychotic) cannot understand why others think they are ill because from their perspective all is well.

In this book we use the term mental health problems as that is a widely used terminology, although specific disorders such as schizophrenia, depression and the like are defined as mental illness using the *International Classification of Disease* (WHO).

The classification of mental illness

The *International Classification of Diseases* (ICD) is the international standard diagnostic classification for all general epidemiological and many health management purposes, research and clinical use. It is used to classify diseases and other health problems recorded on many types of health and vital records such as death certificates. However the way that these diagnostic categories are used in practice varies across the world. The major categories for mental health and behavioural disorders are shown in Box 1.1. The ICD is revised periodically and is currently in its tenth edition with the eleventh edition being planned.

The *Diagnostic and Statistical Manual of Mental Disorders* (DSM) is published by the American Psychiatric Association and provides diagnostic criteria for mental disorders. It is used in the USA and in varying degrees elsewhere. There is some consistency between the two classification systems, especially for mental health. However, the DSM tends to use broader categories and is considered by some too inclusive in some of the disorders it includes. The multi-axial format used by the DSM can be helpful as shown in Box 1.2.

Both classification systems have their limitations but are useful in providing a common language for research and practice and both use the categorical approach as described below.

Entity or dimension?

Kendall and Zealley (1988) present the relative merits of using categories and dimensions with respect

---

Box 1.1: Multi-axial classification often used in child mental health services (ICD-10)

Axis 1 – Mental health diagnosis

Axis 2 – Developmental

Axis 3 – Intellectual

Axis 4 – Organic/physical

Axis 5 – Psychosocial

Mental and behavioural disorders (F00–F99)

F00–09   Organic, including symptomatic, mental disorders

F10–19   Mental and behavioural disorders due to psychoactive substance use

F20–29   Schizophrenia, schizotypal and delusional disorders

F30–39   Mood [affective] disorders

F40–48   Neurotic, stress-related and somatoform disorders

F50–59   Behavioural syndromes associated with physiological disturbances and physical factors

F60–69   Disorders of adult personality and behaviour

F70–79   Mental retardation

F80–89   Disorders of psychological development

F90–99   Behavioural and emotional disorders with onset usually occurring in childhood and adolescence

---

Box 1.2: Multi-axial system used in DSM

The DSM-IV organizes each psychiatric diagnosis into five levels (axes) relating to different aspects of disorder or disability.

- Axis I: clinical disorders, including major mental disorders, as well as developmental and learning disorders
- Axis II: underlying pervasive or personality conditions, as well as mental retardation
- Axis III: acute medical conditions and physical disorders
- Axis IV: psychosocial and environmental factors contributing to the disorder
- Axis V: Global Assessment of Functioning or Children's Global Assessment Scale for children and teens under the age of 18

Common Axis I disorders include depression, anxiety disorders, bipolar disorder, ADHD, phobias and schizophrenia.

Common Axis II disorders include personality disorders and mental retardation.

to mental illness. Typically, medicine has used categories, given its roots in the biological sciences. Categorization allows for easier definitions. It enables recognition of someone's symptoms conforming to a clinical concept. However, a dimensional approach allows for greater flexibility. They conclude that where psychotic illness is concerned then a categorical approach may be preferable, whereas in other conditions, the situation is more likely to be changeable, and perhaps benefit from a dimensional perspective. The categorical approach essentially allows the clinician to make a diagnosis based on the presence or absence of symptoms. There are two possibilities, either the patient has the disorder or not.

The difficulties with the categorical approach are that disorders may not present with the whole range of symptoms needed for a diagnosis to be made. However, the presence of those symptoms may still be sufficient to cause significant impairment. The dimensional approach allows for context and specific factors to be accounted for such as developmental stage and gender, among others.

With respect to emotions and behaviours it can be useful to ask when is a problem a problem, as people may have the same level of anxiety for example but be troubled by it to different extents. Pain is a common symptom in general medicine and may be a helpful analogy. So, we all experience some degree of anxiety but it is only likely to be viewed as a problem that needs help when it occurs frequently and/or is so severe that it interferes with everyday functioning. The symptom may also be identified as a problem when it begins to impact on those around the patient.

One way of distinguishing between distress associated with adverse life events and more severe disorders, which involve physiological symptoms and underlying biological changes, is to distinguish between mental health problems and mental illness, using a multidimensional model. This has an additional advantage in enabling normal 'distress' (e.g. grief following bereavement) to be recognized as part of the 'human condition', rather than being medicalized and possibly classed as 'depression'. It is suggested that a variety of normal human experiences have become medicalized through an ever increasing range of psychological disorders with virtually every type of behaviour eligible for a medical label (e.g. social phobia, over-eating disorder, dependent personality disorder).

Mental health: one of many factors

It is also important to recognize that neither physical nor mental health exists separately; mental, physical and social functioning are interdependent. Furthermore, all health issues need to be considered within a cultural and developmental context. The quality of a person's mental health is influenced by idiosyncratic individual factors and experiences, their family relationships and circumstances and the wider community in which they live. Additionally, each culture influences people's understanding of, and attitudes towards, mental health issues. However, a culture-specific approach to understanding and improving mental health can be unhelpful if it assumes homogeneity within cultures and ignores individual differences. Culture is only one, albeit an important, factor that influences individuals' beliefs and actions. It can be argued that the above are rooted in Western perspectives. However, they provide a useful starting point from which to discuss mental health issues.

Incongruence between personal values, familial and wider societal expectations can be a significant stressor especially for young people. People's cultural backgrounds can affect:

- the way they think about mental health and mental health problems;
- the way they make sense of certain symptoms and behaviours;
- the services they choose to accept;
- the treatment and management strategies they find acceptable;
- the way in which those who have mental health problems are perceived.

Some of these factors are mitigated by others, such as the level of education and personal experience.

Anti-psychiatry

This term was coined in the 1960s in response to a movement led by Laing and Szasz, who essentially questioned the validity of psychiatry and the use of diagnoses that they felt were subjective. Their perspective was that medical concepts were being inappropriately applied to normal human behaviour. There was also considerable opposition to the treatments applied. Since then, the 'movement' has had periods of greater visibility than at other times. Whatever one's perspectives about psychiatry, the suffering that many people experience cannot be dismissed. A major example of a criticism of psychiatry by the anti-psychiatry movement is that earlier versions of the classification systems included homosexuality as a disorder, which many now accept is not the case. However, psychiatry and indeed medicine are very much products of the various societal relationships, so it seems rather strange to single out some disorders over others and deny their existence. Just because we do not understand the aetiology of a disorder does not necessarily mean that the disorder does not exist. There is now a tendency to call anti-psychiatry critical psychiatry.

The scale of the problem

The prevalence of specific disorders will be covered in the chapters relating to those disorders. Here we will outline the scale of the problem in terms of broad figures and also the public health impact of mental illness. We use information provided by the WHO. The purpose is not to overwhelm you with figures but impress upon you that the scale of mental illnesses and the impact of these on individuals and society is not insignificant. Also, psychiatrists treat only a small proportion of those who have mental

health problems, with some treated in primary care, but the vast majority receiving no treatment at all. WHO has consistently argued that the economic and personal costs of mental illness are huge. For example, estimates made by the WHO in 2002 showed that 154 million people globally suffer from depression and 25 million people from schizophrenia; 91 million people are affected by alcohol use disorders and 15 million by drug use disorders (Fig. 1.1).

One in four patients visiting a health service has at least one mental, neurological or behavioural disorder, but most of these disorders are neither diagnosed nor treated. It is also important to note the high prevalence rates of mental illness in those suffering from chronic physical conditions such as cancer, heart and cardiovascular diseases, diabetes and HIV/AIDS. The mental illness can lead to non-compliance with prescribed medical regimens and poorer prognosis. Stress, depression and anxiety are common reasons for absenteeism from work but may often not be addressed as illness and may be hidden to prevent stigmatization.

An often cited figure by the WHO is that one in four people in the world will be affected by mental or neurological disorders at some point in their lives. Unfortunately, this does not emphasize that only a small minority will go on to have enduring and disabling illness. It is well established that mental and behavioural disorders have a large impact on

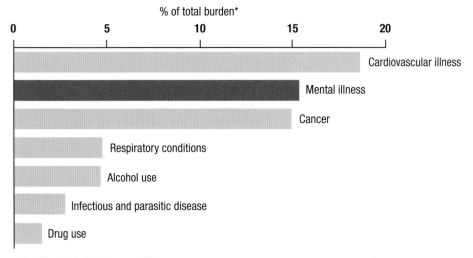

*Disability Adjusted Life Years (DALYs)

Figure 1.1   The burden of disease: established market economies (1990). Murray, C.L., Lopez, A.D. (eds) (1996) *The Global Burden of Disease*. Harvard University Press.

individuals, families and communities. Individuals suffer through the symptoms they experience but also because they may be unable to work when they are unwell and often suffer from discrimination even after they have recovered. There is an associated 'loss of productivity' with economic impact on individuals and society.

Families also bear the burden of mental illness in that they often provide support and care to family members who are mentally ill and also manage the negative impact of stigma and discrimination. The nature of mental illness often means that family relationships are also affected in addition to the stress caused by disturbed behaviour and disruption to normal family life. In many parts of the world the cost of treatment is borne by families and not the state. Costs resulting from mental illness can be viewed as direct (that is the costs related to providing care and treatment for the disorder) and indirect (costs related to loss of productivity in work, school and home).

A number of studies have reported on the quality of life of individuals with mental disorders, concluding that the negative impact is not only substantial but sustained. It has been shown that quality of life continues to be poor even after recovery from mental disorders as a result of social factors that include continued stigma and discrimination. The WHO considers that mental health provision was severely under-resourced in many countries because of stigma, apathy and neglect. Change may be happening but it is slow.

Another cost for those suffering with mental health problems is the negative impact of stigma. Before we discuss this, we highlight some common myths.

Myths about mental illness

Myths about mental illness abound across the world in all societies. The myths often seek to explain the cause of the behaviours exhibited as part of mental illness but also demonstrate the ignorance there is about mental illness. While myths persist, individuals with mental illness often delay seeking treatment or families fail to access appropriate treatment. Box 1.3 highlights some common myths and Box 1.4 gives the facts about the myth. Before moving to Box 1.4, try the exercise in Box 1.3 and see how many myths form your knowledge base about mental health and illness.

Box 1.3: Common myths about mental illness

As you read through these myths, think about which statements you agree with and what basis you have made your decision on.

- Young people and children don't suffer from mental health problems
- A person who has had a mental illness will not recover
- Mentally ill people are violent and dangerous
- Mental illness affects others and cannot affect me
- Mental disorders are caused by a personal weakness in character
- Mental illness is a single, rare disorder
- Psychiatric disorders are not true medical illnesses like heart disease and diabetes
- People who have a mental illness are just 'crazy'
- Schizophrenia means split personality, and there is no way to control it

It is the fear of the unknown that causes such myths about mental illness. The endurance of myths leads to stigma. The Royal College of Psychiatrists' website provides further information on many of these issues (www.rcpsych.ac.uk).

Stigma and mental illness

In this section the aim is to explore the concepts of, and the relationship between, stigma and mental illness. One possible reason for both conceptual confusion regarding mental illness and reluctance to seek help is that the stigmatization of mental illness continues to be a worldwide phenomenon.

Definition of the concept of stigma

The word stigma used to convey the negative views about those with mental illness originates from the Greek tradition of branding slaves with marks to identify them. Social stigma is a 'mark of infamy or disgrace; sign of moral blemish; stain or reproach caused by dishonourable conduct; reproachful characterization' (Webster's Dictionary).

Stigmatization is a social construct, and through this process those with mental illness are identified as being somehow different and having less worth.

Box 1.4: Common myths about mental illness and the facts

Myth: *Young people and children don't suffer from mental health problems*

Fact: It is estimated that between 10 and 25% of young people under the age of 18 suffer from mental health problems impacting on their ability to function at home, in school or in their community (see Chapter 14)

Myth: *A person who has had a mental illness can never recover*

Fact: People with mental illnesses do recover and resume normal activities. Recovery depends on appropriate treatment and psychosocial factors and many people function well between episodes of illness

Myth: *Mentally ill people are violent and dangerous*

Fact: The vast majority of people with mental illnesses *are not* violent or dangerous but are often vulnerable. On average about 55 people a year are killed by someone with a psychiatric illness at the time of the homicide

Myth: *Mental illness affects others and cannot affect me*

Fact: Mental illnesses are surprisingly common and do not discriminate – they can affect anyone. One in four people will experience a mental illness at some point

Myth: *Mental disorders are caused by a personal weakness in character*

Fact: Mental disorders are caused by biological, psychological and social factors

Myth: *Mental illness is a single disorder*

Fact: Mental illness is not a single disease but a broad classification covering many disorders, as shown in this chapter

Myth: *Psychiatric disorders are not true medical illnesses like heart disease and diabetes. People who have a mental illness are just 'crazy'*

Fact: Brain disorders, like heart disease and diabetes, are legitimate medical illnesses. Research shows there are biological factors that can in combination with other factors cause psychiatric disorders, and they can be treated effectively (see Chapter 2)

Myth: *Schizophrenia means split personality, and there is no way to control it*

Fact: Schizophrenia is often confused with multiple personality disorder. Actually, schizophrenia is a brain disorder that causes disordered thinking and perceptual abnormalities (see Chapter 9)

Much of the work about stigma has until quite recently been survey based and focused largely on schizophrenia. Stigma can be seen as an overarching term that contains three components that interlink: problems of knowledge (ignorance), problems of attitudes (prejudice) and problems of behaviour (discrimination).

The extent and impact of stigmatization of adult mental illness

It is difficult to be clear about why we as a society continue to have such negative views about those with mental illness. It may be a way of creating a sense that those with mental illness are different from us and thereby reducing our own fears of becoming like 'them'. It is therefore perhaps not surprising that negative attitudes towards mental illness are largely culturally non-specific and commonplace across the world. Stigmatizing processes can affect multiple domains of people's lives, having a dramatic bearing on the distribution of life chances in such areas as earnings, housing, criminal involvement, health and life itself.

Health care staff attitudes generally tend to be similar to those of the lay public. Medical students have been shown to be critical of those whom they believe play a part in the development of their problems, for example self-harm, eating disorders and substance misuse. Patients are often very critical of general practitioner attitudes. However, they also complain about negativity from mental health professionals, especially those patients with personality disorders and substance misuse problems.

It is worth adding that not only are there negative views about those who have mental health problems but also about staff who work with them.

Exercise

Just reflect on some of the stereotypes and attitudes towards mental illness and psychiatrists you have come across in your medical career

Children, mental illness and stigma

From the sparse literature available on stigma in relation to children and mental illness, it appears that adolescents' attitudes towards mental illness tend to be negative and stigmatizing. Our work in Nigeria with young people shows that such attitudes transcend culture.

Exercise

Think about the last three times you have seen mental illness depicted on TV or in the newspaper. How did the media portray mental illness?

Did the articles

- stereotype people with mental illness (for example assuming they are all violent)?
- minimize the difficulties faced by people with mental illness and/or the illness itself?
- patronize people with mental illness?
- assume that people with mental illness are somehow different from 'normal people'?
- perpetuate other myths?

Media, mental illness and stigma

Popular images of mental illness are both longstanding and stable. Two large-scale literature reviews have suggested that the media can be regarded as an important influence on community attitudes towards mental illness. It is considered that there is a complex and circular relationship between mass media representation of mental illness and public understanding. Negative media images promote negative attitudes and the resulting media coverage feeding off an already negative public perception. It is also thought that negative images will have a greater effect on public attitudes than positive portrayals.

Thornicroft explored newspaper, television and film portrayal of mental illness and found it to be largely negative, although there were occasional exceptions. All media leaned heavily towards depicting those with mental illness as being dangerous. There was a tendency to use mental illness generically as opposed to referring to specific diagnoses. Disappointingly, children's television programmes consistently linked violence to mental illness and use derogatory terms. This may suggest to young children that these are acceptable ways in which to refer to those who have mental health problems. There is an argument that media representations matter because they play an active part in shaping and sustaining what mental illness means as suggested above. Another relevant

factor is that by its very nature, the media is highly visible and hard to ignore. Further, the tabloids' use of derogatory language may legitimize its use in our everyday language.

The media appear to give greater priority to their own needs to entertain and cause headlines. In the process, they may be drawn to using the short cuts that stereotypes provide without challenging the damage they might be causing.

Interventions to reduce stigma

There is generally limited evidence about effective interventions to reduce stigma. Large-scale interventions, such as high-profile campaigns, are often difficult to evaluate. In the UK there have been several such campaigns (e.g. The Royal College of Psychiatrists' campaign, Every Family in the Land). There is little evidence to indicate that these have successfully changed public or personal attitudes. Although much of the work to date has focused on adults, there are increasing efforts to address the issue among younger populations, with some evidence that knowledge and attitudes can be improved.

There is as yet little evidence that anti-stigma work takes place in many medical schools and, where it does, how well it works to reduce the negative views that medical students have about mental illness. We discuss this more in Chapter 4, 'Making the most of your placement'.

It has been argued that the best way forward to tackle stigma may be to focus on discrimination rather than merely knowledge. In a way this also makes sense from the medical student educational perspective. *Good Medical Practice*, published by the GMC, places on doctors a responsibility to provide equitable care irrespective of various patient characteristics, including any diagnosis they may have. So irrespective of your own views you need to ensure you provide good quality care to all patients including those that have mental health problems.

Summary

There is still considerable debate around the terminology used in psychiatry. We suggest it is important to understand the principles of when someone is 'mentally healthy' and when they may have mental health problems that may be severe enough to be defined as a disorder. It is clinically more useful to take a multidimensional approach rather than the traditional categorical approach used in medicine. The impact of mental illness in the broadest sense for individuals, their families and society is significant and cannot be ignored. Yet despite the fact that we are all vulnerable to developing mental health problems, the stigmatization about mental illness pervades all cultures and societies and continues to be a challenge. Efforts are being made to address some of the stigmatization but progress is slow. Perhaps, you might want to conclude this chapter by returning to the exercise at the beginning of the chapter and ask yourself, are you ready to challenge yourself?

Further reading

American Psychiatric Association (1994) *Diagnostic and Statistical Manual of Mental Disorders*, fourth edition. Washington DC: American Psychiatric Association.

Crisp A (2004) The nature of stigmatisation. In A H Crisp (ed.) *Every Family in the Land: Understanding Prejudice and Discrimination against People with Mental Illness.* London: Royal Society of Medicine Press.

Crisp AH, Gelder M, Rix S, *et al.* (2000) Stigmatisation of people with mental illnesses. *British Journal of Psychiatry* 177: 4–7.

Edney DR (2004) *Mass Media and Mental Illness: A Literature Review.* www.ontario.cmha.ca/ (Accessed 14/01/10).

Gureje O, Lasebikan VO, Ephraim-Oluwanuga O, *et al.* (2005) Community study of knowledge of and attitude to mental illness in Nigeria. *The British Journal of Psychiatry* 186: 436–441.

Jorm AF, Korten AE, Jacomb PA, *et al.* (1997) 'Mental health literacy': a survey of the public's ability to recognise mental disorders and their beliefs about the effectiveness of treatment. *Medical Journal of Australia* 166: 182–186.

Kendall R (1988) Diagnosis and classification. In R Kendall and A Zealley (eds) *Companion to Psychiatric Studies.* Edinburgh: Churchill Livingstone.

Rose D, Thornicroft G, Pinfold V, Kassam A (2007) 250 labels used to stigmatise people with mental health. *BMC Health Services Research* 7: 97.

Thornicroft G (2006) *Shunned: Discrimination against People with Mental Illness.* Oxford: Oxford University Press.

World Health Organization (1992) *International Statistical Classification of Diseases and Related Health Problems*, 10th revision. Geneva: WHO Press.

World Health Organization (2001) *World Mental Health Day. Mental Health: Stop Exclusion – Dare to Care.* www.emro.who.int/mnh/whd/WHD-Brochure.pdf (Accessed 30/10/10).

CHAPTER 2

PERSONALITY, PREDISPOSING AND PERPETUATING FACTORS IN MENTAL ILLNESS

Nisha Dogra and Stephen Cooper

KEY CHAPTER FEATURES

- Outline of key aetiological factors
  - biological: e.g. genetic, organic, trauma, physical health problems
  - psychological: e.g. personality traits, developmental stage, attachment and ability to form and maintain relationships
  - social: e.g. environment, culture, family and wider sociopolitical factors
- Disorders of personality

Introduction

Traditionally we like to consider aetiological factors in different disorders; however, this is more difficult in mental illnesses for a variety of reasons, particularly the greater difficulty in measuring what may be subtle biological changes and the difficulties in creating clearly defined syndromes. In this chapter we will outline the key relevant aetiological factors that play a part in the development of mental illness and mental health problems. As raised in Chapter 1, it is unusual in psychiatry to find many disorders that have a single aetiological factor. Mental health problems usually arise out of a complex interplay between the biological, the social and the psychological. Each of these types of factors will be considered in turn. We will also consider protective factors.

It can also be useful to consider whether at a particular point in an individual's illness relevant factors are predisposing, precipitating and/or perpetuating. Biological and psychological factors may be more likely to predispose an individual to particular problems whereas psychological and social factors are more likely to precipitate and perpetuate problems. Aetiological factors are important to consider, as identification can help plan more effective interventions.

It is almost impossible to discuss aetiological factors without the issue of nature versus nurture being raised. Although the academic debate raises interesting points, in practice, especially in psychiatry, it is a combination of these factors. Trying to home in on single aetiological factors is usually unhelpful.

Biological factors

It is perhaps best to consider biological factors in three main groups: (a) physical disorders and insults that may secondarily cause a mental illness; (b) genetic factors; and (c) changes seen in studies of brain structure, neuropharmacology and functional imaging. These will be described in turn. Although it is unusual in psychiatry to have a single aetiological factor, this clearly is the case for some learning disability disorders such as Down's syndrome. A disorder such as Huntington's chorea, which is caused by a specific genetic disorder, can have psychiatric manifestations, but the presentation of these may be influenced by other factors such as the social circumstances and alcohol or drug abuse.

Physical disorders

Table 2.1 provides a list of some situations where a physical disorder or insult may give rise to the presentation of a psychiatric disorder, sometimes as the sole or main manifestation and sometimes as a secondary diagnosis. This is not a comprehensive list and aspects of this are complemented in Chapter 12 on organic disorders.

Genetics

Evidence for genetic factors in the most serious mental illnesses was really the first fairly replicable

Table 2.1   Physical disorders and insults that can be important in the aetiology of some psychiatric presentations

Physical factor	Related disorder or features
In utero and birth problems	
Intrauterine exposure to toxins, e.g. alcohol	Fetal alcohol syndrome
	ADHD
Perinatal, brain injury at birth; premature birth	ADHD
	May impair intellectual abilities
Severe head injury	Mood disorders
	Frontal lobe disorder
Infection	
Syphilis	Dementia
HIV	Dementia; substance misuse; depression
Viral encephalitis, e.g. from herpes simplex virus (HSV-1)	Amnesic syndrome, behavioural disturbances, irritability, depression
Neurological disorders	
Neoplasm and other space occupying lesions	Personality changes
	Mood disorders
Poorly controlled temporal lobe epilepsy	Schizophrenia-like psychosis
Post myocardial infarction (MI)	Depression is common after MI. Important to recognize, because morbidity and mortality are increased in the presence of depression
Endocrine disturbance	
Hyperthyroidism	Anxiety
Hypothyroidism	Depression
Addison's disease	Depression
Cerebrovascular	
Stroke	Depression, mood variability/abnormal emotionality, anxiety
	Changes in personality
Arteriovenous malformations	Depending on the site, may sometimes cause mood disorders or anxiety disorders
Iatrogenic	
Corticosteroids	Elation and depression
Anabolic steroids	Aggression, changes in personality
Methylphenidate	Can cause psychosis (even in very young children)

indication that biological factors were relevant in aetiology. Genetic links were initially established through family and then twin and adoption studies. Table 2.2 describes the genetic risks relating to some common mental disorders.

It is useful to consider the example of schizophrenia to understand the relevance of different types of approach. Initial population and family studies showed that where a family had an affected member the risks were greater for other family members, with first-degree relatives carrying greater risk than more distant relatives. However, this of itself does not prove a genetic link. As well as sharing some genes, families also share the same environment. Thus, it could be argued, and was by some, that aspects of how family members interacted with each other might equally be the cause of the higher risk of schizophrenia in first-degree relatives. (For example, it was suggested that abnormal patterns of communication by parents might lead to behaviours in the children that were similar to features of schizophrenia.) One way to circumvent this problem

Table 2.2   Genetic risk for some major mental disorders

Disorder	Concordance rates for twins and risk to other family members
Schizophrenia	Concordance rate for monozygotic (MZ) twins 46% compared to 14% for dizygotic (DZ) twins Siblings and children of someone with schizophrenia have 8–10 times greater risk of developing schizophrenia than general population. Second-degree relatives are 3–4 times more likely to develop the disorder than general population
Bipolar disorder	Concordance rate for MZ twins is 80% compared to 16% for DZ twins 50% of those with bipolar disorder have one parent with history of depression If a parent has bipolar disorder, child has 25% chance of developing depression. If both parents have bipolar disorder, child has between 50 and 75% chance of developing bipolar disorder. Siblings of those with bipolar disorder are up to 8–18 times more likely to develop bipolar disorder and 2–10 times more likely to develop depression than others with no such siblings
Depression	Concordance rate for MZ twins is 46% and 20% for DZ twins Having a parent or sibling who has had depression increases risk by 1.5–3 times greater than if no family history
General anxiety disorder	Twin studies suggest a genetic contribution One out of four (25%) of first-degree relatives with general anxiety disorder will be affected
Obsessive compulsive disorder	Twin studies suggest a genetic contribution One out of four (25%) of first-degree relatives with general anxiety disorder will be affected
Autistic spectrum disorder (ASD)	Concordance rate between 30% and 60% for MZ twins and between 0% and 6% for DZ twins. Some variants more genetically linked. This is only the case for when the ASD is not linked to a specific genetic disorder such as Angelman syndrome or Prader–Willi
ADHD	Some studies report 82% concordance in MZ twins compared with 38% for DZ twins If a child has ADHD there is a fivefold increase in the risk to other family members

is to study twins. Monozygotic (MZ) twins share 100 per cent of their genetic material whereas dizygotic (DZ) twins share only 50 per cent. However, twins, whether MZ or DZ, are born and brought up in the same environment. Thus, differences in concordance between MZ and DZ twins, when one of a twin pair suffers from schizophrenia, are most likely to be due to genetic rather than environmental factors. Where one twin has schizophrenia the concordance in MZ twins is around 45 per cent whereas it is only around 14 per cent for DZ twins.

Another way to control for environmental factors is through studies following up children one of whose parents had schizophrenia but who had been adopted away from their natural parents almost immediately after birth. Their outcomes were compared with those of adopted children whose parents did not suffer from schizophrenia. Results of such studies indicate the expected population level of schizophrenia in the control children but rates of schizophrenia in those with psychotic parents that would be expected in such first-degree relatives. The rationale here is that there is no reason to suspect any major difference in the nature of the environments into which both groups of children are adopted.

What you will have noticed here is that even for MZ twins the concordance for schizophrenia is considerably less than 50 per cent. This suggests that genetic risk of itself is not always sufficient to cause schizophrenia and that certain environmental factors must also operate. Thus, from a clinical perspective, it is important to emphasize to patients and their families that although major mental disorders carry a genetic risk, there is no inevitability that the children will also have the disorder. When there is a family history of mental illness, especially schizophrenia, behavioural disturbance in children can be misinterpreted and the child given a particular script that is hard to escape.

Approaches such as the above have established that genetic risk is a factor in many mental illnesses. Since the 1980s investigators have turned their attention to use of modern molecular biological techniques to try to identify particular genes that may be involved. This has had a limited degree of success but has perhaps been disappointing given the enormous amounts of funds provided for genetics research in medicine as a whole including psychiatry. Nevertheless, certain genes have been found that seem to be linked to schizophrenia, severe mood disorders and alcohol abuse. However, a problem remains that we do not know the functional effects in the brain of most of these genes. Thus, this knowledge has not yet helped to understand a pathway by which these disorders are caused and thus cannot yet lead to prevention or pre-emptive treatment.

Brain structure, neuropharmacology and functional imaging

Serious consideration of biological factors in mental illnesses (other than those described above) began towards the end of the nineteenth century as interest in neuropathology expanded. Studies were reported of the examination of post-mortem brain samples from patients who had suffered from various types of psychotic disorders as well as from those who had suffered from dementia and other neurological conditions. Whereas studies of the dementias began to reveal the neuropathology of these conditions, studies of the so-called 'functional' psychiatric disorders were unsuccessful. (Psychiatric disorders without clear evidence of neuropathological abnormality were for many years described as 'functional' disorders because they could only be recognized as disorders of brain function without measurable evidence of physiological or other biological abnormality as was possible with organic disorders such as dementia.) This type of approach was hampered by inadequate techniques for measurement of what we now know are subtle abnormalities, by a lack of clear diagnostic criteria and by the complicating effects of brain injury, vitamin deficiencies and other such factors that often afflicted patients with chronic mental illnesses.

The early twentieth century saw a preoccupation with psychological factors and psychoanalytical approaches. However, the development of effective biological treatments (ECT in the 1930s; antipsychotics in 1952; antidepressants in 1957), improvements in chemical/biochemical techniques and increased understanding of biochemistry led to a steady resurgence of interest in biological investigation of mental illnesses during the 1950s, which accelerated exponentially over the following five decades.

Initially many studies were aimed at trying to find biological markers for various mental illnesses. For example, patients with schizophrenia were examined for putative psychotogenic substances that could theoretically be produced in the brain, from known metabolic pathways, and which, if in excess, might cause psychotic symptoms. The transmethylation hypothesis suggested the possibility of increased concentrations of 3,4-dimethoxyphenylethylamine, which Friedhoff and van Winkle identified on chromatography of urine samples, from patients with schizophrenia, as the famous 'pink spot'. Although many interesting results were initially found, these were generally not able to be replicated by different investigators with their own patients and sometimes turned out to be secondary effects of drug treatments (as was probably the case for the 'pink spot').

During the late 1950s and early 1960s, however, a more fruitful approach emerged of trying to understand how the now available effective drugs worked. For example, in 1957 Arvid Carlsson had demonstrated that dopamine (DA) was a neurotransmitter, a finding later developed into the first effective treatment for Parkinson's disease. Of relevance to psychiatry, he also demonstrated, in 1963, that antipsychotic drugs had profound effects on the dopamine system. This finding began the cascade of research leading to the dopamine hypothesis for schizophrenia proposed by a number of scientists in the early 1970s. (In 2000 Carlsson received the Nobel Prize for Physiology and Medicine for his lifetime of work on various aspects of dopamine function.) Similarly, working from the effects of antidepressant drugs, Schildkraut proposed a noradrenergic theory for depression and Coppen a serotoninergic theory for depressive illness. Although current knowledge suggests that the early versions of these hypotheses require considerable modification, this approach has led to greater interest in trying to understand neurochemical processes in the brain and into how these might be disrupted in mental illnesses.

Success in demonstration of the relevance of particular neurotransmitter pathways, the development of more sophisticated brain imaging techniques and the development of molecular approaches to neuropathology encouraged renewed attempts to understand other types of biological factors in the aetiology of mental illnesses. For example, although early pneumo-encephalographic studies demonstrated increased lateral ventricular volumes in patients with chronic schizophrenia it was not until the advent of computed tomography and magnetic resonance imaging in the 1970s and 1980s that this type of finding could be properly and safely investigated in large numbers of patients at different stages of illness. This has led to the establishment of consistent evidence of brain structural changes in schizophrenia, to the resurgence of neuropathological and molecular studies of post-mortem brain tissue from patients using modern techniques, and to hypotheses suggesting disturbance of brain development as an aetiological factor in schizophrenia.

Schizophrenia

A wide range of biological and cognitive disturbances has been found to be associated with schizophrenia. Table 2.3 summarizes some of the structural brain changes found that have been relatively consistent in recent neuroimaging and neuropathological studies. These changes are small in absolute terms, and sizes of the brain structures involved overlap considerably with those in non-schizophrenic subjects. Thus, such changes are only seen when comparing a large number of patients with control subjects and cannot be used to help make a diagnosis of schizophrenia. These structural abnormalities have been demonstrated in

Table 2.3 Brain structural changes found in schizophrenia

Finding	Comment
Reduced overall brain volume	Meta-analysis of 58 studies suggests 2% reduction in cerebral volume
Increased volume of cerebral ventricles	Particularly the temporofrontal aspect of the lateral ventricles
Reduction in volume of the hippocampus	Possibly greater on the left side
Reduction in volume of the hippocampus	In discordant monozygotic twins, the affected twin has reduced hippocampal volume
Reduction in volume of parts of the frontal and temporal cortices and possible alterations in gyral folding	Findings in some studies relate to particular symptoms

patients with established illness but some appear to be present at the onset of the illness and to progress over time. Along with other evidence, for example increased obstetric complications during the gestation of people subsequently developing schizophrenia, the effects of maternal influenza during pregnancy to increase the risk of schizophrenia in the child (by 1–2 per cent) and the presence of increased frequencies of a number of minor physical anomalies that are determined *in utero* (e.g. palmar creases and craniofacial abnormalities), these findings suggest that in many cases an important factor may be neurodevelopmental disturbance.

Other studies have suggested disturbances of physiological function (Table 2.4). These changes are often best demonstrated when patients are asked to perform specific cognitive tasks (such as certain memory tasks or verbal tasks) which will normally activate particular brain regions. It is also clear that patients with schizophrenia have a variety of cognitive impairments. These are particularly in the areas of executive function (planning and decision-making), attention and memory. Such impairments have often been found to correlate with both the 'negative' symptoms of schizophrenia and poor outcome in terms of social functioning.

During the 1960s and 1970s a combination of laboratory studies, clinical observations and post-mortem studies suggested that the 'positive' psychotic symptoms of schizophrenia (see Chapter 9) might be due to overactivity of the DA system and primarily to an underlying increase in dopamine type 2 (D2) receptors (Table 2.5). The advent, in the 1980s, of techniques such as single photon emission tomography and positron emission tomography, which allow measures of neurochemical function in live human beings, did not provide consistent confirmation of the first version of the dopamine hypothesis, which suggested an underlying increase in DA receptors.

However, subsequent, more sophisticated studies have suggested that there may be an underlying tendency for DA overactivity in the striatum and underactivity in the prefrontal cortex in schizophrenia. Linked with the knowledge that DA is key to how we attach importance, or 'salience', to events or thoughts this fits well with evidence that patients with schizophrenia demonstrate inappropriate salience compared with healthy subjects. Such abnormal salience could form the basis of delusional thinking. These findings also suggest a mechanism by which cannabis abuse might increase the risk of developing schizophrenia as cannabis can induce release of DA and may thus alter the salience attributed to events.

There has also been evidence of dysregulation of the excitatory neurotransmitter glutamate. For example, drugs such as PCP, which block glutamatergic NMDA receptors, can induce psychotic states. Glutamate is the main excitatory neurotransmitter in the brain and general dysfunction of this, or dysfunction of certain major pathways, could affect functioning in many brain regions and secondarily disrupt other transmitter systems, such as DA. Post-mortem studies have shown alterations in the glutamatergic system in the hippocampus.

The second-generation antipsychotic drugs have potent effects at serotonin (5-HT) receptors, principally 5-HT_{2A} receptors. This may account for some of their benefits and has stimulated research into the 5-HT system in schizophrenia. At present, there is no conclusive evidence for any specific abnormality but it may be a system through which other transmitters can be modulated in certain brain regions relevant to particular symptoms.

Table 2.4   Disturbances of brain function

Finding	Comment
Reduction in amplitude of some 'event related' potentials, such as P300 and MMN	These are complex EEG measures that indicate disturbances in how individuals process information
Disturbances in regional cerebral blood flow measured using PET or functional MRI	Evidence that some of these changes relate to particular groups of symptoms
Altered pattern of blood flow when performing specific cognitive tasks	Suggests some alteration in the normal pattern of connections between different brain regions

Table 2.5   Evidence suggesting altered dopamine transmission in schizophrenia

Finding	Comment
Potency of antipsychotics in binding to dopamine (DA) receptors correlates with their clinical potency	Ability of these drugs to bind to other receptors (e.g. serotonin, histamine) does not correlate with clinical potency
Amphetamine abuse can induce some schizophrenia like symptoms	Amphetamine stimulates the DA system
Clinical trial in schizophrenia of alpha- and beta-isomers of flupentixol showed benefit only for the alpha-isomer	Only the alpha-isomer blocks DA receptors. This isomer reduced positive psychotic symptoms
Increased density of DA receptors in post-mortem brain tissue from patients	Initial studies agreed but then evidence emerged that this effect might be caused by the long-term antipsychotic treatment most patients had received. Little or no change seen in most studies of patients free of antipsychotic drugs for some time before death
Studies using positron emission tomography (PET) to measure DA receptors in vivo in drug-naïve patients fail to find consistent increases	Problem of small size of many of these studies. Meta-analysis suggests there may be a small increase
SPET and PET studies used to show that patients release more DA than control subjects when given amphetamine	Suggests some dysregulation of the DA system in patients with schizophrenia
PET studies show greater increase in DA receptor binding in patients with schizophrenia after depletion of DA	Confirms dysregulation of the DA system in patients with schizophrenia
Cannabis induces release of DA in the striatum	Increasing evidence that cannabis abuse increases the risk of developing schizophrenia

Depression

Until the 1990s, the main focus of investigation into the biological aetiology of depressive illness was into disturbances of neurotransmitter function, particularly 5-HT and noradrenaline (NA). Table 2.6 summarizes much of the evidence in favour of a serotoninergic dysfunction. Like the schizophrenia story, this comes from a variety of laboratory, clinical and post-mortem brain studies. A useful paradigm used to investigate mood change, in both patients and healthy individuals, has been the tryptophan depletion paradigm (experimental approach). This paradigm depends on the fact that the amino acid tryptophan is the essential precursor for the formation of serotonin. An important enzyme in this process, tryptophan hydroxylase, is unsaturated with tryptophan so any reduction in availability of tryptophan will result in a fairly rapid fall in serotonin levels in the neurone and synapse. Subjects are asked to drink a mixture of amino acids, normally acquired from the proteins we eat, which do not contain tryptophan. This results in a dramatic, short-term fall in brain serotonin and will induce a temporary relapse of depression in recovered patients (rapidly reversed on being given tryptophan in a normal meal) and in some individuals with a familial genetic risk of depression.

The paradigm of tryptophan depletion is also used in a variety of other ways to help us understand what may be happening in depression. In conjunction with measures of cerebral blood flow it is found that reducing serotonin function in the brain, by tryptophan depletion, alters activity in the orbitofrontal cortex, an area also implicated in other studies of brain structure and function in depression (Table 2.7). It has also been

Table 2.6   Evidence suggesting altered serotonin function in depression

Finding	Comment
Reserpine may induce depression	Reserpine depletes neurones of 5-HT and noradrenaline
Patients respond to SSRI antidepressants	These drugs have fairly specific effects on the 5-HT system
CSF levels of 5-HIAA (the main brain metabolite of 5-HT) are reduced in depression	This suggests reduced release of 5-HT. It is particularly found in those with previous suicide attempts
Tryptophan depletion may induce depressed mood in recovered patients	Artificial reduction in serotonin induces depressed mood lending strength to the idea that 5-HT function may be reduced in those with depressive illness
Reduced secretion of the hormone prolactin following stimulation of the 5-HT system	Suggests altered function of 5-HT receptors controlling this
Post-mortem brain studies suggest reduced 5-HT_{1A} receptors and increased 5-HT_{2A} receptors	
Molecular imaging studies using PET suggest reduced 5-HT_{1A} receptors in depression	
PET studies less consistent with regard to 5-HT_{2A} receptors	

Table 2.7   Disturbances of brain structure and function in depression

Findings
Reduction of grey matter volume in the orbitofrontal region of the cortex
Reduced volume of the hippocampus in patients with a long history of depression
Reduction of blood flow in orbitofrontal cortex
Increased orbitofrontal cortical blood flow following tryptophan depletion
Reduced blood flow in the caudate nucleus

demonstrated that subjects who have been tryptophan depleted may show changes in emotional processing similar to those that may occur in depression.

A similar but smaller body of evidence also suggests that there may be dysfunction of the NA system in patients with depression, although this may be more specifically linked to particular symptoms or types of presentation.

A further interesting series of findings relate to the hypothalamic–pituitary–adrenal (HPA) axis. It has been known for many years that patients with depression have elevations of plasma cortisol compared with a healthy population, although not sufficiently high to make this diagnostically useful. A large proportion of these will fail to suppress cortisol after administration of dexamethasone. Magnetic resonance imaging (MRI) studies indicate enlargement of the adrenal glands in depression. There is also a blunted ACTH response to CRH. This suggests some abnormality of receptor function normally designed to detect elevated cortisol secretion and from this a dysregulation of the HPA axis. Stress will normally cause activation of the HPA system and can be a precipitant of depression. Thus it may be that there is an inability of the HPA system to switch off following stress, and hypercortisolaemia could thus play a part in the development of depression. Elevated cortisol may also be damaging to the hippocampus and thus MRI findings of reduced hippocampal volume in some patients are consistent with this.

Bipolar disorder

Intensive investigation of the biological changes in bipolar disorder began a little later than such studies in schizophrenia. However, the last 10 years have seen consistent evidence emerging for brain structural changes that seem to differ a little from the pattern seen in schizophrenia. In particular, there has been evidence for reduction in the grey matter volume of parts of the prefrontal cortex, enlargement of the lateral ventricles and enlargement of the globus pallidus. Like the situation in depression, there is also evidence for reduced cerebral blood flow in the orbitofrontal cortex and anterior cingulate gyrus. However, in a state of mania patients seem to experience an increase in blood flow in these regions.

All three monoamine neurotransmitters have been implicated in bipolar disorder. There is evidence for an underlying underactivity in the 5-HT system. In states of mania, there is evidence for overactivity in both the DA and NA systems. Disturbance of the HPA axis has also been demonstrated, with evidence of more marked change in the depressive phase of bipolar disorder than in unipolar depression.

Anxiety disorders

Over the last 20 years, evidence has accumulated for the importance of biological factors in some types of anxiety disorders. It is more difficult to study this group of disorders because of diagnostic overlaps and co-existence of different anxiety disorders in many patients. However, it is clear that benzodiazepines (BDZs) and a variety of antidepressant drugs are effective in treating anxiety in many, though not all, patients. The effectiveness of BDZs led to investigation of the possibility of altered sensitivity of the GABA–BDZ receptor complex in some anxiety disorders. In patients with panic disorder the GABA–BDZ receptor antagonist flumazenil has been shown to induce feelings of anxiety and panic while having no effect in non-anxious control subjects. This suggests that there may be some alteration of function of GABA–BDZ receptors in these patients. This effect is not seen in patients with post-traumatic stress disorder (PTSD). However, in PTSD as well as panic disorder patients the drug yohimbine (an alpha-2 noradrenergic receptor agonist) can induce feelings of panic, while

only inducing milder anxiety in control subjects, suggesting altered function of the NA system.

These are examples of the evidence for biological abnormalities in anxiety disorders. It is not feasible here to summarize the principal evidence for biological factors in all of the anxiety disorders. However, it is important to recognize that while many developmental, social and psychological factors are also important we must remember that for many mental illnesses it is an interplay of all of these potential aetiological factors that is important – an interplay where the balance of each will differ from patient to patient.

Psychological factors

Individual personality traits and personality types are significant factors in the development of mental health problems. This encompasses temperament type, which is often used for children. The individual's early development and attachment to carers may influence their ability to develop appropriate and meaningful relationships and may be significant aetiological factors. The developmental life stage that someone is at may also be an important factor.

Personality types

Temperament is used to describe the way individuals and especially children behave. It does not attempt to explain what causes the behaviour. Temperament is present from birth and influences how we behave towards people and how we see our environment. This helps understand why some individuals are able to manage many stressors whereas others develop problems in the face of what others may see as minor stressors. It is also important to note that our behaviour may lead others to behave in particular ways which may then establish helpful or non-helpful coping strategies. There is strong evidence that some temperament types in children, which become personality traits as they mature, are more strongly linked with some mental health problems than others. Problems in childhood are more likely when the child has a temperament that fits less easily with parental styles.

In terms of thinking about personality types, it may be helpful to use the ICD categories of personality disorder (Box 2.1). That is not to say that

Box 2.1: ICD classification of personality disorders

F60 Specific personality disorders

Paranoid – includes previous categories such as sensitive and querulant personality

Schizoid – not the same as schizotypal disorder (related to schizophrenia)

Dissocial – more used term is antisocial, psychopathic or sociopath

Emotionally unstable – either impulsive or borderline type

Histrionic (was hysterical)

Anankastic (was obsessive)

Anxious (also called avoidant)

Dependent (was asthenic, inadequate or passive)

Other specific personality disorders, including narcissistic personality disorder

F61 Mixed or other personality disorders

everyone with those traits develops problems, but identifying the types of personality disorders helps relate the personality characteristics to the most likely mental health problems. (Issues around personality disorder are discussed in Chapter 15.) Young people under the age of 18 years cannot be diagnosed as having a personality disorder, and the term emerging personality disorder may be used. However, given that adolescence is a stage of life when young people are establishing a sense of who they are, some of the behaviours, especially those of the emotionally unstable type, may be transient.

On the whole, personality traits are enduring but that does not mean individuals cannot learn ways of managing the behaviours around certain traits. Now, most of us will not fit the full criteria for a specific personality disorder but most, if not all of us, will have some of these traits. A helpful way of looking at these is to use broad categories:

- odd/eccentric types, such as paranoid or schizoid
- emotional, erratic type (such as dissocial, histrionic, emotionally unstable)
- anxious/fearful types (dependent, anxious, anankastic).

Individuals in the first category tend to be loners and can struggle with relationships. Individuals with such traits (as opposed to the disorder) are more likely to present with problems when these personality traits interfere with daily living. They may present with depression and/or feelings of persecution. The emotionally unstable group of traits are most likely to present with deliberate self-harm, aggression, substance misuse and comorbidity. Unsurprisingly, those with anxiety and obsessive traits are more likely to present with anxiety and phobic type of disorders. However, just because they are predisposed to these types of disorders does not mean that these are the only disorders they may have. There are other recognized types of personality, although not classified as disorders, such as depressive (unsurprisingly characterized by chronic moroseness, worry and negativity) and passive aggressive types. The latter can be very difficult to deal with in practice as they will not openly raise or address issues but instead act out their hostility. For example, they may disagree with a management plan suggested by the doctor. However, rather than say so they will not comply with the treatment and then claim it is ineffective. The way we think about personality has come some way from when the way people looked was used to define their personality!

It is important to recognize that someone with anxiety traits who is supported by addressing some of the issues may learn to manage their anxiety (even though it is unlikely ever to completely go away). However, if the anxiety is managed with excessive reassurance and support of avoidance strategies, the situation is likely to be exacerbated. Particular personality types may be more prone to use particular kinds of defence mechanisms as discussed in Chapter 3, but we all use different defence mechanisms to manage situations.

Attachment

It was after the Second World War that Bowlby wrote about attachment of babies with their mothers thus reflecting that at the time he wrote mothers were the primary caregiver. Attachment refers to a specific type of biologically based relationship which provides a secure base from which children can explore the world. Attachment relationships can be classified as either secure or insecure. Essentially with secure attachment, the child learns that their needs are met by their caregiver and thereby learns trust. This is not the case for insecure attachments. Three types of insecure relationships have been identified: ambivalent, avoidant or disorganized. Insecure attachment relationships, coupled with high levels of parental anxiety, are associated with increased risk of anxiety disorders in children. Those with ambivalent insecure attachment may develop relationships with strong passive aggressive patterns of behaviour. Disorganized insecure attachment may lead to short-term superficial relationships in which there is little trust.

Individuals who have secure attachment and a good model for functional relationship are more likely to develop and maintain healthy relationships. Over time it has become clear that the particular person the child develops the relationship with is less important than the nature of the relationship itself. That is, the relationship does not have to be with the biological mother as first hypothesized. A relationship that is warm and positive with someone familiar may be enough.

Self-esteem

The way we view ourselves can influence how we view what happens to us. Individuals with a good sense of who they are and positive self-esteem are less likely to be impacted on by some environmental factors. If they experience a life event, they are less likely to feel persecuted or picked on and more likely to see it as just one of those things. Children and adults with poor social skills find it difficult to develop relationships, so may find themselves excluded and socially isolated. Social skills can be improved through training.

IQ

Generally, children with lower cognitive levels are at increased risk of antisocial behaviour. Research suggests that lower IQ is a risk factor because such children have poorer problem-solving skills and are more vulnerable to family adversity. This risk is carried on into adulthood. Having special skills can sometimes mitigate for other risk factors. For some individuals talent is also a way of escaping socioeconomic disadvantages and the risk inherent within them, which is discussed later.

Life stages and life events

The life stage is important to consider as some behaviours are appropriate at some stages but become a problem if they continue. This can be developmental stages or following life events.

Life events could arguably be environmental factors but are included here as we all experience them. Whether a life event becomes a precipitating or perpetuating factor will depend on the interplay between the life event, an individual's personal characteristics and other factors. The most stressful life events are bereavement, divorce and moving house or job.

The experience of success or failure at dealing with expected life events can also shape our world view. If one set of events such as exams are managed well, we learn that exams are okay and are less likely to be stressed by future exams. However, if we manage events ineffectively and are distressed by the experience, the next time we come across the same event we are likely to remember our previous failing. It can also be the case that being mugged reinforces our predisposition to believe that the world is a dangerous place and thereby reinforces any anxiety traits. Although having an episode of mental illness does not inevitably mean problems will recur, the likelihood of further problems is increased.

Social factors

There are a variety of social factors with many subcategories (Box 2.2). The major categories are environmental, life events, cultural and sociopolitical factors. Each will be considered in turn. Disentangling genetic from environmental influences is not easy.

Box 2.2: Aetiological social factors
Culture
Religion
Family
Neighbourhoods and social networks
Work and school
Socioeconomic disadvantage
War/conflict

Bronfenbrenner's model of layered contexts is a fairly widely used model to help understand social factors. The layers are the microsystem, mesosystem, exosystem and the macrosystem. The first layer (microsystem) is relationships that the individual is actively involved in, for example parents, siblings and peers. However, these interactions depend on context and personal characteristics. The mesosystem describes how the different components of the microsystem come together. The exosystem is the wider local community such as the neighbourhood. The macrosystem is usually remote from any specific individual but may still be a major social influence, for example socioeconomic policy regarding child rearing, benefits for those who are ill, education and health policies, wider cultural and political contexts. It is worth noting that various factors may influence differently at various stages of an individual's life. Some adverse family factors may be mitigated by external factors in older children. The broad political and cultural aspects are not covered in detail in this chapter as they vary from context to context. However, it is important to recognize their potential significance.

Environmental factors

There is a wide range of environmental factors and the influence of these will be individually and contextually variable.

Cultural factors

One of the difficulties in thinking about culture is that it can often mean different things to different people. It is beyond the scope of this text to enter into the debates about the meanings of culture. In this context culture is not predefined but takes into account the various aspects of an individual's life that are important to them, so can include ethnicity, geographical identification, religious perspectives.

Culture in itself (no matter which definition is used) does not cause mental health problems. However, it can strongly influence what is perceived to be a mental health issue, what treatments are sought and potentially even the support provided. There is some evidence that the prevalence in some groups is higher in one context than in another. For example, Afro-Caribbean migrants in the UK have higher rates of schizophrenia than the same population group in the West Indies. This suggests that the risk is neither entirely genetic or social but an interplay of the two that manifests itself differently dependent on context.

Religion

Religion can be a protective factor against developing mental health problems but this has to be understood in context. For many people, if religion challenges their sense of who they feel they are it can be considerably stressful, especially when there are strong differences within the family. A very obvious example of this is homosexuality.

Families

Families are a crucial social factor as they can provide enormous support to those with mental health problems but they can also be causes of considerable stress. It is not that long ago that parents were thought to be responsible for their children developing autism and schizophrenia. As with culture, families do not cause problems *per se* but may be significant factors in the development of problems. The nature of what a family is varies considerably. As more and more families move away from the traditional nuclear family, the stresses that families bring change. The reconstitution of step-families brings challenges within that process. An additional factor to consider is extended families, and the various supports and stresses that this type of arrangement might provide. Our relationships with our parents and families often form the template for all our other relationships, no matter how much we might wish they did not.

The impact of families will be considered for children, working age adults and older adults as the relationships differ. For children parents can be significant factors through:

- parenting styles
- parental relationships (parental hostility rather than whether parents live together or not seems to be a key factor)
- parental mental or physical illness. Maternal postnatal depression may be particularly relevant, as if untreated may impact on bonding and attachment
- abuse (children who experience abuse may externalize their hostility and develop aggression whereas others may internalize their feelings and self-harm, and present as anxious or depressed)

- unresolved parental issues related to their own upbringing
- differing expectations of what the child wants and what might be expected of them.

Other factors for children will be if there are siblings who have chronic physical health problems or learning disability. Sibling relationships can also be relevant, although relationships in childhood do not always indicate the type of relationship siblings will have as adults.

For working adults, families can be relevant aetiological factors through:

- their relationship with their partner
- relationships and demands of their children
- relationship with their own parents, especially when their parents become less independent or suffer loss.

For older adults families are relevant in:

- issues around ageing and whether older people feel supported by their family
- bereavement and loss of partners and siblings.

It is often the case that staff working with children identify that parents need to address their issues. Staff working with adults may feel that if child services just got the child sorted, their patients would be less stressed. The reality is that the key issue is how this dynamic plays itself out. How each player in the scenario can be helped to understand their role and the impact it has on others may be a more productive way forward. Another way of looking at it is that a depressed mother may not be able to respond warmly to her child and the child then responds by defiance, which then makes it even more difficult for the mother to respond. Breaking such a cycle can be difficult but identifying the relevant factors is important to devise an appropriate intervention plan.

The way that families interact and communicate can affect all members of the family and it is often the case that what impacts on one person has some degree of influence on other family members. It is generally agreed that clear communication, direct style and being emotionally responsive to family members while allowing them some autonomy is ideal. Few families achieve this on an everyday basis and go through life finding mutually acceptable ways of managing.

It can be easy to dismiss the impact of families on adults. Work in the latter part of the twentieth century found that families who were overly expressive played a part in the relapse of schizophrenia. The family members may have unwittingly been factors in perpetuating the illness. This is not the same as saying the family is responsible for the illness.

Families are an important factor in how we view ourselves and the parts we are allowed to play. It can be very difficult to change the narrative, so if you have been labelled as shy within the family context it may be difficult to be anything else.

Domestic violence in families can cause mental health problems for the abused partner (usually female) and for the children. Males may especially model their behaviour on their aggressive fathers.

Exercise

As you go through your psychiatry placement, consider how people describe their families and whether they identify them as a strength or stressor. Think about how you feel about your own family and how that influences your expectations of patients and their families. In your placement after psychiatry, repeat the exercise and see if there is any difference in the range of ways people view their families.

Neighbourhoods and housing

The places in which people live can have significant impact on their mental health. As discussed later, poorer people live in less desirable areas and may have to tolerate high levels of crime, violence and risk to their personal safety. Neighbourhood disadvantage is associated with higher rates of major depression and substance abuse disorder. Those suffering from mental illness may also experience a loss of financial security and be over-represented in poorer areas.

However, this is also dependent on social networks and support within the neighbourhood. Social isolation can be a risk factor for depression, especially in older adults. Migrants may find living in areas with high levels of similar migrants more of a support than those who are not migrants, as for the latter it may represent greater and more enduring socioeconomic disadvantage. The value of support networks should not be underestimated. Such support may help mitigate the consequences of poverty, disadvantage and discrimination.

Work and school

Individuals spend a considerable amount of time in either work or school. Many manage this without any problems. However, the demands of work or school can provide considerable stress, as can having to develop working relationships with colleagues and peers. For older adults the loss of work may bring other losses such as a purpose and a sense of being valued, social contacts as well as reduced financial security.

Life events (which are not a normal expected part of life)

Trauma, sexual assault and being a victim of crime may all decrease the threshold for someone developing mental health problems, especially anxiety and depression. However, most people who experience trauma do not suffer from PTSD or develop other problems.

Sociopolitical factors

Socioeconomic disadvantage

A key factor is socioeconomic disadvantage, which brings with it a range of stressors that in turn impact on the development of some mental health problems. This factor is significantly associated with development of mental health problems in children and adults and is relevant across cultures. It is not within our scope to discuss what constitutes poverty. However, whichever way it is measured or defined, there is no doubt that poverty is linked to social inequality and these factors coupled together impact on the overall health of individuals. There is higher mortality and morbidity in deprived communities than in less deprived ones. Being poor means that meeting tasks of daily life can be challenging. Poor people have less access to safe neighbourhoods, decent housing and jobs, and to health and education. The disadvantage therefore becomes cumulative. Poverty can cause mental health problems but may also be a consequence of them. Children from disadvantaged backgrounds are less likely to perform well in schools, are more exposed to unstable family life and are more likely to have behavioural problems. Adults from disadvantaged contexts are more likely to develop mood disorders and may experience more anxiety (which may well, for example, be justified if they live in violent neighbourhoods). Substance misuse problems are also more prevalent among lower social classes but it may be that spending what money they have on substances leads to greater problems than substance misuse in more affluent groups.

War and conflict

Besides causing considerable anxiety, war and conflict also lead to refugees and asylum seekers. The potential trauma experienced (not just from bombings but associated insults such as rape and torture) and the following displacement (and associated losses) are considerable stressors and increase the risk of mental health problems. War and conflict may also lead to oppression and denial of human rights, which increase the likelihood of developing mental health problems. War also carries a risk of PTSD for those actively involved as soldiers.

Stress

Is stress a cause or a consequence?

Resilience

Helping individuals build on the factors that promote resilience may be helpful (Box 2.3).

> **Box 2.3: Factors promoting resilience (modified from Ahmed, 2007)**
>
> **Personal characteristics**
>
> Positive self-esteem
>
> Secure attachments with an ability to trust others
>
> Have experienced authoritative parenting which gives the individual a sense of mastery and self-sufficiency
>
> Experiencing success
>
> Interpersonal abilities such as social skills, problem solving skills, impulse control and a range of coping strategies
>
> **External factors**
>
> Being safe
>
> Positive and supportive relationships
>
> Sense of belonging through religious or other affiliations

Summary

In this chapter we have reviewed the major aetiological factors that play a part in the development of mental disorders and mental health problems. There is no single aetiological factor in any major mental disorder. Rather, it is the complex interplay between the biological, psychological and social factors that leads to problems. In terms of understanding what causes mental health problems, despite the progress made, we still have some way to go. From a practical perspective because individuals are different and see the world in such different ways, the environmental factors will always influence people differently. In your clinical practice, remember that whatever the genetic risks, anyone with enough environmental challenges can develop problems.

Further reading

Ahmed AS (2007) Post traumatic stress disorder, resilience and vulnerability. *Advances in Psychiatric Treatment* 13: 369–375.

Kendler KS, Prescott CA, Myers J, Neale MC (2003) The structure of genetic and environmental risk factors for common psychiatric and substance use disorders in men and women. *Archives of General Psychiatry* 60: 929–937.

Murali V, Oyebode F (2004) Poverty, social inequality and mental health. *Advances in Psychiatric Treatment,* 10: 216–224.

CASE STUDY

Clare is 16 years old and presents to her GP with anxiety about her upcoming exams. She is struggling to concentrate and focus on any revision. She will often begin by making a list but then becomes overwhelmed by what lies ahead. She is often tearful and relates this to her recent loss. Six months ago her paternal grandmother to whom she was very close passed away after a long and painful time suffering from terminal breast cancer.

Clare was a normal pregnancy and delivery. There were no early concerns regarding her development and she started school without any major problems though took a while to settle. Her father has struggled to cope with the loss of his mother harbouring feelings of guilt as he does not feel he helped his mother as much as he could. Over the last few months he has tended to shut himself off from the family and started working longer hours. He has been more irritable and his relationship with Clare has suffered. There is no family history of mental illness although Clare's mother reports she can struggle with new situations and that her husband finds change difficult. The family do not really talk about the grandmother although when she was alive they had frequent and regular contact.

Who in this scenario has mental health problems?

From Clare's perspective, what are the possible aetiological factors?

Once you have identified the factors draw a table outlining what type of factor it is and whether it is predisposing, precipitating and/or perpetuating.

What would change if her father has developed an alcohol misuse problem?

What might be the aetiological factors to consider in this case?

CHAPTER 3

ASSESSMENT AND ENGAGEMENT WITH PATIENTS

Brian Lunn and Nisha Dogra

KEY CHAPTER FEATURES

- Key elements of psychiatric history
- Mental state examination
- Cognitive examination
- Physical assessment and investigation
- Explaining the importance of integrating cultural issues into the assessment and management process
- Establishing effective working relationships with patients
- Outlining principles that are useful in developing therapeutic relationships with patients
- Defence mechanisms
- How you can develop your own communication style

Introduction

The first part of the chapter deals with the content of psychiatric history taking and mental state examinations. The second part of the chapter deals with some of the principles of developing rapport with patients and also looks at the process of developing a therapeutic relationship. First encounters with patients with mental health problems are often daunting for medical students. One significant concern is that taking a psychiatric history is in some way different from assessment in other areas of medicine. It is actually the case, however, that the psychiatric history has much in common with taking good histories in any area of medicine. The history needs to be taken in a systematic way using good interview techniques and with a desire to understand the patient's experience. Histories will only be comprehensive if they are taken by someone who has a sound knowledge of the signs of mental illness, such as delusions and hallucinations, and knowledge of how to clarify exactly what the patient is presenting with.

History

In whatever setting it occurs, history taking is a process of obtaining information and testing out hypotheses with the aim to fully understand the nature of the patient's experience. This is only possible when the focus is not too narrow, as in many cases, psychiatric and physical problems are present at the same time and interact with each other: physical disorders may have a significant psychological component and psychiatric disorders may present first to a non-psychiatrist. It is therefore important that psychiatric symptoms are explored in all patients and that physical and psychiatric disorders are considered together. All doctors must therefore be comfortable asking about psychiatric symptoms.

The basic principles of taking histories in patients with psychiatric symptomatology are set out in Box 3.1.

Box 3.1: Basic principles of history taking

Begin with open questions

Shift to more directive (closed) questions to clarify what the patient means and what their symptoms are

Establish a timeline setting out the sequence of the patient's experiences and relevant events

Allow the patient to talk

Try and obtain an understanding of the patient's experience

Be empathic

Every history should start in as open a format as is possible as this is the only way that a patient can explain what is concerning them. It is important not just to accept what the patient says at first at face value as there may be things they are embarrassed about or not realize the significance of. Questioning patients about information can be a delicate learning process between patient and doctor, as patients may feel they have already given you the key facts. However, it is often helpful to explain that you need to ensure a shared understanding of how they are using terms, given that terms such as depression may be used differently by the public and health professionals. Once you have identified what you think the main issues are, summarize this list and check that you have identified everything and understood what the issues actually are.

Once the problems have been identified there needs to be a shift to the use of more directive questions to test out hypotheses about what the patient is experiencing and to seek clarification of their symptoms. To use an analogy that may be more familiar to medical students, if a patient complains of pain the student would normally ask about the nature of the pain, its site, any radiation, how the pain varies in response to stimuli such as exercise and certain foods, etc. As they get more experienced they would include questions about psychosocial factors, e.g. if the onset of the pain coincided with significant life events. This does not imply that the pain is solely of psychogenic origin, but acknowledges that several factors may be relevant. In the same way, if a patient complains of hearing voices the student would need to ask where the voices were heard, what was the content of the experience, when it occurred, what was the quality of the voice, and so on.

Establish a timeline

As psychiatric disorders quite often have an insidious onset, establishing a timeline is vital. Patients and their relatives may confuse the chronology of illnesses, mixing up what were consequences of early illness with potential causes. The most useful tool for a historian here is to constantly clarify and use fixed time markers, e.g. birthdays, annual holidays such as Christmas, to identify symptom onset and progression.

Time to talk

This is common to all histories, as the key to all effective histories is not making the patient feel they are not valued or able to talk about their experiences in full. The person taking the history acts as a facilitator, directing the conversation to allow a full elucidation of the patient and their issues. This also enables the patient to build up trust, as we will discuss later.

Understand the patient

This is the whole point of the history. Without understanding the patient's experience there can be no successful intervention. It is all too easy to jump to conclusions about what patients mean. An example might be the use of the term 'paranoid'. Laymen (and many professionals) may misuse this term to mean 'anxious', e.g. 'I'm feeling paranoid about my exams'. So even when you think you know what a patient means you will need to clarify this to ensure that you actually do. It is also important here to consider cultural issues, for the manner in which symptoms are expressed can vary with language and culture, making history taking more complex. This is covered in more detail later in the chapter.

Be empathic

Empathy can be difficult when those with psychiatric disorders have experiences that are so far removed from life experiences of the person taking the history. Ensuring understanding and non-judgemental responses can be difficult. An awareness of this and a willingness to challenge one's own emotional responses and prejudices is therefore essential.

Finally, one of the most important points for any historian is to gain verification or alternative views regarding what they have learned from the patient. The best way to do this is to seek out collaborative histories from those who have witnessed the patient's presentation. This need not be restricted to relatives or the patient's partner but may include a work colleague, ambulance staff or a police officer. When the informant is emotionally involved with the patient or the consequences of the patient's behaviour, the principles of history taking outlined above apply.

The key areas for inquiry are contained in Box 3.2.

Box 3.2: Key components of a psychiatric history

Mode of presentation

How did the patient present? For example, self-referral, referred by a professional, brought by police, etc.

Legal status

Are they informal or detained under mental health or other legislation?

History of presentation

What is the problem, what is the timeline, what events have occurred in the preceding period and subsequently?

Patient perspective

How does the patient conceptualize the problem?

Family history

Might include not only medical and psychiatric histories of family members as appropriate but also comments on their personalities, work history and relationships with the patient and others

Personal history

This covers the development of the patient including such elements as the patient's gestation and birth, early childhood, including developmental milestones, schooling

Box 3.2 continued

Work history

Relationship history, including sexual history

Forensic history

Current circumstances

Previous psychiatric and medical history

Collect all information about current and previous health problems including a medication history

Use of alcohol and recreational drug use

Persistence is often required to get as accurate a picture as possible. Questions about money spent can be useful. Ensure that symptoms and signs of dependence are asked about

Premorbid personality

This can be difficult as patients often focus on how they are in the 'present'. Asking about how they were prior to the onset of problems is useful as is asking them how others see them, not just how they see themselves

Current medication

Make sure that both prescription and self-prescribed medication/remedies are included

Corroborative history

This should be obtained from more than one source if possible and can include family members, friends, carers, the police and other health professionals

Mental state examination

Examination of the mental state is one of the core skills that all doctors need to develop. It is the way in which the patient's clinical signs are explored and classified. Table 3.1 sets out the key domains of the mental state examination along with a list of some possible signs that fall under each domain. A brief explanation of each of these is given below but a full exploration of psychopathology is beyond the remit of this textbook. Video examples can be found on YouTube (www.youtube.com/user/psychiatryteacher) and at Newcastle University (http://mbbs-psychiatry.ncl.ac.uk/video/index2.html).

Appearance and behaviour

Observation of a patient's behaviour can reveal a great deal about a patient's mental health. Poor self-

Table 3.1   Key aspects of a mental state examination

Areas of examination	Example signs
Appearance, behaviour and engagement with the interviewer	Impaired self-care Poor eye contact Restless/anxious Withdrawn/inappropriate
Speech	Socially appropriate or not, e.g. too loud Vocal intonation Poverty of amount Slow Pressured Perseverative
Affect and mood	Depressed Elated Incongruous Blunted
Suicidal ideation	Thoughts of suicide Plans of action
Thought form	Flight of ideas Knight's-move thinking Neologisms Echolalia
Thought content	Poverty of content Obsessional thoughts Overvalued ideas Delusions Thought alienation
Perceptions	Distortions of size, colour or intensity Illusions Hallucinations
Other	For example unusual movements such as dyskinesias or tics

care may be present due to depression, schizophrenia, dementia, etc. In addition, depressed patients may make poor eye contact and move slowly. Conversely, a manic patient may appear to have boundless energy and have difficulty sitting still, make flamboyant, expansive gestures and not respect social boundaries during the interview. Alternatively, they may be irritable, hostile and/or condescending.

Speech

Through observation of a patient's pattern of speech and mode of conversation, insight can be gained into underlying thought processes. An example is slow speech, which may reflect slowing of thought (e.g. in depression or frontal lobe disorders). Speech may also be slowed or hesitant secondary to distraction by internal experiences such as hallucinations or when thoughts are so fast that the patient struggles to keep up verbally with them. Rapid speech can represent rapid thoughts, which manifest in mania and can be termed 'pressure of speech'. Here one may have difficulty interrupting the patient. Remember that when anxious anyone can talk more rapidly and pressure of speech needs to be differentiated from this normal experience.

Other abnormalities of speech include automatic repetition of a phrase (echolalia), word (pallilalia) or syllable (logoclonia) just spoken by the person speaking to the patient. These may be found in organic brain disorders and mental illnesses such as schizophrenia.

Patients may also be reluctant to speak because of other factors such as paranoia. They may also be fearful in case of reprisals, for example in cases where there is domestic violence or child abuse.

Mood

A common mistake in describing mood is to note 'subjective' mood and 'objective' mood. A much more logical way of describing mood is to talk of mood as described by the patient and mood as observed by the examiner respectively. This does not add spurious value to the latter simply by labelling it 'objective'. Typically mood can be 'low' (depressed), 'high' (elevated, elated) or 'normal' (euthymic) but can also be rapidly changing (labile) or out of keeping with what the patient is describing, e.g. smiling when discussing the death of a loved one (incongruous). Depressed and elevated mood states are typically associated with mood disorders but abnormal mood states can occur in other conditions, particularly dementia and schizophrenia. The patient's mood may be incongruous, particularly in schizophrenia. Mood disorders may be accompanied by other concomitants of disturbed mood, e.g. anxiety symptoms in depression and irritability in mania. Lability of mood can be a sign of a rare variant of bipolar disorder, an organic disorder or borderline personality disorder.

It is vital in enquiring about a patient's mood to ask about suicidal thoughts and plans. This should take place for all patients and should include full exploration of any specific plans together with protective and exacerbating factors. There is a common misconception that doing this can lead to an increased risk of suicide. This is not the case.

Thought form

Abnormalities of thought form need to be clearly distinguished from abnormalities of thought content. Through careful listening to the patient's conversation, the interviewer may pick up abnormalities of form of thought, which may have diagnostic relevance. Pressure of speech, which was described above, can be associated with 'flight of ideas', when the patient skips rapidly from one thought to another one that is related in terms of content, meaning or sound (rhyme). The last one is known as 'punning' and is more typical of mania. Flight of ideas needs to be differentiated from 'loosening of associations', where there is no association between successive thoughts. An example of this is 'knight's-move thinking', which at its most extreme can lead to 'word salad' (an incomprehensible jumble of words) that may have some meaning to the patient but not anyone else. Formal thought disorder of this type is highly suggestive of schizophrenia. Neologisms are literally 'new words' that have no generally recognized meaning. They tend to be either completely new or condensations of existing words and are mainly seen in those patients with schizophrenia or structural brain disease.

Thought content

Disorders of thought content include preoccupations, obsessional thoughts, overvalued ideas and delusions. A preoccupation in itself need not be pathological but can be present in mental illness, and if observed should be described. Delusions in contrast are by definition pathological. These are beliefs that persist despite evidence to the contrary and that are out of context with the individual's religious, cultural and educational background. Delusions can be defined as set out in Box 3.3 below.

Obsessions, in contrast to thought insertion, (Box 3.3) are recognized as being the patient's own thoughts. They are recurrent, persistent thoughts, images or impulses that enter the patient's mind unbidden. They often involve fear of contamination or concerns that something has not been done correctly. In the early stages of suffering from these, the patient classically tries to resist the thoughts but as time goes on they may be unable to do so. These thoughts lead to anxiety, which is often reduced by means of compulsive behaviours. Typically these relate to the nature of the thoughts, e.g. fears of contamination can lead to compulsive cleaning and hand washing. Compulsive behaviours often have a ritualistic nature and are conducted in a 'magical' manner. Obsessional thoughts and compulsive acts are most typically seen in obsessive compulsive disorder, but can also occur in other psychiatric illnesses including schizophrenia and depression.

Overvalued ideas are thoughts that a patient believes in firmly in certain circumstances but about

Box 3.3: Classification of delusions

Delusions can be classified as primary or secondary. The latter arise from another pathological experience, for example delusions that develop to explain the experience of auditory hallucinations. In contrast, primary delusions arise *de novo*. This is usually difficult to be certain of. The various subtypes of primary delusion are:

- delusional perceptions in which a normal perception is suddenly interpreted in a delusional manner, e.g. a patient may see a red traffic light and immediately realize that he is the son of God
- sudden delusional ('autochthonous') ideas in which an idea suddenly enters the patient's consciousness like a 'brainwave', unrelated to previous real or psychic events
- delusional mood which is a state of perplexity in which the patient has some sense of some inexplicable change in his environment. He senses 'something going on' which he cannot identify, but which has a peculiar significance for him. This can then be explained by a sudden delusional idea

which the individual can be reassured when in a more neutral context. They are most commonly paranoid in nature. In some senses they fall between preoccupations and delusional thoughts. An example would be someone who strongly feels that when on a bus the other passengers are talking about them but when they are made to look at this in retrospect can accept that it was not really so. These are ideas that frequently cause anxiety to the individual.

Delusions can be further be classified by their content but particular delusions do not suggest particular diagnoses. Certain delusions are, however, more common in particular conditions. Examples include:

- Persecutory delusions where the patient believes that others are out to do them harm.
- Thought alienation, which can take the form of thought insertion, thought withdrawal or thought broadcasting. In thought insertion, the patient believes that thoughts are being put into his or her head. Conversely, in thought withdrawal, the patient believes that thoughts are being 'taken away' by an external agency. In thought broadcasting, the patient's thoughts are being passively broadcast. Although patients sometimes describe this using the term 'telepathy' it should be ascertained whether they believe their thoughts are being broadcast or actively read. The latter is a persecutory delusion rather than thought broadcasting.
- Somatic passivity phenomena are delusions of physical control, i.e. the patient believes that an external agency is controlling or manipulating his or her body or mind.
- Nihilistic delusions (which include delusions of worthlessness, guilt and poverty) are delusions where the belief is centred on loss. At its most extreme, the patient may believe that they are actually dead.
- Grandiose delusions are where the patient has an overexaggerated absolute belief in their self-worth or abilities. Although classically seen in mania these also occur in schizophrenia.

Perceptions

Abnormalities of perception include distortions of real perceptions, false perceptions in the presence of a stimulus (illusions) and false perceptions in the absence of a stimulus (hallucinations). Disorders of perception include disorders of size (smaller – micropsia; larger – macropsia; lopsided – dysmegalopsia) or colour. There are various causes, but typically these are organic and include drug use. Note, however, that transient non-psychiatric disorders such as migraine can cause these symptoms. Equally, illusions can occur in health and illness and on their own have little diagnostic value. They are most common when consciousness is altered (e.g. delirium), when sensory input is reduced (e.g. in the dark) or when the individual is distracted or anxious. Understanding this has particular therapeutic value as it highlights the need to nurse patients with delirium in a well-lit environment.

True hallucinations have the quality of a normal perception (and to the patient are indistinguishable from such) while arising in the absence of a stimulus. They may occur in any sensory modality (Box 3.4) but auditory hallucinations are the most common.

Other

Patients may show dyskinesias (a wide variety of movement patterns, e.g. choreoathetosis, rocking, pouting, etc., which may be related to antipsychotic

Box 3.4: Classification of hallucinations

Auditory hallucinations can take any form from simple, elemental sounds to complex speech or music. The most common experience of hearing voices is of second-person voices, i.e. talking to the patient. These are not associated with particular disorders, but in mood disorders will typically be mood congruent (i.e. in keeping with the patient's mood). Voices that speak the patient's thoughts aloud, give a running commentary on his/her actions, or speak about him/her in the third person are suggestive of schizophrenia. Other types of auditory hallucination can occur in organic disorders, mood disorders and schizophrenia, and sometimes in borderline personality disorder (in which they are usually experienced in internal space, do not have the quality of normal perception and are often termed 'pseudohallucinations'). Visual hallucinations should always raise the possibility of an organic disorder such as epilepsy, delirium, dementia or drug intoxication but can occur in schizophrenia and mood disorders

Somatic (or touch) hallucinations can be a result of withdrawal states (cocaine, alcohol) and include 'formication', which is the sensation of insects crawling over or under the skin. Hallucinations of joint movement (kinaesthetic) occur in benzodiazepine withdrawal. Deeper body hallucinations are often of a sexual nature and can occur in organic disorders and schizophrenia

Olfactory (smell) and gustatory (taste) hallucinations often occur together and should always raise the suspicion of temporal lobe epilepsy

medication) and stereotypies (which are repetitive, non-goal-directed movements). The latter are perhaps most commonly seen in schizophrenia.

Cognitive assessment

A description of how to perform a full cognitive assessment would require a chapter on its own and is beyond the remit of this book. Here only general principles are set out.

It is important to realize that in testing a patient the results of a 'memory' test do not in themselves indicate the nature of a patient's memory but merely allow the tester to infer information about how the patient's memory might be. Of the various factors that influence test performance most are outwith the tester's control but being aware of them allows appropriate interpretation of the results and potentially minimization of them. Factors include the environment (temperature, noise level, interruptions), time of day (this is particularly relevant in mood disorders), the patient's physical state (e.g. pain, breathlessness) and their compliance with testing (e.g. wilful non-cooperation, difficulties with the test). It is important therefore to be aware of these before beginning testing.

All testing must include:

- conscious state
- language difficulties
- concentration and attention
- auditory/verbal new learning (sometimes misleadingly termed 'short-term memory').

There are a number of commonly used screening tests that can pick up on these areas. A prime example is the Mini Mental State Examination (MMSE). In using this, as in all tests, the examiner must be aware of the range of correct answers to the chosen tests and the range of scores in a 'normal' population, as well as how to deliver the tests in such a standardized way that the results can be compared with these normative data. One important issue is that the examiner should not be critical and not respond to 'poor' performance by a patient, for this may also reflect other factors, such as cultural relevance of the information being tested. It is important to understand what tests actually measure. An example is the three-item word list from the MMSE, which assesses more than just memory. Performance is also influenced by factors such as language (comprehension and expression), executive function, concentration and attention. Scores are affected by age and education, and, as a consequence, false-positive results can be achieved in less well-educated patients and false-negative results in the well educated. It is worth remembering that 'absence of evidence is not evidence of absence'; a patient who performs well on a test providing information about memory (e.g. 30/30 in the MMSE assessment of auditory/verbal new learning) does not necessarily have an unimpaired memory.

Physical assessment and investigations

As discussed above the separation into physical and psychiatric illness is artificial at best and carries risks of missing diagnoses and the full range of a patient's problems. It is therefore important that assessment of physical health is not neglected in patients presenting with psychiatric problems. It is doubly important because patients with mental health problems are at high risk of physical health problems because of lifestyle factors (high rates of smoking and obesity and low levels of physical activity), side-effects of medication (increased appetite, sedation) and poor adherence to medication. Health care services and clinicians are at risk of further stigmatizing these patients by ignoring or unduly minimizing the importance of physical health care monitoring and providing appropriate levels of interventions.

Physical examination

All patients require a comprehensive physical examination, which in psychiatric patients does not differ materially from that required in patients presenting with any other health problem. When there are concerns about substance misuse, particular attention should be paid to possible signs of such behaviours, including needle marks and injection site abscesses.

Blood tests

A range of routine tests should be considered at first presentation. These include urea and electrolytes, random glucose concentration and full blood count. Thyroid problems are associated with mood and anxiety disorders so thyroid function tests should be undertaken. Liver function tests (particularly γ-glutamyltransferase) along with the previously mentioned full blood count (particularly mean cell volume) can reveal harmful use of alcohol. There may be a need for more specific tests where particular disorders are suspected. In eating disorders, electrolyte balance and calcium can be affected. Tests to consider in specific clinical presentations may be syphilis serology, copper levels for Wilson's disease and testing for HIV.

When patients have been on psychiatric medication, again particular tests are required. For example if they are taking antipsychotic medication prolactin levels, plasma glucose and lipid profiles should be carried out or if taking lithium assessment of lithium levels and renal and thyroid function is required. Use of clozapine requires regular full blood counts because of the risk of neutropenia.

Urine testing

Dipstick testing of urine has routine value. In addition, there may be cases when a urine drug screen may be useful.

Electrophysiology

Electrocardiograms (ECGs) are a routine investigation because of the recognized link between psychiatric illness, treatments and cardiac risk factors. Of particular concern is QTc prolongation with antipsychotics. Electroencephalography (EEG) has value when seizure disorders are suspected.

Imaging

Brain imaging can be used to exclude certain organic disorders but is not indicated in all cases. Functional imaging is particularly useful in patients with degenerative disorders.

Integrating cultural issues

There can be an assumption that cultural issues only need to be considered in minority and non-white patients and families. Taking this approach clearly limits the quality of care that other patients receive. Everyone including patients has culture, and a good history needs to incorporate relevant aspects as an integral part of the assessment.

Using culture in its broadest sense as defined for example by the American Association of Medical Colleges may help us deliver tailored care to all patients. The definition used is:

> Culture is defined by each person in relationship to the group or groups with whom he or she identifies. An individual's cultural identity may be based on heritage as well as individual circumstances and personal choice. Cultural identity may be affected by such factors as race, ethnicity, age, language, country of origin, acculturation, sexual orientation, gender, socioeconomic status, religious/spiritual beliefs, physical abilities, occupation, among others. These factors may impact behaviours such as communication styles, diet preferences, health beliefs, family roles, lifestyle, rituals and decision-making processes. All of these beliefs and practices, in turn can influence how patients and health care professionals perceive health and illness and how they interact with one another.

(AAMC 1999: 25)

It has been argued that this definition is patient centred and enables patients to decide which of these factors that make up culture are relevant to them.

In delivering care to patients, doctors need to consider the following points:

- They should reflect on their own biases and prejudices to ensure that these do not consciously or subconsciously justify lesser quality for some patients.

- As many factors influence the individual's understanding of mental health and mental health services, at the outset of any assessment the patient's understanding of what they think is going to happen should be checked. Their explanation or understanding for how things are may be very useful for the interventions that are planned.

- Do not be afraid of asking if you are not sure – you just need to ensure you ask respectfully without judgement.

- Do not be intimidated into avoiding difficult questions just because someone is from a visibly different background. Don't assume that because someone superficially looks as though they may be from a similar background that this means they view the world in a similar way.

- Do not assume that because the last person from a particular background believed that mental illness is caused by spirits so will the next patient from a similar background.

- If there are a number of treatment options, do not assume which option the individual will choose. Discuss all the options and ensure the patient and/or family are able to make an informed choice. Different people will need different levels of explanations and time. Working with interpreters can increase the time needed.

- Ensure that you do get the patient's perspective. At times of distress and stress, family members may speak for the patient and make choices that they would make for themselves rather than think about what the patient might truly want.

Using interpreters

It is beyond the remit of this book to focus on this in detail. However, it is important to make sure that the interpreter is an appropriate person. It is usually not good practice to use children and/or family members as interpreters, except in emergency situations. There

---

Exercise

Practitioner cultural and patient cultural influence on the health care encounter

What is it about you and your patients that might influence the health care encounter?

Annotate the diagram below with the factors that might influence the encounter

Exercise answer

Every single factor that makes you the person you are may influence the encounter. There may be advantages or disadvantages to this. All of the factors below and possibly more influence the encounter. You are not a neutral presence in the encounter.

Dress	Gender	Decoration
Age	Religion	Verbal behaviour
Colour	Politics	Non-verbal behaviour
Previous stereotypes	Space	Fear
Projection	Touch	Personal histories
Attitudes	Language	Personality disposition, i.e. introvert,
Level of knowledge	Disability	extrovert, open, etc.
about the other	Power	Empathy
Greeting behaviour	The situation in which they meet	Why are they meeting?
	Is there a previous history?	

are issues about appropriateness of the content covered but also confidentiality. It can also be stressful, as the presentation will be causing concern for family members too. Using staff who speak the language is preferable to using family members. It can be difficult to find trained interpreters, especially for languages that are not widely spoken. There may be concerns that confidentiality will be maintained in small communities. It also takes practice to be aware when the interpreter is interpreting what the patient is saying or when they are 'reinterpreting' what the patient has said. When using an interpreter it is important to talk to the patient and not just work through the interpreter. Remember non-verbal language is also important and you can make only make sense of this if you communicate with the patient directly.

Diagnostic summary

Having collected all of this information, which may take more than one meeting and include talking with one or more informants, what should happen next? You need to write a structured summary (approximately half an A4 page) in which you identify the key presenting features, an outline history of these, relevant background factors and significant mental state findings. These are then used to construct your differential diagnosis and you should indicate which you think is most likely and why. This then should support your plan of investigation and initial management plan. New information, as it emerges, is then used to review the initial diagnosis and plan of management. This is also known as a case formulation.

Establishing effective working relationships with patients

In this section we consider developing working relationships with patients. Our own sense of culture and our personal values strongly influence our communication styles so it is relevant to be aware of how some of these factors can interplay with each other to impact on working relationships. We consider different stages of the clinical relationship and how these might be facilitated. We also consider some concepts, such as transference and defence mechanisms, that can influence the working relationship with patients.

Engagement

Engagement is the process by which the clinician establishes a working relationship with the patient and/or their family. Effective engagement is an important aspect of all clinical relationships but absolutely crucial in psychiatry. Although patients may tell you about their physical complaints even if they do not feel engaged with you, they are less likely to share personal details about themselves unless they feel they can trust you and that you are sensitive to their potential difficulties. This means that unless they are engaged with you, you may not get all the information you need.

There is much that can be done to increase the likelihood of effective engagement. Some of the suggestions below may sound as though they are basic common sense and in some ways most of them are. However, they are often the things that students forget to do especially when under pressure or feeling uncomfortable. These are essential in psychiatry, but they are also relevant in the practice of medicine in general. Appearing warm and friendly but professional at the same time is important in gaining patient confidence. Research has shown that patients generally liked doctors to be formally dressed. This suggests that although the relationships between doctors and patients are changing, with doctors less paternal than they might have been in the past, there are certain expectations that remain. Appropriate dress also extends courtesy to the patient as it reflects to some extent the pride you take in your role.

During the introduction it is important not just to say who you are, and what you intend to do, but it is equally important to check out with the patient what they think is going to happen. It is also important to explain to them at an early stage what information you are obliged to share so no false expectations are set up.

Active listening

This is more than just listening to what someone is saying. Active listening is the process by which the listener makes the person who is talking feel comfortable and valued. The listener gives the other person the time and space to be able to say what they need to say. When you are trying to take a history and know that you need specific information, it can be very tempting to interrupt too early and make the patient feel as though you are not really listening to them or worse dismissing their views. It takes practice to sensitively bring someone back to your agenda but still be mindful of giving them the time to tell their story.

Reflecting and summarizing

Summarizing (paraphrasing) is the skill of repeating back what someone has said and is a way of checking that you have understood what has been conveyed. Reflecting is the process by which you consider what has been said and may acknowledge how the person feels. It is usually best to be speculative rather than presumptive, e.g. 'that sounds like it was a difficult time' rather than 'that must have been a difficult time'.

Question types

Open questions that encourage more than simple categorical responses are more appropriate to begin with. It is important to give patients the time and space to be able to relate their experiences, so using statements like, 'Tell me what has been happening over the last few days' may be a useful way of beginning. In psychiatry, towards the end of the history, it can be useful to use closed questions to fill any gaps in the history but rarely are such questions effective at obtaining a rich history.

Endings

Finishing a conversation takes skill. It can be particularly difficult for students as they may feel that they have taken and learnt from the interview process but not given anything in return. If the interview has been long and difficult, acknowledge that the person might be tired and thank them for their time. After the interview, it will be useful to reflect back on your performance and also pay some attention to how you felt doing the interview. This will help improve your interviewing skills but also help you become more comfortable tackling difficult issues.

Responses to patient histories

Some patients' stories touch us for various reasons and some stay with us. It is important to be able to deal with any issues this raises for you, even if only by chatting to your peers. There are always patients we find difficult; again think it through. The difficulties may be because we are not functioning at our best and/or the patient is difficult. If it is the latter, don't take it too personally as distress can make people less reasonable and cooperative than they might otherwise be.

At times patients may describe events or experiences that resonate personally with you for whatever reason. In these situations, it is even more essential to be aware of the issues of transference and counter-transference discussed below. If the interview is too difficult to continue because of this, as a student it is appropriate to terminate it or at least take a break while you collect your thoughts.

All patients have the potential to reveal histories that are painful and distressing, and as students learning how to manage this effectively without detriment to your own health but retaining compassion is important.

Finally, our own state of mind can strongly influence the outcome of our working relationships with patients. It is consistent with good medical practice to be professional and not allow our personal issues to impact on professional roles. However, pretending that there are no personal issues is not an effective way of addressing this. Being aware of your own issues and feelings is important so you can recognize the potential impact of these when you communicate with patients and colleagues.

Other aspects to consider

Rapport

This refers to the development of a relationship where there is a sense of understanding about each other.

In the professional relationship when a rapport is established there is a sense that both parties are vested in the relationship (in the professional sense) and they are working together towards achieving a shared goal.

Boundaries

Boundaries are a way of defining your personal space and limits, both physically and emotionally. Physical boundaries are limits around physical contact. It goes without saying that physical relationships with patients are inappropriate, as they may compromise the professional relationship. Different people have different levels of comfort around physical contact from unfamiliar people. It is important to be able to offer patients comfort but be aware that their boundaries may be different from your own. It is probably best to do no more than offer tissues or move closer if someone cries as both will demonstrate that you are attending to the distress but are not running the risk of being misinterpreted. Even taking someone's hand or touching them on the shoulder may be seen as an intrusion by some patients. You should check that it is okay to touch a patient before you do so, but that can remove the element of comfort. It is important to be very aware of the cues the patient gives you about their comfort levels regarding personal space. Experience teaches you much about when physical contact is acceptable or not.

Emotional boundaries are the limits you set around how much of your thoughts and feelings you choose to share with others. This can be more difficult as a student as you may be asked personal questions by patients but feel unable to express a preference not to discuss the issues. Any student undergoing their own personal issues (such as bereavement, relationship difficulties) may find that dealing with psychiatric patients' distress over similar issues has an exaggerated effect on their own emotional world. This may be because it becomes difficult to be clear about which feelings are your own and which belong to the patient.

Boundaries are important for your protection and also that of patients, so think very carefully before you breach them. Patients have a right to expect that you take responsibility for ensuring that professional boundaries are maintained. They may challenge them, but it is up to you to ensure you are clear about the limits. Social engagements with patients are inappropriate while you are in any way involved in their care. Given you know sensitive information about them, relationships even after the placement may be inappropriate due to the vulnerability of the patient.

Sharing personal information

Sharing personal information may cross some emotional boundaries. It is perfectly acceptable to chat with patients about subjects other than their psychiatric histories. However, it is advisable to keep conversations non-personal. Sharing personal information in therapeutic contexts can be incredibly powerful but requires skill and experience. The outcomes may not be as expected and knowing how to deal with any fallout from sharing personal information should be anticipated. Watch carefully during your placement to see when colleagues share personal information and how this is done. Sensitive personal information should only be used in a planned manner and not just because you are unable to contain your emotions.

Working collaboratively with patients and their families

Societal and political changes have led to increased expectations that patients now have greater say in their care and management. This applies equally in psychiatry, although psychiatry faces greater challenges than many other areas of medicine with movements (such as the anti-psychiatry movement) that contest the validity of psychiatric disorder, arguing that it is nothing more than a social construct designed to empower doctors.

Within appropriate constraints around confidentiality, in psychiatry there is often a need to collect third-party information as so much of mental illness changes the way people think and understand the world. When interviewing other informants, it is important to keep in mind that people give information that is coloured by their own experiences. This does not mean that they are being untruthful or saying that the patient is incorrect, but that their perception differs. Information about what the person was like before they became ill is information that can often only be provided by family or friends, especially if someone presents acutely unwell.

Useful concepts to help develop therapeutic relationships

Transference

Transference occurs when a person takes the perceptions and expectations of one person and projects them on to another person. Projecting is when you project your own feelings, emotions or motivations into another person without realizing your reaction is really more about you than it is about the other person.

Typically, the pattern projected on to the other person comes from a childhood relationship. This may be from an actual person, such as a parent, or an idealized figure or prototype. This transfers both power and expectation. This can have both positive and negative outcomes. In which situations and whom we place our transference on reveals and illuminates our motives and our thoughts that would otherwise not be expressed to others or perhaps even acknowledged to ourselves. Our acts of transference provide a window into what we want and what we might be trying to avoid, and our hopes and fears. What we read into other people reveals our own prejudices and unfulfilled wishes. Transference occurs on a regular basis and in all relationships, but is particularly useful as a therapeutic tool to promote understanding.

Counter-transference

Counter-transference is the response that is elicited in the recipient (therapist) by the other's (patient's) unconscious transference communications. The transference generated by patients may evoke responses in clinicians that they need to be aware of. Transference also provides a good idea of what the patient might be expecting from you.

Feelings are easier to identify if they are not congruent with the doctor's personality and expectation of his or her role. Doctors may struggle with transference, as often they need to feel needed and they may encourage this and only realize the impact once a degree of dependency has been created. If they lack awareness they may react emotionally with irritation, rather than consider the role they might also have played in establishing this dynamic. Awareness of the transference–counter-transference relationship allows a more considered response. Being aware of the subconscious patient agenda may help the doctor recognize some of the patient's wishes and fears and address these openly and sensitively. It may also help explain certain behaviours from both the patient and the doctor. Understanding this also means that the doctor is able to step back and prevent themselves from feeling overwhelmed by excessive patient demand as they have greater awareness of what might be happening.

Transference happens in most relationships and not recognizing transference and counter-transference can have a negative impact on the doctor–patient relationship.

Defence mechanisms

These are discussed here as they are important factors that play a part in clinical and other relationships. Although much of Freud's work may now be considered out of vogue, except in very specific contexts, understanding defence mechanisms can really help understand human functioning. It is worth highlighting that we all use defence mechanisms, and they can be effective coping strategies in the short term. However, over-reliance on them and an unwillingness to explore deeper meanings can impact on relationships and how we feel about ourselves. Freud considered that defence mechanisms are used to deal with anxiety and actions that we may find unacceptable either to ourselves or may be unacceptable socially. There was also an emphasis that at the heart of it lay sexual or violent tendencies. For the purposes of explaining them here, this emphasis is not made.

The most commonly described defence mechanisms are:

- **Denial** – the refusal to accept the reality of a situation, thought or event. An example of this can be when something that someone does not want to happen has happened, e.g. bereavement, a relationship break up. The initial response can be a denial that the event has taken place.
- **Projection** – this is placing the feelings an individual has on someone else. So instead of acknowledging that you feel angry, you say someone else is angry because you are unable to own your feelings of anger.

- **Rationalization** – this is the mechanism whereby we try and explain something logically as the feelings we have may not be feelings we feel are acceptable or logical. An example might be saying that you were justified in being cross with a colleague as they were late for a meeting when the real reason might be that you do not like that person.

- **Sublimation** – this is when the energy from feelings about one issue is channelled into another activity. Being angry with someone at work and then using the aggression when you play sport is an example of sublimation.

- **Reaction formation** – this is expressing the opposite of what you might feel or think because to acknowledge the real feelings or thoughts may be unacceptable (either socially or to yourself).

- **Displacement** – this is placing the feelings for one person (or a situation) on to another person or situation because it may be unacceptable to have the feelings for the original person. This may be being attracted to someone who is unavailable and thereby displacing those feelings on to someone else who may be available. It is also often done when an individual is angry with someone in authority but cannot communicate that so takes out their anger on a peer or someone who is less senior.

- **Regression** – this is when someone reverts to a coping style from an earlier stage of development. A temper tantrum in an adult is a very good example of this.

- **Repression** – highly stressful events that led to particular feelings are 'locked' away into our unconscious self. They may impact on our response to other situations but we are not aware of this as we do not 'recall' the event. An example might be someone who was bullied at school but repressed the recall of this. In their workplace or other relationship, they may function in such a way that anticipates they may be bullied because of the earlier events.

It is also important to note that we all use defence mechanisms, and they are a useful means of understanding the way we communicate our feelings to others. However, if defence mechanisms, transference and counter-transference are considered together, sometimes what a person is saying is exactly what they are saying. The fact that we are unable to hear this may be because we are using particular defence mechanisms and are unable or unwilling to hear what the person is saying. A student may say they were badly taught as an explanation of poor academic performance when in fact they had failed to study effectively (rationalization, if we consider defence mechanisms). However, as a tutor it is worth noting that the student may not be rationalizing but may well have not been well taught.

Exercise

Having read about defence mechanisms, think about your own life in the last week or so. Denial, projection and displacement are very commonly used in everyday life. Can you think about if you used them and when?

It may also be helpful to think about when the people you have come across during this time used them or not

What are the emotions you find most difficult to own?

How might this impact on your future practice as a doctor?

Developing your personal communication style

As a student you have opportunities to watch many different professionals at work. When you observe them, reflect on what works and what is less effective. As you develop your own skills, consider which aspects of good practice you can incorporate into your style. It is rarely effective to simply 'copy' someone else, as patients can tell whether your communication flows or not. Communication is a skill that requires continued refinement even after many years in practice. Developing your own style that incorporates your personal style with good professional practice means that you will inevitably make mistakes but this is an important learning opportunity if you leave yourself open to change. It is also useful to consider which areas you find most difficult to talk about and how this might impact on the way you communicate with patients. It is not necessarily that these issues need to be addressed but knowing about them enables you to be a more reflective clinician.

Summary

In this section we have considered the stages of developing an effective working relationship with patients and some of the factors that may influence this. Communication by its very nature means that there is more than one perspective to take into account. The interview enables you to learn about the patient. Reflection and discussions with peers and staff enable you to learn about yourself. Knowing yourself is useful to help effectiveness at interviewing patients and developing productive working relationships.

To finish this chapter you may find it useful to repeat the first exercise.

Further reading

Casey PR, Kelly B (2007) *Fish's Clinical Psychopathology: Signs and Symptoms in Psychiatry*. London: Royal College of Psychiatrists.

Oyebode F (2008) *Sims' Symptoms in the Mind: An Introduction to Descriptive Psychopathology (Made Memorable)*, 4th edition. Edinburgh: Saunders Elsevier.

CHAPTER 4

MAKING THE MOST OF YOUR PLACEMENT

Nisha Dogra

KEY CHAPTER FEATURES

- Preparing for the placement
- Maximizing opportunities during the placement
- What teachers expect from you and what you can expect from your teachers
- Passing your exams
- Service provision

Introduction

In this chapter we begin by considering how you can make the most of your clinical placement in psychiatry. We discuss some of the issues related to safety, stigma and fear that often accompany the placement and have been shown to be a concern among students. There is a section on passing psychiatric exams, although we are aware that few medical schools now have end of clinical block exams. The final section considers how you might look after your own mental health and that of your colleagues. We also provide evidence of why this is important as a student and once you are practising. We then provide a framework for mental health service provision focusing on those aspects that may influence your placement.

Preparation for the placement

Before you start your placement, it may be useful for you to reflect on your views about psychiatry and patients who have mental health problems. Before you dismiss this as typically 'touchy-feely' psychiatry, just consider recent evidence. There has always been good evidence that non-mental health professionals have negative views about patients with mental health problems and often their views are as stigmatizing as those of the general public (the work of AF Jorm and colleagues is particularly useful in this area). A study at one UK medical school found that students had negative views about patients with mental health problems even after their clinical placements. They also had more negative views about those with mental illness than for patients with diabetes. This suggests that clinical placements reinforced rather than challenged their views. A study led by Simon Budd at Leeds found that students agreed that they often felt uncomfortable during their placements and had difficulties communicating with patients in psychiatric services. Most students also agreed that it can be harder to deal with patients who have mental health problems, but despite this did not consider psychiatry to be stressful. However, we are aware that many students can find the psychiatry placement to be a challenging experience.

As Dixon and colleagues highlight, some of the concerns may be justified. However, you need to address these concerns, as it is important to ensure that your care of patients with mental health problems is not poorer because of your views. Not doing so means you are unlikely to comply with the General Medical Council's Good Medical Practice guide.

Dixon *et al.* argued that although patients with mental health problems may as a group be more difficult to manage than other patients, this does not mean that all or even the majority will be difficult to manage. Indeed in psychiatry you may learn more about managing the range of human presentations than in any other specialty and this skill will come in useful whatever area of medicine you ultimately end up practising in.

Patients with mental health problems are likely to need more time than other patients, but that should not mean that they receive a lesser quality of care. The media are also likely to fuel the stereotype that patients with mental health problems are more violent. The evidence for this being the case is more questionable but, rather than remain fearful, it may be better to find out when this is more of a possibility so that you are effectively prepared.

In preparation, think about what your concerns or fears are and how you can address them.

Write down a list of what you hope to learn and take it to discuss with your clinical team (or consultant if there is a named individual). This will also be good practice for when you graduate and will be expected to take more responsibility for your learning. It is also worth reviewing your earlier learning, as some of the basic sciences foundation will be very useful for the clinical placement.

Psychiatry is a specialty in which your clinical skills, including communication skills, are going to be your strongest asset. There are few diagnostic tests so you really have to use the clinical skills you have. Consider how you might develop your clinical skills and which aspects warrant particular attention.

Read any preparation material you have been sent or asked to read, and before the placement check out the practical details such as where to go and when.

On the day

- Help make a good impression by turning up on time.

- Dress appropriately – this does not necessarily mean formally. You should however be smart and well groomed.
- Comply with your university and hospital regulations regarding badges.
- Be sure you know what the issues are with respect to consent and confidentiality.
- Check out what's expected of you (and if you are not sure, ask).
- Be reassured by the knowledge that most of those involved in teaching you psychiatry actually do enjoy it!

During the attachment

You are likely to meet lots of people, try and remember their names. Try and look like you are interested and most clinicians are happy to help you gain the clinical exposure you need. Clinicians may at times be protective of their patients but if you are enthusiastic they are likely to try and ensure you get to see as many patients as you can. You will impress clinicians if you take the time to be mindful of the efforts made on your behalf.

Prepare for clinical sessions by reading about the conditions you may see. In doing this you are likely to gain more from meeting the patient. You will find that the same condition can have varying impacts on people's lives. This is true for every medical condition but very well illustrated in psychiatry. There are also great opportunities for seeing the interplay of biological, psychological and social factors in action. However, although textbooks are useful in helping you prepare, textbooks cannot substitute for real experience. It is also worth using the resources of the clinicians you see during your placements. Feel confident enough to ask them questions to help your learning. Most will welcome the opportunity to discuss their work and appreciate your enthusiasm and willingness to learn. They will appreciate that you may have had limited opportunities to see clinical psychiatry in action and will do their best to support your learning. Most clinical teachers will be busy but clinical teaching is an important part of their job and most enjoy it, so make the most of it.

It is unacceptable to access notes of people or colleagues you know personally unless you are directly involved in their care. Make yourself familiar with the relevant local protocols so that you practise safely.

Health and safety

Personal safety

There is some evidence that there is a small increased risk of violence among patients who have schizophrenia. This is likely in younger men who are not treatment compliant and lack social support. If a patient is acutely psychotic, their perceptual difficulties make them more vulnerable but can also increase the risk to others. Any time you feel concerned or unsafe or are not sure, ensure you take steps to make yourself safe. Take the time to familiarize yourself with the safety protocols in place. It is important to realize that the skills learned in assessing risk in a psychiatric setting will be useful in all clinical environments. Rates of assault on staff are higher in A&E units than in general psychiatric settings.

Paying regard to the safety of others

If a patient discloses to you that they are considering hurting someone else or themselves, you need to ensure you share this information with the clinical team. Do not assure the patient that they have confidentiality, as you are not able to guarantee this. It is a legal obligation to share information that may put another person at risk; for example, thoughts of violence towards another; potential abuse of others (especially children and other vulnerable groups). As a student, you should ensure you communicate what you have been told clearly and in a timely manner. If a patient asks you about the limits of confidentiality, be honest about this and state the parameters within which you are expected to work.

Attendance

Clinical placements rely on attendance to be able to make the most of clinical opportunities and learning. If you are finding the placement difficult discuss this, as just avoiding it does not help your learning or your future patients.

What to expect from clinical teachers

There are efforts afoot to set baseline standards for clinical teachers in psychiatry. You should reasonably expect teachers:

- to be prepared
- to make time to meet with you to discuss your placement and what you hope to achieve from it
- to provide support regarding the clinical subject by answering questions you may identify when reading about the subject
- to be obliged to report their concerns if they identify problems with your attitude or behaviour.

It will help your teachers if you understand that teaching you is often one of many roles that they undertake and even the best laid plans can go awry.

Most of your clinical teachers will understand your fears and/or concerns. They would much rather you discussed them as that can help you deal with them rather than just pretending everything is okay.

Patient expectations

Most psychiatric patients are usually happy to talk with students about their illnesses and the impact of this on their lives. They often value the opportunity of having extended time to be able to share their story and help your learning. Do not take it personally if they decline to be interviewed as they may just not be well enough to do so but may be willing to do so when their health has improved. Even if they have previously consented to talking to you, it can be helpful to check again at the time of the interview. Talking to as many different patients as you can enables you to see the breadth of psychiatric disorders but also how the aetiological factors interplay to lead to similar diagnoses with different outcomes. Patients can help you see that there is a person beyond the diagnosis and that many of them when not ill have hugely varied and fulfilling lives.

It goes without saying that patients need to be courteously approached. Explain what you would need to do and ask what their expectations are. It can be useful at the outset to say what you plan to do with any information you obtain so that the patient is aware of the parameters of confidentiality and is assured that their details are not shared beyond the clinical context. Given that it will take you some time to take a detailed history, check how much time the patient expects to spend with you and if they are happy for you to also talk to accompanying family members if relevant and appropriate. Talking to carers can provide valuable learning experiences. Some patients and/or their carers may want to recount difficult situations to ensure that as a student you learn from this so you will hopefully provide better care than they might have experienced.

Worries or problems during your placement

In the first instance, any worries or problems should be discussed with your lead consultant. If the worries are about the consultant, then share them with your personal tutor and/or the lead person who is in charge of the psychiatry programme. This may be a clinical academic or an NHS consultant with a particular role for undergraduate education.

Passing your exams

It goes without saying that being prepared increases the likelihood of passing your exams. For clinical psychiatry exams as with others, you will be examined on the process and the contents of your interviewing and examinations. Passing exams is a lot easier if you have had practice of interviewing patients. The best practice opportunities will come on the wards, in day hospitals and in clinics, not through reading textbooks. Try and ensure that you balance your learning in terms of the knowledge, skills and attitudes. Patients will usually be quite happy to provide useful feedback and are well placed to say what you could have done to help them open up more or feel more comfortable.

The process

As part of good medical practice, you are expected to treat patients and colleagues with courtesy and respect. It is important that this is demonstrated in your exams. Sometimes under pressure you may fail to do fairly straightforward things that you usually do without thinking, e.g. asking the patient their name. Should you omit some questions, don't panic. Just take a deep breath and remedy the error. In OSCEs for example you will often have 7–10 minutes to collect quite a lot of data. Under pressure, you may not attend to the patient, as you are preoccupied with getting the information to pass the exam. Examiners will mark you down if you fail to respond to the patient in an appropriate way, e.g. if you don't follow up on their

cues, do not acknowledge distress. Remember that clinical examinations are focused on assessing clinical skills rather than simply being designed for you to exhibit your knowledge.

Contents

A mental state examination should be part of all medical assessments, even if it might often only be very brief. Avoid making any judgemental or pejorative comments, as that is inappropriate.

Looking after your own mental health and that of colleagues

Your own mental health

It is often speculated that one of the reasons that there are negative perceptions of those with mental health problems is that it raises concerns about our own vulnerabilities. Apart from psychosis, many of the problems experienced by people with mental health problems are on the range of 'normal' human experiences but vary in frequency and intensity. Differentiating people with mental health problems as different from ourselves may enable us to apply denial and thereby minimize our own risk.

As we discussed in Chapter 1, mental health problems are common. Doctors may not have as many of the social risk factors at play as the general public but they may have psychological and professional factors that increase their vulnerability. It is worth noting that more than 90 per cent of cases referred to the General Medical Council relating to the health of doctors and concerns about their practice are to do with mental health problems. Doctors and students cope with stress in different ways. It is useful at this stage for you to consider what coping strategies you use and how effectively these work. It is also important to think about how you recognize that you are becoming stressed and how you deal with this early on.

The mental health of colleagues

If you know or suspect that a colleague has mental health problems, try talking to them and encourage them to seek appropriate help. It can be helpful to keep a careful eye on them but be wary of stepping in too often to bail them out as you may just be avoiding the inevitable. If a colleague's problems (for example substance misuse) are potentially or actually impacting on their job, you have a responsibility to report this. Avoid being tempted into misguided loyalty by keeping quiet; you will ultimately be doing your colleague and patients a disservice. By not raising concerns you may be jeopardizing patient safety and your own career. As a student, there is no need for you to carry anxieties about your colleagues as there are senior staff with whom to share concerns.

Psychiatry as a career

If you are interested in psychiatry as a career visit the Royal College of Psychiatrists website at www.rcpsych. ac.uk and find out more. Also take the opportunity to talk with clinicians on your placement – your enthusiasm will be rewarded.

Mental health service provision

Mental health service provision will vary across the UK and internationally. Service developments are dependent on local context (including local history, local health priorities, politics and local staff interest), national policies (where these exist, but in many countries there is little policy regarding mental health) and resources available (staff expertise as well as financial resources).

The UK has had a dramatic reduction in beds available over the last few decades as the focus has increasingly moved from inpatient care to community-based services. The support that patients actually receive in the community is highly variable.

It is most likely that the community mental health teams that you will come across are multidisciplinary in nature. Very few psychiatric services in the UK do not have such teams. Working out the roles of various members of the team can be quite confusing, so ask if you have any questions. Most teams will have a psychiatrist, community psychiatry nurses (who have trained in mental health but may also have general nursing qualifications), nursing assistants (who take on some nursing duties but have not completed a nursing qualification), occupational therapists, psychologists (in some areas the psychology service will be independent of the psychiatric service), social workers (it may vary whether these are an integral part of the team or work alongside it dependent on local arrangements), specific therapists who may have a range of different professional backgrounds and administrative support.

Over the last decade or so there has been a proliferation of specialist teams such as crisis intervention, early intervention services for psychosis, assertive outreach and deliberate self-harm teams. This will vary locally and it is worth discussing with patients and clinical staff how such teams have influenced service delivery and impacted on factors such as continuity of care.

Summary

In summary, as with any other placement, you will get more out of the placement if you prepare effectively for it. The psychiatry placement may be more challenging than other placements, especially if there are areas you have anxieties about. Being willing to acknowledge and address these difficulties will mean that whatever your future specialty, you will acquire skills that will benefit your patients and ensure high-quality care.

Further reading

Dixon RP, Roberts LM, Lawrie S, Jones LA, Humphreys MS (2008) Medical students' attitudes to psychiatric illness in primary care. *Medical Education* 42: 1080–1087.

Jorm AF (2000) Mental health literacy: public knowledge and beliefs about mental disorders. *British Journal of Psychiatry* 177: 396–401.

Jorm AF, Korten AE, Jacomb PA, *et al.* (1997) 'Mental health literacy': a survey of the public's ability to recognise mental disorders and their beliefs about the effectiveness of treatment. *Medical Journal of Australia* 166: 182–186.

MENTAL HEALTH LEGISLATION

Brian Lunn

KEY CHAPTER FEATURES

- An introduction to the principles of mental health legislation
- An overview of compulsion in the treatment of mental illness
- An overview of capacity in mental illness
- Common principles in mental health legislation
- A brief overview of the English and Welsh Mental Health Act (1983)

Introduction

One of the most contentious and complex issues in psychiatry is the compulsory detention and treatment of patients with mental disorders for assessment and treatment. The issue raises important questions such as 'To what extent should a person suffering mental disorder be held responsible for their behaviour (e.g. is it fair to punish a man who smashes a window in response to 'voices' over which he has no control as they are part of a mental illness)?' If they are not fully responsible then should their freedom be limited 'for their own good' (i.e. should the same man be taken to hospital against his will if he cannot be held accountable for his actions)?

The law must provide practical responses to this type of question and has to balance the needs of the individual with the needs of the community. So, for example, if through a mental illness the man represents a risk to himself or others, is it reasonable to detain him for his protection and/or the protection of others? Before we consider these issues, it is worth highlighting that the definition of what is a mental disorder or illness is contentious. Historically there have been models of illness used throughout the world that today seem at best bizarre

and at worst prejudiced and oppressive, whether used for political reasons or because they were based on what was understood and believed at that time. The importance of defining mental illness within a legal framework is that it protects people regarded as 'odd' or a 'nuisance' from inappropriate and unnecessary compulsion. People should surely not be considered mentally disordered simply on grounds of 'immoral' conduct, sexual choices or dependence on alcohol or drugs. It is important to remember that psychiatric diagnoses do not necessarily correspond to legal definitions!

Before reading further it is worth considering:

- Are there circumstances in which compulsory admission/treatment are justified?
- If so, when might this be appropriate?
- If not, what are the alternatives?
- Should mental illnesses be treated differently from other illnesses?
- If so, what would be the justification?
- Who should decide whether compulsory detention is indicated?
- How can the individual's rights be protected even if they are detained?

Why is this important for you?

Whilst it is unlikely that more than a few of you reading this will become psychiatrists, why is it important that you know about mental health legislation? It is likely that even in your Foundation years you will come across patients with mental disorders and/or loss of capacity. Understanding the principles of legislation is therefore important for all doctors. It is also possible that you will be in a position where you will be treating patients already detained under the Mental Health Act and understanding the limits of the Act is therefore important.

Case studies

Consider each of the four case histories below and consider how you think the patient should be managed. For each case, it might be helpful to consider the justification for your decision. They will be revisited at the end of the chapter with some comments about how they might be managed within current legislation.

CASE STUDY 1

A 47-year-old single woman with multiple sclerosis is referred to local mental health services by her mother. She is concerned that her daughter has voiced an intention to commit suicide. The patient, having been brought up in a very religious household, rejected her family's religious beliefs in her late teens, when she left home to go to university. She and her parents have been estranged until a few years ago when her father had a serious myocardial infarct (MI). Six months after their reunion her father died from a second MI.

Just after university, the patient developed blurred vision. It was on presenting for investigation that her multiple sclerosis was diagnosed. Her illness has followed a relapsing/remitting course, but over the last 5 years the decline has been steadily accelerating. Currently she is just recovering from another relapse and now needs to look at moving into living in a more supported environment. Her mother has suggested she moves home.

The patient has always said that when she lost her independence she would choose to end her life rather than live beholden to others. She has recently discussed this with her younger sister who revealed her confidence to their mother. Suicide is an anathema to the rest of the patient's family. They consider her to be depressed, given that she is having such thoughts. As such, they have asked that the patient be assessed and detained for treatment if she cannot be persuaded that suicide is wrong.

CASE STUDY 2

A 23-year-old man is stopped by the police as he was noted to be wandering the streets muttering to himself. On stopping him, the police found that he was carrying a knife. He is being assessed in the cells by a duty psychiatrist following referral by the police surgeon.

The young man's flatmates describe a gradual pattern of deterioration in functioning that they feel might be related to recreational drug use. The young man talks of his fears of a vague group of 'officials' who are monitoring him and he feels that they will ultimately try to make him a victim of 'extraordinary rendition', taking him away to Pakistan to be tortured. He has told the police that he is carrying a knife for his own 'protection'.

CASE STUDY 3

A 38-year-old musician with bipolar affective disorder is in hospital nearing the end of his stay. His admission was compulsory as he had developed another manic episode that had resulted in him running up significant debts and displaying increasingly disinhibited behaviour, culminating in him running down the middle of the main shopping street naked apart from a 'Santa' hat.

He is grateful that he was detained and admitted and is now euthymic. He has had successful spells at home and is ready for discharge but has stated that although he believes medication helped with the acute phase of his illness he intends stopping everything within 3 months of discharge, as he believes that lithium, which he is currently on, blunts his creativity. He no longer requires inpatient treatment.

CASE STUDY 4

A 55-year-old man with recurrent major depression is found in his home by his CPN in a state of squalor. He is emaciated and in poor physical health. Assessment reveals that he has a severe depressive illness with psychotic features, including profound nihilistic delusions, e.g. the belief that his internal organs have rotted away. He refuses to eat or drink and pulls out any intravenous or nasogastric tube inserted. He will not take medication. In line with treatment protocols, it is felt by his treating team that the most appropriate treatment is ECT. His family are supportive of this recommendation but the patient refuses saying that is pointless as he is already dead.

Compulsory treatment

The whole area of compulsion in health is a contentious one. There isn't even commonality in the legislation between the various legal jurisdictions in the UK. Over the past few years significant changes in legislation have taken place in Scotland, and England and Wales. At the time of going to press, proposals for new legislation in Northern Ireland are being consulted upon.

It is beyond the remit of this chapter to consider all the complexities of the various pieces of legislation in the UK, even if they were not changing. Instead it is intended to introduce some basic principles and then illustrate one approach by describing the various elements of the Mental Health Act as currently enacted in England and Wales.

Consent

It is a fundamental principle of ethical medical practice that patients are only treated with their consent. There are, however, some circumstances where this principle cannot be easily adhered to, for example if the patient lacks capacity because they are unable to communicate their wishes or understand what treatment is being offered. The key elements of capacity to be able to consent are that:

- the patient understands the information presented to them;
- the patient can retain the information;
- the patient can weigh the information in the balance and come to a decision based on this;
- the patient can communicate their wishes.

If the patient cannot fulfil the above criteria, their capacity to give consent is questionable. It is important to remember that the default position under the Mental Capacity Act (2005) is that all adults (i.e. people aged 16 years and older) are assumed to have capacity to make their own decisions, to consent to or refuse treatment unless there is evidence to the contrary. Obviously issues of consent can come up in any area of medicine but as this book focuses on mental health that is where discussion of principles will be focused here.

The inter-relationship between the Mental Health Act and the Mental Capacity Act is complex and currently being tested by case law. Most recently, judgement has been delivered emphasizing that when there is the possibility to invoke both Acts the Mental Health Act has priority. Capacity is more likely to be regained if the mental disorder is treated.

Compulsion

There are three key areas where patients with mental health problems may find themselves being considered for compulsory treatment. These are:

- when they present an actual or potential risk to others as a result of a mental disorder (e.g. if they are having auditory hallucinations telling them to harm someone; if they are paranoid and believe others are out to harm them whether they are or not);
- when the mental disorder they present with results in them posing an actual or potential risk to themselves e.g. suicide, harm from impulsive behaviours (such as overspending in a manic illness) or self-neglect. Hopelessness in post-natal depression can present significant risks to babies as severely depressed mothers may believe that it is kinder to kill the child than for them to be in a bleak and hopeless situation;
- when the risk of deteriorating mental health results in the potential for either of the two conditions above developing.

Now of course it is possible that an individual may meet one or more of these three criteria and still have legal capacity, and it is in such circumstances that compulsion is most controversial. In a 1999 Department of Health review, an expert committee chaired by Professor Genevra Richardson highlighted this inequality and suggested it be addressed along with strengthening the rights of patients to act autonomously in any new Mental Health legislation. Unfortunately, this opportunity was missed and the subsequent drafts of a new Mental Health Bill in 2002 and 2004 were seen by a broad alliance of patients' groups, mental health professionals (including the Royal College of Psychiatrists) and lawyers, who mounted a successful campaign against the proposed legislation, which led to it being abandoned. Meanwhile many of its principles were adopted in new Scottish legislation. Subsequently the 1983 Mental

Health Act of England and Wales was amended following a 2007 amendment bill that came into force in November 2008. This incorporated many of the elements resisted in the draft bills, including a change in definition of mental disorder that is now broader. It is now defined as any disorder or disability of mind. Previously exempted were 'immorality, promiscuity and sexual deviancy' but now the only exemption is 'dependence on alcohol or drugs'. Additionally, patients with a personality disorder were required to have a 'treatable' disorder to be detained. The requirement of treatability has now been abolished. This however raises questions of what the functions of detention are? Should doctors be involved in detaining patients for whom there are limited effective treatments and the main justification is to detain them to limit their freedom so they cannot harm others? Or should this be a non-medical and purely legal decision? Also, how reasonable is it to detain someone on the possibility that they may harm others?

Common principles

Across the various legal jurisdictions, a variety of principles hold true. These include:

- more than one person making the decisions: any decision about detention of any duration, or treatment, is not taken by one person alone and there is no conflict of interests affecting those people making decisions;
- defined periods of detention: periods of detention are not 'open-ended'. That is patients can only be detained for a set period and if extension of that period is sought then independent review is required;
- rights to appeal: patients once detained have the right to appeal to an independent authority which has the right to discharge the patient from their compulsory admission;
- discharge when appropriate: once detained that period of detention should be terminated when the patient no longer meets the legal conditions justifying detention, i.e. compulsory treatment ends when the patient recovers;
- change from informal to formal status: a patient who is admitted to hospital voluntarily can be detained if they withdraw their consent for the

admission or treatment and their condition has deteriorated such that they meet the criteria required for detention;

- police responsibilities: police on coming into contact with a patient who appears mentally ill are required to make obtaining suitable assessment and treatment a priority whether or not an offence has taken place;
- consent when detained: patients while detained should still be approached for their consent and treatment plans should, where possible, be agreed upon rather than just imposed;
- offenders: those convicted of offences, no matter how serious, have the same right to treatment as non-offending patients. Most mental health legislations have separate but usually overlapping, systems for offenders.

Having read the above discussion how does this influence (if at all) your original answers to the questions posed above?

Summary of Mental Health Act (1983), England and Wales

Who can detain patients?

One of the fundamental changes of the Mental Health Act amendments was that mental health professionals other than doctors can now take on the responsibility for managing detained patients. Detaining a patient requires the involvement of more than one doctor and another professional in the majority of detention orders. For the longer orders (Sections 2 and 3) the requirement is for two doctors to make the recommendation and an Approved Mental Health Professional (AMHP) to make the application. The two doctors need to be one who is recognized by the Secretary of State as having expertise in the diagnosis and management of mental disorders (known as a Section 12 approved doctor). The other is typically a registered doctor who knows the patient (most often the patient's GP) but when they are unavailable a second Section 12 approved doctor can provide a recommendation so long as they are not in a relationship (financial, personal or in a subordinate role) with the first doctor. The AMHP is most commonly a specially trained social worker.

The exceptions to these rules about the above make-up of the assessing 'team' are the emergency Sections 4 and 5. In the case of Section 4, there can be one of the two doctors who would normally make up the assessing team and an AMHP. In the case of a Section 5(2) there only needs to be the doctor in charge of the patient's care or their nominated deputy. This means that on a medical ward the patient can be detained only by their consultant or someone nominated by them from within the same employing organization. This means that a psychiatrist cannot be called to detain a patient in a general medical ward on a 5(2). Finally a Section 5(4) is applied by a Registered Mental Nurse.

The sections

- Section 2: An assessment order allowing compulsory detention for up to 28 days that can be used either in the community or in hospitals.

- Section 3: A treatment order allowing detention for up to 6 months that can be used either in the community or in hospitals.

- Section 4: An emergency order to admit a patient to hospital from the community for up to 72 hours if waiting for the second doctor to complete a Section 2 or 3 would result in a delay that might cause difficulties for the patient or others.

- Section 5(2): An order that allows detention for up to 72 hours of inpatients. This section applies to hospital inpatients and authorizes the detention of an informal patient for up to 72 hours allowing an assessment, which may lead to an application for admission under Section 2 or 3 if necessary.

- Section 5(4): An order that allows detention of a patient in a psychiatric unit for up to 6 hours to enable them to be assessed for detention by a doctor. Typically, this means that the next section considered would be a 5(2).

- Section 135: An order that allows the police to force entry to allow a Mental Health Act (MHA) assessment of an individual believed to be mentally ill.

- Section 136: An order allowing the police to remove a person believed to be mentally ill from a public place to a 'Place of Safety' to allow an MHA assessment to take place.

Supervised Community Treatment: This is administered by a Community Treatment Order. The aim is to allow some patients to live in the community whilst still subject to powers of the Act. These patients remain under compulsion and can be recalled to hospital for treatment. Only those patients who have been detained for treatment (see Section 3 above) are eligible for Supervised Community Treatment.

Patients involved in criminal proceedings

The Mental Health Act allows courts to deal with mentally disordered offenders. Whereas court sections require medical recommendations, the decision whether the prisoner 'deserves' punishment or treatment is for the court.

There are seven court sections: the two most important examples are:

Section 37: This allows a person convicted of an imprisonable offence to be detained and treated in hospital. The patient is discharged when well regardless of the length of prison sentence they may have been given if they had not been detained in hospital.

Section 41: This restricts discharge of 'dangerous' patients detained under Section 37 by requiring permission from the Home Secretary.

Some criminal law also involves psychiatric reports, for example the verdict of 'not guilty by reason of insanity' or 'unfit to plead' (person too mentally disordered to know right from wrong) results in the individual's detention as if under Section 37 with Section 41 restrictions. The verdict of 'diminished responsibility' can reduce a murder verdict to one of manslaughter.

Vulnerable groups

For young people under 16 years of age parental consent may be sufficient to detain their children if they fulfil the criteria above. However, it is considered better practice to use the Mental Health Act in some contexts given the safeguards that fall into place for detained patients if the Act is implemented.

Individuals with learning disability may not be able to understand or retain information in which case it is unlikely they have capacity to consent to treatment.

Treatment

The MHA applies only to treatment of mental disorder and cannot be used in treatment of physical conditions. Unconscious patients are treated under authority of Common Law, which recognizes a duty to save life etc. (Doctrine of Necessity). Restraint of a potentially violent or suicidal informal patient, whether in a general medical or a psychiatric ward, would be justified on the same basis. For less urgent cases where the patient lacks capacity the Mental Capacity Act applies.

There are several key principles involved in treating mentally ill patients for their mental illness:

- Voluntary patients cannot be treated for a psychiatric disorder without informed consent.
- Patients detained under Sections 4, 5(2), 135, 136 (72-hour sections) and guardianship cannot be treated without informed consent except in emergencies when the principles outlined above apply.
- Patients detained under Sections 2, 3 and 37 may be given some treatments without consent under the conditions detailed below.

General treatments

There are no conditions applied here to general care and treatments except as outlined below. Nursing care, occupational therapy and other care may be given to detained patients without consent.

Medication and ECT

Consent or a second opinion is required. To be given ECT or prolonged medication, i.e. for more than 3 months, either the patient must give consent certified valid by the consultant (remember their wish to leave hospital is considered invalid!) or agreement to the treatment plan must be obtained from a doctor appointed by the Mental Health Act Commission.

Urgent treatment

If urgent, a course of ECT or medication may be started with a detained patient while waiting for the second opinion.

Irreversible treatments

This includes treatment such as neurosurgery for psychiatric disorders and hormone implants. Here consent *and* a second opinion are required. For these treatments, the second opinion appointed doctor must agree with the plan and the patient must give consent which is considered valid by a three-person panel.

Summary

This chapter has outlined the principles behind mental health legislation, although it should be clear that this is in no way as straightforward as it may initially sound. Although the detail varies within the UK and also elsewhere, the guiding principles are usually similar and aim to protect both patients who have mental illness and the community if there is risk from such patients. The key points to remember are when the MHA can be applied and when it cannot. If there is no evidence or high suspicion that a patient has a mental disorder, the MHA cannot be used. When the MHA is applied there are certain safeguards in place to ensure that patients' rights are protected.

Further reading

Mental Health Act (England and Wales) www. dh.gov.uk/en/Healthcare/Mentalhealth/Policy/ InformationontheMentalHealthActs/index.htm (Accessed April 2010).

Mental Health Act (Scotland) www.scotland.gov.uk/ Topics/Health/health/mental-health/mhlaw (Accessed April 2010).

CASE STUDY 1

A 47-year-old single woman with multiple sclerosis is referred to local mental health services by her mother. She is concerned that her daughter has voiced an intention to commit suicide. The patient, having been brought up in a very religious household, rejected her family's religious beliefs in her late teens, when she left home to go to university. She and her parents have been estranged until a few years ago when her father had a serious myocardial infarct (MI). Six months after their reunion her father died from a second MI.

Just after university, the patient developed blurred vision. It was on presenting for investigation that her multiple sclerosis was diagnosed. Her illness has followed a relapsing/remitting course, but over the last 5 years the decline has been steadily accelerating. Currently she is just recovering from another relapse and now needs to look at moving into living in a more supported environment. Her mother has suggested she moves home.

The patient has always said that when she lost her independence she would choose to end her life rather than live beholden to others. She has recently discussed this with her younger sister who revealed her confidence to their mother. Suicide is an anathema to the rest of the patient's family. They consider her to be depressed, given that she is having such thoughts. As such, they have asked that the patient be assessed and detained for treatment if she cannot be persuaded that suicide is wrong.

POSSIBLE OUTCOME

The patient if found, as is probable, to still have capacity to make such decisions and if there is no evidence of a mental illness such as a mood disorder is not liable to be detained.

CASE STUDY 2

23-year-old man is stopped by the police as he was noted to be wandering the streets muttering to himself. On stopping him, the police found that he was carrying a knife. He is being assessed in the cells by a duty psychiatrist following referral by the police surgeon.

The young man's flatmates describe a gradual pattern of deterioration in functioning that they feel might be related to recreational drug use. The young man talks of his fears of a vague group of 'officials' who are monitoring him and he feels that they will ultimately try to make him a victim of 'extraordinary rendition', taking him away to Pakistan to be tortured. He has told the police that he is carrying a knife for his own 'protection'.

POSSIBLE OUTCOME

This patient appears to be suffering from a paranoid psychosis. This is a new presentation and it is unclear whether it is due to intoxication with drugs, a drug-induced psychosis or a more chronic illness such as schizophrenia (see Chapter 9). He is therefore liable to be detained for assessment, i.e. a Section 2 as described above. Criminal proceedings are unlikely.

CASE STUDY 3

A 38-year-old musician with bipolar affective disorder is in hospital nearing the end of his stay. His admission was compulsory as he had developed another manic episode that had resulted in him running up significant debts and displaying increasingly disinhibited behaviour, culminating in him running down the middle of the main shopping street naked apart from a 'Santa' hat.

He is grateful that he was detained and admitted and is now euthymic. He has had successful spells at home and is ready for discharge but has stated that although he believes medication helped with the acute phase of his illness he intends stopping everything within 3 months of discharge, as he believes that lithium, which he is currently on, blunts his creativity. He no longer requires inpatient treatment.

POSSIBLE OUTCOME

If this was a repeated pattern with the patient being admitted regularly following discontinuation of medication the clinical team may seek to impose a Community Treatment Order with conditions around his use of medication, accepting monitoring of his mental state and investigations required for mood stabilizers (see Chapter 16). If, however, this was early in his illness it is likely that he would be discharged with an attempt to negotiate a plan involving close monitoring of his mental state and a negotiated phased withdrawal of medication.

CASE STUDY 4

A 55-year-old man with recurrent major depression is found in his home by his CPN in a state of squalor. He is emaciated and in poor physical health. Assessment reveals that he has a severe depressive illness with psychotic features, including profound nihilistic delusions, e.g. the belief that his internal organs have rotted away. He refuses to eat or drink and pulls out any intravenous or nasogastric tube inserted. He will not take medication. In line with treatment protocols, it is felt by his treating team that the most appropriate treatment is ECT. His family are supportive of this recommendation but the patient refuses saying that is pointless as he is already dead.

POSSIBLE OUTCOME

As this is a presentation of a patient with a recurrent illness needing admission for treatment he is liable to be detained under a treatment order (Section 3). His illness is life-threatening and so ECT is a logical and potentially life-saving treatment. A Second Opinion Approved Doctor's opinion would be sought for this. If there was no chance to wait for this emergency treatment using Section 62 might be used.

MOOD DISORDERS

John Eagles

KEY CHAPTER FEATURES

- Depression: history, prevalence, risk factors, clinical presentations, assessment and management
- Depression in older patients
- Bipolar affective disorder: history, prevalence, risk factors, clinical presentations, assessment and management
- Seasonal affective disorder
- Childbirth and affective disorders

Introduction

It is very important for all doctors to be competent in the diagnosis and management of mood disorders. Although patients with bipolar affective disorders will be managed predominantly by psychiatrists and general practitioners, depression will be seen by all doctors who work with conscious patients. This chapter will deal first with depression, then with bipolar affective disorders and will conclude with brief accounts of other mood disorders. Childhood mood disorders are covered in Chapter 14.

Why is this relevant to you?

Mood disorders (most notably depression) are very common and will be seen frequently by nearly all doctors. When a patient is depressed, almost by definition, the quality of their life is markedly impaired. Depression often goes unrecognized, and untreated, and the opportunity is lost to effect a very significant improvement in the quality of that patient's life.

Depression

History

The term 'melancholia', commonly used until the early twentieth century and still used occasionally to describe severe depression, dates back to ancient Greece, when it was believed to arise due to the accumulation of black (melan) bile (chole). Depression has been diagnosed retrospectively in many historical figures, including Kings Saul and David (from the text of the Bible), Rembrandt, Mozart and Abraham Lincoln. For thousands of years opinions varied as to whether melancholia was essentially a religious or a medical affliction, and it was only in the nineteenth century that a medical model of depression began to hold sway. Some would assert that this process has now extended too far into the 'medicalization of unhappiness' and this possibility will be mentioned below. Depression of clinical significance is now termed depressive disorder.

Prevalence

It is difficult to provide definitive rates for the prevalence or incidence of depression for two main reasons. First, as in the diagnosis of hypertension or diabetes, many depressive symptoms exhibit a continuous variation across the population, giving rise to difficulties in knowing where to draw the line between distress and unhappiness on one hand and mild depressive illness on the other. Second, the results of population-screening studies will reflect the accuracy of the screening questionnaire deployed, the skills of the interviewers, especially where symptoms are more subtle and are observer rated, and the proportion of the community who agree to participate.

Despite these caveats, enough good studies have been conducted to yield reliable data on prevalence rates of depression. For example, in 1996 Weissman and colleagues deployed tight criteria for depression in 10 countries, finding overall lifetime prevalence rates of 9 per cent and annual incidence rates of 4 per cent. There were wide international differences in lifetime rates ranging from 1.5 per cent in Taiwan, through 9 per cent in Germany to 19 per cent in Beirut. In 2001, Ayuso-Mateos and colleagues screened both urban and rural populations in five European countries, using more inclusive criteria for depression. They found an overall point prevalence rate of 8.6 per cent for depressive disorders. Again, there were marked international differences, ranging from a rate of 2.6 per cent in Santander, Spain, to 17.1 per cent in Liverpool. This may reflect psychosocial disadvantage.

The message from these figures is that depression is a common condition in many societies, it causes much suffering (as discussed in Chapter 1) and it constitutes a hugely important challenge to the medical profession.

Risk factors for depression

The main 'risk factors' for depression are summarized in Table 6.1. It is important to note that although these factors are associated with depression, and may often act as predisposing factors, they are not necessarily causative. For example, although depression may well result from the break-up of a marriage, pre-existing depression may have contributed materially to the separation in the first instance. Milder cases of depression may be related to psychosocial factors alone, whereas more severe cases are likely to have a greater biological component. Also, some individuals may develop severe depression in the absence of any social problems (although these may occur secondary to the illness) but as discussed below it can be difficult to separate out environmental from non-environmental factors.

Sociodemographic factors

Rates of depression in childhood exhibit no gender difference, but from puberty onwards, females begin to predominate, outnumbering males during their reproductive years by at least two to one, with rates tending to equalize again among older adults. Possible reasons for this female preponderance may include factors associated with pregnancy and childbirth (leading to postnatal onsets that do not occur in males), lower self-esteem coupled with self-blaming cognitive styles and more difficult sociocultural roles (which may also include an increased vulnerability to adverse life events). Widowed, divorced and separated people have higher rates of depression, but marriage seems to be more protective for men than it is for women. Single men are more likely to be depressed than married men, but several studies have found that single women have lower rates than married women. People in lower socioeconomic groups suffer something of a 'double whammy' in that not only do they experience higher rates of depression but their outcomes are less good. This probably relates to a combination of later recognition or non-recognition, being subject to more perpetuating factors, lesser likelihood of receiving appropriate treatment and lower levels of treatment adherence.

Psychosocial factors

It can be helpful to think in terms of distant and current adverse psychosocial factors. Among distant factors, there is good evidence that the death of one's mother before the age of 11 years increases the likelihood of future depression. As a corollary, any event that adversely affects parent–child emotional bonds is likely to be a risk factor, for example parental separation or dysfunctional parenting. Such factors are difficult to disentangle from the effects of childhood

Table 6.1 Factors associated with an increased risk of depression

Sociodemographic factors	Physical illnesses
Female gender	Viral infections
Adult age groups	HIV/AIDS
Marital status (see text)	Cancer
Unemployment	Diabetes
Lower socioeconomic status	Cardiovascular disease
Urban area of residence	Stroke
Born after 1950	Epilepsy
Biological factors	Multiple sclerosis
Genetic predisposition	Asthma
Low birth weight	Chronic obstructive lung disease
	Arthritis
	Cystic fibrosis
Psychosocial factors	**Prescribed medication**
Early loss of mother	Steroids
Childhood sexual abuse	Calcium channel blockers
Bereavement	Beta-blockers
Other adverse life events	Digoxin
Lack of a confidant(e)	Opiates
Social isolation	
Psychiatric comorbidity	**Miscellaneous**
Alcohol misuse	Chronic pain
Generalized anxiety disorder	Use of cannabis or psychostimulants
Panic disorder	Smoking
Agoraphobia	Gambling
Social phobia	Pregnancy/childbirth
Somatoform disorders	Obesity
Eating disorders	

abuse (sexual, physical or emotional), which are also more likely to occur when family function is abnormal or parenting is poor.

Of current and recent factors, adverse life events are of clear importance in precipitating depression. The magnitude of the effect of life events ranges downwards in severity from the death of a spouse, and many of these events are linked by the common theme of loss; this could be loss of relationships (through bereavement, separation or moving house), loss of physical health, loss of livelihood or loss of prestige/self-esteem. Social relationships, in terms of having both at least one close person in whom one can confide and a broader network of social support and contacts, are important buffers against depression.

At this point, it is perhaps worth commenting on the terms 'reactive' and 'endogenous' depression, which fell out of common usage during the 1990s. Students should avoid using these terms, although they may hear them used on the wards or read of them in older literature. The term 'reactive' depression was applied to patients whose depression seemed to be secondary to adverse circumstances, whose symptoms were often less severe and who lacked the somatic, or biological, symptoms that often go along with more severe depression. The term 'endogenous' depression implied something caused by the person's innate biology, arising without clear external cause, and generally associated with greater severity and somatic symptoms. It became clear that it was not possible to clearly separate two such types of depression using either symptom profiles or the presence or absence of precipitating stressful life events, which were found to occur in both. Thus, we now refer to depressive disorders as a single category. Nevertheless, the history of research and debate around the issue of whether there are distinct subtypes of depression exemplifies one of the main difficulties psychiatry faces in attempting to develop clinically meaningful classifications that are of utility in communicating to others the nature of a patient's presentation as well as saying something about appropriate treatment and likely prognosis.

Biological factors

As in hypertension and diabetes, the risk of adult depression is higher among infants with low birth weight, possibly due to dysfunction of the hypothalamic–pituitary–adrenal axis. The size of this effect is relatively small and the genetic component of the aetiology of depression is also small in comparison with environmental factors. No specific gene has yet been found to play a major role and inheritance is very likely to be polygenic. In broad terms, major depression in a first-degree relative effectively doubles the risk of experiencing depression. That being said, the genetic component of aetiology rises with more severe depressive disorders, with a concomitantly increased risk among relatives. In practice, it can be difficult to disentangle the genetic factors from environmental ones.

Psychiatric comorbidity

Comorbidity of depression and alcohol use is particularly common. It is often very difficult to know which arose first, with alcohol offering temporary relief from depression before exacerbating the condition in a vicious circle. Primary chronic alcohol abuse may also lead to persistent chronic low mood. All of the anxiety disorders listed in Table 6.1 are more than twice as common in depressed people as in a control population. The importance of recognizing comorbidity is that treatment of both conditions has an additive effect, reversing the types of vicious circle mentioned above.

Physical illnesses

As shown in Table 6.1, many physical disorders are associated with raised rates of depression underlining the need for vigilance in general medical settings.

Miscellaneous factors

Of these, the association with smoking, gambling and illicit drug use may be underpinned by abnormal function in the brain's reward mechanisms. The link with obesity is again a complex 'chicken and egg' vicious circle situation. Mood disorders in pregnancy and childbirth will be discussed separately below.

Presentation

Given the high prevalence of depression among adults, and the tendency for many people to deny psychological symptoms, doctors should maintain a high index of suspicion, particularly when someone has associated risk factors for depression. For example, a recently bereaved middle-aged woman with painful arthritis has a high risk of developing a depressive disorder.

Clinical features

Many systems for classifying depression have been in vogue at different times and in different countries over the last 60 years. None has been without its strengths and weaknesses and the ICD-10 criteria for a depressive episode are summarized in Box 6.1.

Before these symptoms, and others, that may occur in depression, it is important to emphasize that individuals can present with mild to extremely severe depression. Mild depression has fewer symptoms as indicated in Box 6.1 and the mood itself is less likely to impact on every aspect of the individual's life and general functioning is less impaired. In severe depression, not only is a low mood pervasive, the individual is unlikely to function effectively in any

Box 6.1: ICD-10 criteria for depressive symptoms

Minimum duration of 2 weeks (unless very severe)

Core symptoms	Depressed mood
	Loss of interest and enjoyment
	Reduced energy with increased fatigability
Other common symptoms	Reduced concentration and attention
	Reduced self-esteem and confidence
	Ideas of guilt and unworthiness
	Pessimistic view of the future
	Ideas or acts of self-harm or suicide
	Disturbed sleep
	Diminished appetite

Mild depressive episode requires at least two core symptoms plus at least two of the other symptoms

Moderate depressive episode requires at least two core symptoms plus at least three of the other symptoms, and symptoms are likely to be 'present to a marked degree'

Severe depressive episode requires all three core symptoms plus at least four of the other symptoms

area. The other symptoms are also more likely to be severe so that for example there will be a greater disturbance of sleep and appetite or more pervasive thoughts regarding suicide.

Depressed mood is, of course, the central feature of depression. It is distinguished from dejection and unhappiness by its persistence and its intensity. Unlike unhappiness, depressed mood tends not to improve in response to positive events such as the visit of a friend or a victory by one's football team. Uncharacteristic tearfulness is common, and anxiety is a frequent concomitant. When people are depressed for the first time they may find depressed mood difficult to recognize, and irritability may be a more evident affect, especially to family and friends. Diurnal variation of mood, whereby depressed people feel at their worst in the morning and improve as the day progresses, is often evident especially in those more severely ill.

Loss of interest in activities such as work and hobbies is characteristic, coupled with a lack of

pleasure and enjoyment from previously pleasurable pursuits (anhedonia).

Loss of energy (**anergia**) is a common presenting complaint in depression, giving rise to a differential diagnosis that includes the various physical causes of energy loss and fatigue. The anergia and easy fatigability of depression tend to be coupled with subjectively impaired motivation, whereas an anergic physically ill person will typically feel that 'the spirit is willing but the body is weak'. As a related symptom, **loss of libido** is common in depression.

Impaired concentration and attention are common. For example, patients are often unable to follow a TV programme or focus on a book. Depressed people will often feel that their thinking is fuzzy and inefficient, and will encounter short-term memory difficulties.

Reductions in self-esteem and confidence result from the negative cognitions associated with low mood (mentioned under 'Aetiological models of depression'), and it needs to be clear that low self-esteem did not pre-date other features before it should be deemed to be a depressive symptom. A pessimistic view of the future is also typical of negative depressive cognitions, as are feelings of personal guilt and unworthiness. There are significant gradations in the degree of negativity of such thinking from mild/moderate depressions through to severe depression with psychosis. For example, a moderately depressed person may think it likely that he/she will lose his/her job because he/she has not worked hard enough, whereas a severely depressed patient may hold a delusional conviction that he/she faces redundancy and destitution because he/she was late for work on one occasion.

Self-harm and suicide are intimately linked with depression, at all levels from transient thoughts of taking an overdose through to completed suicide.

Sleep disturbance is an important symptom of depression. Early-morning wakening (sometimes defined as 2 hours or more before one's usual wakening time) is characteristic, especially in more severe depressions. Wakening during the night with difficulty falling asleep again (middle insomnia) and problems falling asleep (initial insomnia) are also common patterns.

Loss of appetite, often coupled with weight loss, is a common depressive symptom that again needs to be distinguished from possible physical causes. In depression, eating is often one of the activities that has ceased to be pleasurable. Some people with (usually milder) depressions may gain weight through 'comfort eating'.

Psychomotor changes tend to occur with more severe depression. Retardation refers to apparent slowing of movement and speech, while patients may report a slowing of their thinking processes. Agitation comprises excessive motor activity, often coupled with anxiety. Patients are fidgety and restless, and can find it almost impossible to stay still.

Obsessive compulsive symptoms (see Chapter 7) occur commonly in depression, often as an exacerbation of pre-existing obsessional personality traits.

Psychotic symptoms occur only in severe depression. Most commonly, these comprise **delusions** that can generally be understood as extreme extensions of depressive thinking. Typical depressive delusions relate to guilt, impending catastrophe, poverty, hypochondriasis or persecution (usually as a result of wrongly perceived misdeeds). When auditory hallucinations occur, unlike in schizophrenia, they tend to be relatively brief and in the second person. The content is usually derogatory, consistent with depressed mood. Visual hallucinations do occur (e.g. of threatening faces or the devil) but they are rare and should generally lead to consideration of organic causation (see Chapter 9).

ICD-10 also classifies depression as to whether or not 'somatic' symptoms are present. These are sometimes termed the 'biological' symptoms of depression, and do tend to point towards more biological, as opposed to psychosocial, causation and can indicate a greater likelihood that physical treatments will prove to be successful. The somatic/biological symptoms of depression are as follows: loss of interest or pleasure in usually enjoyable activities; lack of emotional reactivity to normally pleasurable events; early-morning wakening; depression worse in the mornings; psychomotor retardation or agitation; marked loss of appetite; weight loss; marked loss of libido.

An episode of depressive disorder may be a single event in a person's life. However, for many people further episodes ensue and it is then appropriate to describe the individual as suffering from recurrent depressive disorder. This is classified separately in ICD-10 because recurrence may have implications for future management. This category excludes people with a history of significantly elevated mood, and recovery between distinct episodes differentiates it from chronic depression.

Dysthymia refers to a syndrome of chronic mild depression that does not meet the severity criteria for depressive episodes or recurrent depression. Its onset is often in adolescence. The pervasively negative and pessimistic cognitive style has sometimes given rise to the description of 'depressive personality disorder'.

Depression in older adults

Modest increases in rates of depression have been reported to occur in females at the time of menopause and there has been much debate regarding the aetiology of this and whether it represents a distinct syndrome of post-menopausal depression. Marked hormonal changes cause physical symptoms but no clear link has been established between these hormone changes and mood changes. The menopause also constitutes a psychological landmark signalling the end of a woman's reproductive years. Socially, it may coincide with life events such as children leaving home, perhaps precipitating 'empty nest syndrome'. Thus, depression at this phase of life may be no different in its causation from that at other times but, as for the postnatal phase, there may be unique psychosocial factors that make females more vulnerable.

In old age, somatic symptoms tend to be more common when depression presents. Prevalence rates are similar to those in younger adults, but there are significant differences between old people living independently and those in institutions. Prevalence rates are high in nursing homes, perhaps largely because risk factors tend to cluster in residents: they are more likely to be bereaved, socially isolated and suffering from concomitant (often painful) physical illnesses. Such factors may serve to perpetuate depression in older people, and depression *per se* will also increase the likelihood of, and the necessity for, admission to institutional care. There is a significant association in old people between depression and early mortality.

There is also a complex association between depression and dementia, with each apparently giving rise to an increase in the chance of developing the other. Dysfunction in the hypothalamic–pituitary–adrenal axis may predispose to both disorders. When elderly people become significantly depressed, as many as 15 per cent can develop 'depressive pseudo-dementia'. This presents with cognitive impairments suggestive of dementia but actually represents a severe slowing of cognitive function caused by severe, but often unrecognized, depression. Effective antidepressant treatment results in return to normal.

Making the first diagnosis of depression

A large proportion of a GP's consultations are with patients diagnosed as depressed; Scottish government statistics for 2006–7 estimated that 503 700 such consultations occurred that year, compared with 180 650 for asthma and 122 050 for coronary heart disease. However, although more severe cases are usually detected, there is consistent evidence that only about half of the depressed patients who consult in primary care are actually diagnosed with that condition. There are several reasons for this low detection rate.

Older depressed people are less likely to be diagnosed in primary care. Men, although being less likely than women to consult their GP when they become depressed, if they do consult are more likely to be diagnosed. Somatic presentations may hinder the diagnosis of depression. A World Health Organization study screened primary care attenders across 14 countries, and found that some depressed patients reported only somatic symptoms, with rates that varied from 45 per cent in France, through 60 per cent in Manchester to 95 per cent in Turkey. There was a general increased tendency for patients in developing countries to present somatically, as there is for less educated patients in Western societies. Somatic symptoms in depressed patients occur across all bodily systems, with non-specific symptoms (headaches, lower back pain, weakness and tiredness) being particularly common. In general, the more physical symptoms of which a patient complains, especially when such symptoms remain medically unexplained, the more likely they are to be depressed. This also applies to hospital outpatient clinics.

Assessment

Patients may present complaining of some sort of mood or affective disturbance but, as discussed earlier, it is important to maintain a high index of suspicion and consider whether risk factors for depression are present. The diagnosis is made on the basis of the history and mental state. A corroborative history from a family member is usually valuable.

Patients may equate 'mood' with anger or irritability and studies also indicate that many people cannot clearly distinguish between anxiety and depression in their descriptions of symptoms. Underlying these problems are issues of vocabulary as well as the way people conceptualize abnormal emotional states. Thus, it can be better to ask 'How have your spirits been recently?' It is good practice to develop a 'checklist' of depressive symptoms to run through with patients. This should comprise inquiry about mood, sleep, appetite, weight change, loss of interest/enjoyment, energy/motivation, diurnal variation and concentration. One should always ask about suicidal ideation, and a sensitive way to commence this area of inquiry would be: 'Have things sometimes got so bad lately that you've felt life isn't worth living?' An affirmative response would lead to inquiries about possible suicidal plans and recent acts of self-harm (see Chapter 3). It is important to elucidate the timescale of the current symptoms and thus to know if these have endured long enough (usually 2 weeks) to make a diagnosis and whether they represent a change from usual functioning. If they do not, then consider dysthymia.

Other useful areas to consider in the history include:

- recent life events
- difficult ongoing life circumstances
- more distant precipitants (e.g. childhood trauma, relationships with parents)
- possible previous episodes of depression and their management
- recent physical health
- family history of psychiatric disorders and suicide
- comorbid psychiatric conditions (most notably anxiety and alcohol misuse).

Mental state examination includes observation for possible signs of self-neglect and for psychomotor changes in terms of retardation (unusual slowing of movement or speech) or agitation (fidgeting or restlessness). Tearfulness or irritability may be observed. If the patient's mood appears depressed, it is important to note whether this is consistent throughout the interview or if it is reactive to you and to the topics being discussed. To access possible negative cognitions, it can be helpful to ask: 'How do you see the future?' and 'How have you been feeling about yourself as a person?' In more severely depressed patients, one should routinely inquire about psychotic symptoms.

Differential diagnosis

When patients present with overt psychological symptoms at the mild end of the spectrum of severity, a stress reaction will be the common differential diagnosis. The brevity of symptoms and the clear relationship to stressful life events or circumstances will be important pointers. With more severe and enduring symptoms the psychiatric differential diagnosis will include anxiety disorders, dysthymia, alcohol misuse, dementia (in older patients) and eating disorders (notably in younger females). The commoner medical disorders that can present with depressed symptoms are hypothyroidism and adrenal dysfunction. Among prescribed medication, steroids most often cause depression, with the other drugs listed in Table 6.1 being less commonly implicated.

Aetiological models of depression

Aetiological factors in mental illness were described in Chapter 2. To place management of depression in a logical context, I shall very briefly review three prominent models of causation.

Psychodynamic/interpersonal

Psychodynamic theories of the aetiology of depression usually emphasize the importance of loss, especially when the person was ambivalent about the loss (e.g. early death of one's mother with whom there was a poor relationship). Loss of self-esteem coupled with negative expectations of relationships are deemed to be important. Disturbed emotions and relationships are considered to be central issues.

Cognitive

Rather than interpreting negative thoughts as the result of depression, cognitive models perceive them to be the primary cause. Underlying negative beliefs are thought to give rise to pessimistic expectations of the future, of relationships, of oneself and of the world in general. This pervasive pessimism leads to depression and withdrawal in a self-perpetuating pattern.

Neurotransmitters

Whether or not it is a primary phenomenon, there is a wealth of evidence to support the link between depression and disturbed neurotransmitter function. As just one example, depletion of tryptophan (a precursor of serotonin) gives rise to lowered mood in both depressed and non-depressed people. The picture is complex, but serotonin and noradrenalin are the neurotransmitters most closely linked to depression.

Management

General principles

Society's views of, and attitudes about, depression can be contradictory and are often reflected by patients and sometimes doctors. It may be seen as a transient state of lowered mood out of which people who wish to can ascend by strength of character and a positive state of mind. To allow oneself to wallow in self-pity can be seen as a self-indulgent weakness, certainly not as an illness. Such perceptions will often delay or prevent presentation of depression to health services. For milder presentations, a doctor may not wish to overemphasize an 'illness model', since it is helpful to promote an attitude of 'active mastering' of problems. However, for more severely depressed patients it is often a relief to hear that a doctor considers them to have illness rather than weakness.

In managing depression, it is essential to beware of the fallacy of 'understandability'. As an example, one might form the view that 'The chap lost his job and then his wife left him, no wonder he's depressed' and then having 'understood' the situation a doctor may decide that treatment of depression is unnecessary. This is not too different from saying 'The chap had a bad head injury, no wonder he's got epilepsy' and thus deciding not to treat the epilepsy. If someone has symptoms of depression, these need to be treated, whether or not they are 'understandable'. Nowhere is this more important, arguably, than when people are depressed in the context of a physical illness. In the 'heart and soul' study of over 1000 patients with cardiovascular disease, quality of life did not correlate with any measure of cardiovascular incapacity but correlated strongly with depressive symptoms. Similarly, a study in Calgary found that, among patients with cerebral tumours, depressive symptoms were the most important predictor of quality of life.

Mild depression

If the symptoms are of recent onset, and especially if they seem to have arisen in the context of an adverse (but not enduring) life event, the general practitioner is likely to engage in 'watchful waiting'. An initial sympathetic and supportive consultation may be therapeutic in itself. If symptoms have not resolved at a subsequent appointment 2 weeks or so later, then specific therapies would usually be discussed.

Psychological interventions will usually be the first option considered. When disturbed emotions and adverse life circumstances are prominent, counselling and/or problem-solving therapy may be most appropriate. When negative thinking is a predominant component, cognitive behavioural therapy (CBT) may be optimal. Self-help programmes, both through books and the internet, have been used increasingly over recent years, and can be seen as a convenient, cost-effective addition or alternative to direct person to person therapy. Self-help interventions for depression (at the milder end of symptom severity) are of established efficacy, and effectiveness is associated with their incorporating CBT techniques and by ancillary contact with a therapist ('guided self-help'). Self-help programmes usually also contain educational components and attempt to assist with 'behavioural activation', through which patients address helpless inactivity.

NICE guidelines advise a structured exercise programme within the routine management of mild depression. Thirty minutes of aerobic exercise, three times a week would be a standard 'prescription'. Support and supervision are usually important since adherence, particularly among depressed patients, may well be a potential problem. The mechanism of the antidepressant effects of exercise is unproven, but the most plausible hypotheses relate to effects on central noradrenergic function, to enhanced feelings of 'self-efficacy' and as a form of behavioural activation.

Antidepressants are not usually indicated as a first-line treatment in milder cases. However, they should be considered when symptoms endure and have not responded to other interventions or if patients have previously responded well to antidepressants when moderately or severely depressed.

Moderate/severe depression

When patients have moderate or severe depression, the first choice of treatment will usually be antidepressants. Selective serotonin reuptake inhibitors (SSRIs), such as citalopram, fluoxetine or sertraline, are preferred since (compared with the older tricyclic antidepressants) they cause fewer side-effects, treatment adherence is better and they are hugely less likely to cause death when taken in overdose. Perhaps self-evidently, the danger of overdose should be remembered with all depressed patients and realistic doctors appreciate that they cannot predict which of their depressed patients might overdose at any level of satisfactory accuracy. Safe prescribing and frequent reviews in a context of 'suicide awareness' thus constitute appropriate care. Patients should be alerted to some of the more common unwanted effects, as this can help compliance. For SSRIs, for example, these are nausea, headache and sweating, which will usually resolve within 1–3 weeks. Although most recent evidence suggests that a therapeutic effect within days is not uncommon, it is standard practice to inform patients that they may well notice no improvement during the first 2 or 3 weeks. Again, this advice should enhance adherence. Once patients have recovered, the risk of relapse is high if therapy is stopped, and antidepressants should be continued for at least a further 6 months, and 12 months for more severe cases. Withdrawal effects, such as headache, anxiety and influenza-like symptoms, are quite common with SSRIs and the dose should be tapered when they are discontinued. Other pharmacological treatments will be mentioned under 'Secondary care' below.

In moderate depression, psychological approaches (of the types described for mild depression) will often be deployed in tandem with antidepressants and it is helpful for patients to feel that they remain active participants in their own recoveries. CBT and interpersonal therapy are of established efficacy in moderate depression but are not effective for severely depressed patients.

Secondary care

General practitioners will generally refer a depressed patient to psychiatric services when:

- treatment has failed (usually this will comprise non-response to two treatments), or
- treatment options (usually psychotherapeutic) are not available in primary care, or
- there is perceived to be a significant risk of suicide, or
- psychotic symptoms are present, or
- bipolar affective disorder is suspected.

The vast majority of referred patients will be treated as outpatients and admission to hospital is generally reserved for people deemed to be at high risk of suicide or self-harm or those with psychotic symptoms.

The psychiatric management of depression is increasingly sophisticated and evidence based. A full account is given in a review by Anderson and colleagues, and what follows is a skeletal outline.

A detailed appraisal of biological, psychological and social factors will give rise to a treatment plan that may well be multidisciplinary. Partially responsive patients will often be engaged in any of the various psychotherapies, in tandem with medication. Involving partners and families, in both clarifying background and symptoms and assisting with therapy, will often be appropriate. Patients referred to secondary care will usually have failed to respond to an SSRI and/or another of the newer antidepressants in primary care. After attempting to ensure that this has been prescribed in an adequate dose and that non-response has not occurred due to poor treatment adherence, alternative antidepressants will include:

- venlafaxine (a serotonin and noradrenalin reuptake inhibitor)
- mirtazapine (a novel antidepressant with sedative and anxiolytic effects) or
- a tricyclic antidepressant

If patients do not respond to such changes, then pharmacological alternatives include the addition of lithium carbonate, as an augmenting agent, or the use of one of the monoamine oxidase inhibitors such as phenelzine.

Electroconvulsive therapy (ECT) is reserved for severely depressed patients, usually those who have failed to respond to several other treatments or when improvement is urgently necessary. In practice, this applies to people who are at risk either through suicide or through inability to eat and drink adequately. Psychotic symptoms and severe retardation are symptoms that may respond to ECT more readily than to other treatment approaches. ECT will be discussed at greater length in Chapter 14.

Recurrent depression

Depression is frequently a recurrent illness. Following a moderate depressive episode the lifetime risk of recurrence is approximately one in two. After two episodes the likelihood of recurrence is about 80 per cent and rises to over 90 per cent after three episodes. When several episodes occur over a short space of time, or when there have been many episodes over a longer period, long-term, prophylactic antidepressant treatment is usually advised. Patients with recurrent episodes should usually receive CBT since this has been found to have prophylactic efficacy.

Are doctors prescribing too many antidepressants?

Doctors are often criticized for 'medicalizing unhappiness' and then prescribing antidepressants for people who do not need them. However, many people in the community who are depressed and would benefit from antidepressants do not receive them; epidemiological studies confirm that unnecessary prescriptions are far outnumbered by the people who would indeed benefit from therapy (either pharmacological or psychological) that they are not receiving. Unfortunately, policy-makers may be unduly influenced by simplistic public perceptions ('pills bad, talking therapies good') that stigmatize antidepressant therapy and prevent depressed people from presenting for assessment and accepting treatment. The NICE guidelines (2009) provide a useful overview of the different perspectives and may be useful further reading.

Bipolar affective disorders

As well as experiencing episodes of depression, some patients also experience episodes of mania (or the less severe hypomania), in which the principle features are elevated mood, increased energy and pressure of speech. Bipolar affective disorder is characterized by separate episodes of mood disturbance at the two 'poles' of depression and mania. In comparison with (unipolar) depression, it is less common and management tends to be initiated and supervised predominantly by psychiatrists. For these reasons, although it is important and fascinating, it will be accorded less space than depression.

History

The origins of the term 'mania' are obscure, but typical clinical pictures were described by Greek physicians as early as the fifth century BC. It was in the first century AD that Aretaeus explicitly linked mania with melancholia, but this link seems to have been lost until the latter half of the nineteenth century, when various terms including 'folie circulaire' and 'manic-depressive insanity' emerged. Manic-depressive illness became the established diagnostic terminology until quite recently, but now the terms bipolar affective disorder, or simply bipolar disorder, are preferred. Although it may be slowly diminishing, stigma persists, despite the knowledge that prominent people have functioned very well while suffering from bipolar affective disorder (e.g. Winston Churchill). Bipolarity is linked to creativity and has contributed (among a long list) to the work of Van Gogh, Tchaikovsky, Shelley, Byron, Sylvia Plath and Spike Milligan.

Prevalence

Estimates of the prevalence of bipolar affective disorder vary depending on the differentiation of illness from normality. Cyclothymia (sometimes referred to as cyclothymic personality) describes a picture of persistent periods of mild depression and mild elation. This 'disorder' (if indeed it is a disorder) sits between 'normality' and bipolar affective disorder. The prevalence of bipolar affective disorder does not vary greatly between countries or between socioeconomic groups, suggesting that the aetiology is more biological and less psychosocial.

The lifetime risk of tightly defined bipolar affective disorder with episodes of mania (bipolar I disorder) is slightly less than 1 per cent. If one includes less severe cases, with hypomania rather than mania (bipolar II disorder), then the lifetime risk doubles to nearly 2 per cent. For bipolar I disorder males and females are affected with equal frequency, although there is a slight preponderance of women among people with bipolar II disorder. The commonest age of onset

(quite often identified retrospectively) is between 18 and 25 years. Younger age at onset may be associated with a higher genetic loading and there may also be a much smaller peak of onset in old age associated with organic brain disease.

Associations and risk factors

It is difficult to disentangle whether some factors have a causal role, result from the disorder itself or are comorbid due to a common aetiological link. For example, alcohol misuse can result from self-medication for mood swings but can also cause or exacerbate mood swings, or the two conditions could have a shared genetic predisposition.

Genetic predisposition is the most important risk factor. Monozygotic twins have a concordance rate of over 50 per cent for bipolar affective disorder, and the risk among first-degree relatives is between 5 and 10 per cent. The pattern within affected families fits with a model of multigenic inheritance rather than one of specific genes with major effects. Much research has been conducted and although there are areas of promise (e.g. polymorphism in the gene encoding for the enzyme catechol-*o*-methyltransferase, which is involved in the degradation of monoamines), genome scans have detected no consistent sites of genetic linkage.

Table 6.2 lists several conditions through which intracerebral pathology can predispose to manic episodes. If there is a common anatomical site of importance, then this may well be the prefrontal cortex and other limbic structures.

The role of adverse life events in precipitating mania is not clear cut since these may not be independent of the illness itself: when someone is becoming manic they may be an active instigator of a life event rather than its passive victim.

The association between childbirth and affective disorders will be covered below, and the link with circadian rhythms will be mentioned under seasonal affective disorder.

Presentation

When people with bipolar affective disorder are not in a phase of normal mood (euthymia) they are less likely to be manic or hypomanic than they are to be depressed; spells of depression are usually more common and tend to last longer. The clinical features

Table 6.2   Bipolar affective disorder: risk factors and associations

Genetic predisposition	Medication
	Corticosteroids
Medical conditions	L-dopa, dopamine agonists
Hypothyroidism	Thyroid hormones
Cushing's disease	MAOI and tricyclic antidepressants sometimes precipitate mania
Multiple sclerosis	**Miscellaneous**
Epilepsy	Circadian rhythm disruption
Cerebrovascular disease	Insomnia/sleep disruption
Cerebral tumours	Travel across time zones
Head injuries	Shift work
Substance misuse	Childbirth
Alcohol	Adverse life events
Psychostimulants	Summer months of the year
Cannabis	Pathological gambling

of depression are as described earlier and the features of mania/hypomania will now be described.

Clinical features

Summarized ICD-10 criteria for mania and hypomania are shown in Box 6.2. The distinction between mania and hypomania is made (somewhat arbitrarily) on the basis of duration and severity. When patients are manic they are clearly unwell but hypomania can be difficult to detect. Hypomanic patients will be cheerful, optimistic and energetic, and, especially if they are not known to you, can seem to be positively healthy and within the limits of normality. This possible blurring of the 'illness–wellness boundary' should be borne in mind in the descriptions that follow.

Mood is persistently elevated, most usually with excessive cheerfulness and extraversion, less commonly with predominant irritability. Subjectively, patients characteristically report feeling extremely well and their good humour is often infectious at interview. Excessive drive and optimism, when thwarted, can lead readily to confrontation and aggression.

Energy levels are high and overactivity is often apparent. Characteristically, patients will rush around starting new tasks or projects, but tend not to bring these to satisfactory conclusions.

Box 6.2: Summarized ICD-10 criteria for mania and hypomania

Mania

(A) Elated mood (occasionally predominant irritability)

(B) Increased energy

(C) Several of the following: decreased need for sleep, grandiosity, excessive optimism, pressure of speech, loss of social inhibitions, inability to sustain attention, impulsivity, extravagance, aggression

(D) Episode of at least 1 week's duration

(E) Severely disrupts work and/or social activities

(F) Psychotic symptoms may be present

Hypomania

(A) Mild elevation of mood (or irritability)

(B) Increased energy

(C) Symptoms as in (C) above, but *not* to the level of severe disruption in work or social contexts

(D) Duration of 'at least several days on end'

(E) No psychotic symptoms

Patients report decreased sleep requirement without this causing fatigue. Manic patients may go several consecutive days and nights without sleep.

Thinking is positive and optimistic, with patients considering new plans and ventures to be brilliant ideas despite their clear irrationality. At the severe end of the spectrum, plans and self-belief can reach the level of grandiose delusions, e.g. resolving the world's energy problems by harnessing the power of ants' colonies. Patients may come to believe that they have special powers (e.g. telepathy).

Impulsivity is characteristic, frequently becoming evident in overspending and/or in promiscuity. Risks tend to be taken more readily and, coupled with difficulties in sustaining attention, this makes manic patients particularly dangerous behind the wheel of a car.

At **interview,** dress may be bright and gaudy or inappropriate and idiosyncratic in other ways. Self-neglect may be apparent. Patients will usually talk loudly and quickly (pressure of speech). They may describe subjectively speeded thinking and may jump from topic to topic with only tenuous links between one topic and the next (flight of ideas). Elated mood, irritability, grandiosity and overactivity may all be observed. If delusions or hallucinations arise, these are consistent with elation and grandiosity (e.g. messages from God). Manic patients often lack insight into the fact that they are ill.

Mixed affective states

People with mania can often exhibit emotional lability, being moved quickly to tears or anger and then recovering with equal rapidity. In mixed affective states the depressive affect is more enduring but is combined with other manic symptoms such as increased energy and decreased sleep requirement. These mixed states are now being recognized more commonly, making up perhaps 10–20 per cent of presentations of mania/hypomania, and appear to be a time of increased risk of suicide. In relation to management, they should be treated in the same way as a manic/hypomanic state.

Neuropsychological dysfunction

Evidence has accrued over recent years that many patients with bipolar disorder exhibit neuropsychological impairment even during periods when they are well. These difficulties are mainly with attention, memory and executive function (problem

solving, decision-making). Their severity is associated with more severe bipolar disorder in terms of numbers of manic episodes and hospitalizations.

Older adults

Bipolar affective disorder is rather less common among older adults, perhaps due to excess mortality among younger sufferers; it does not appear to 'burn itself out' in old age and episodes may become more frequent and more severe over time. As many as 10–20 per cent of older people with bipolar disorder can have a first episode of mania after the age of 50 years, although many will have a history of previous depressive episodes. Compared with patients who have an earlier age of onset, mania in old age is associated with a lower likelihood of a family history but increased rates of cerebral organic disorders and neurological comorbidity. In old people, the possibility of 'secondary mania' should be strongly considered, noting particularly the physical and pharmacological risk factors listed in Table 6.2.

Course and outcome

Follow-up studies find that the 'average' person with bipolar disorder is well (euthymic) for 50 per cent of the time, manic/hypomanic for 10 per cent and depressed (to varying degrees of severity) for as much as 40 per cent of their lives. The fact that (often mild) depressive symptoms are so common has only recently been recognized. This may contribute to indifferent social outcomes with high unemployment, reduced rates of marriage and high rates of divorce. Suicide occurs in as many as 10 per cent of people with bipolar disorder. Factors associated with poorer outcomes include:

- longer time spent depressed
- psychotic symptoms
- early onset
- alcohol/drug misuse
- poorer social support systems
- low socioeconomic status.

Assessment

When patients are seen (in whatever setting) with a depressive episode, it is important to establish whether the pattern is of unipolar depression or of bipolar disorder, since the subsequent assessment and management may diverge significantly, although at the first depressive episode it may not be possible. Manic symptoms usually necessitate referral to specialist services. That said, a community prevalence of around 2 per cent means that doctors in all specialties will encounter patients with bipolar disorder and thus need to be able to recognize the symptoms.

The interview

Interviewing manic patients can be difficult as their flight of ideas and pressure of speech can take the interview rapidly off course; skill and judgement are required to retain appropriate control over the consultation. The patient needs to talk enough for the mental state and history to be clarified, and if one tries to exert excessive control then unnecessary confrontation can ensue (especially if their mood is labile and they are irritable). Given that a manic patient may well be grandiose and insightless, negotiation regarding treatment is rarely straightforward.

Different issues are presented by hypomanic patients in whom changes of mood and mental state are more subtle. Questions will focus on the symptoms listed in Box 6.2, with particular emphasis on mood ('too cheerful to be healthy?'), energy ('more active than usual without feeling tired?'), reduced sleep requirements and new ideas/interests. Hypomanic people with insight can often 'hold it together' for the duration of a medical consultation, leading to a diagnosis of 'happiness', and an informant should also be interviewed whenever possible and appropriate.

In the history, it is important to establish the temporal pattern of mood changes. The duration of the current episode is of clear importance as is the nature and frequency of any previous episodes of depression or elation. This also affords an opportunity to assess the possible effects of these mood swings on the life of the patient and on those around him or her, especially if a family member is present. Family history can often be further elucidated during an interview with a relative. A history of possible substance misuse should always be taken carefully. Remember also that abuse of alcohol and other substances may be secondary to the impulsivity and loss of normal social awareness that occurs in mania. A corroborative history can be crucial.

Differential diagnosis

In known patients with bipolar affective disorder, diagnosis of elated mood is seldom problematic, but it may not be so clear in a first episode of mania. 'Secondary' mania, caused by factors listed in Table 6.2, should be considered and a history of physical symptoms and medications along with a physical examination should be conducted. A urine drug screen is the most important routine investigation.

The main psychiatric differential diagnoses in adults will be schizophrenia, schizoaffective disorder and substance misuse (see Chapters 9 and 10). The first rank symptoms of schizophrenia can occur in psychotic mania and, by definition, symptoms of both schizophrenia and affective disorder occur together in the same episode in schizoaffective disorder.

Management

The initial diagnosis and management of patients with bipolar disorder will be undertaken, almost always, by psychiatric teams. Once management strategies are established, care will be undertaken by, or shared with, primary care teams; ongoing shared care may be optimal, as patients' quality of life can be enhanced by skilled management and continuity of care.

Manic episodes

In acute mania, rapid symptom control is required to ameliorate behaviour, which can often be dangerous to the patient and very disruptive to others. Admission to hospital will very often be necessary, with or without compulsory detention. Patients with mania are easily overstimulated, worsening their mental state, and it is helpful to attempt to redress this within as quiet and consistent a setting as possible.

In mania, a combined pharmacological approach with a mood stabilizer and an antipsychotic medication is usual. Lithium or valproate would be the commonest mood stabilizers deployed in the acute situation. Second-generation antipsychotics (e.g. olanzapine, risperidone, quetiapine) are effective antimanics and are now the usual first-line treatments. A high-potency benzodiazepine, such as lorazepam, can be helpful as an adjunctive sedative to promote behavioural control, and these are often used in the first few days of treatment. When intramuscular medication is required (in practice when the patient refuses oral medication or this is proving to be ineffective) haloperidol and/or lorazepam are often used.

In hypomania, the situation is much less acute and can often be managed on an outpatient or day treatment basis. A mood stabilizer alone, often the one on which the patient might continue prophylactically, usually suffices. In both mania and hypomania, it is helpful to re-establish a normal sleep–wake cycle, and the temporary prescription of a hypnotic can be therapeutic.

Depressive episodes

Management of bipolar depression differs in two respects from that of depression. Tricyclic and MAOI antidepressants are best avoided since they can induce mania. There is growing evidence that mood stabilizers may be more therapeutic than antidepressants when people become depressed in the context of bipolar affective disorder.

Prophylactic medication

Although it may be ideal to instigate prophylactic treatment after one episode of mania, patients will rarely agree to long-term medication until they have experienced at least one recurrence. Lithium (see Chapter 17) has been used for over 40 years and is of known effectiveness, rather more so in the prevention of mania than depression. The emergence of side-effects and the need for long-term monitoring and blood tests are factors that discourage patients from embarking on treatment, which is advised to be for an absolute minimum of 2 years. The anti-epileptic drug valproate is also used extensively and there is a growing case for lamotrigine, which is more effective at preventing depression than manic recurrences. Second-generation antipsychotics such as olanzapine, risperidone and quetiapine all have prophylactic efficacy, although these too are not without disadvantages especially with long-term use (see Chapter 17). Not infrequently, mood stabilizers are used in combination if patients do not respond adequately to one alone.

Psychological/psychosocial therapy

Psychological therapies have no place in the acute management of mania, but can have a role in the non-acute phases of bipolar disorder, albeit a less central one than in depression. The approaches are, however, less well evidenced.

Common to almost all psychological approaches in bipolar disorder is a strong component of 'psychoeducation', through which patients acquire knowledge about treatments and insight into their illnesses. This is often vital if patients are to adhere adequately with prophylactic medication. The identification and avoidance of factors, such as work stress or sleep disturbance, that may precipitate a relapse is part of this process. Patients can be encouraged to identify their own individual 'early-warning signs' that are the first symptoms heralding a relapse (e.g. irritability, two consecutive sleepless nights), so that hopefully illness can be 'nipped in the bud' at an early stage.

Seasonal affective disorder

Seasonal fluctuations in health and mood have been described by doctors for literally thousands of years, but the term seasonal affective disorder (SAD) has been in use only since the 1980s. The picture varies near the equator, but at temperate latitudes SAD is fairly synonymous with recurrent winter depression. Symptoms characteristically commence in the autumn and remit in spring and around one-third of people with SAD become mildly hypomanic during the spring and summer months. Many winter symptoms are those of non-seasonal depression but, in contrast with the picture of somatic syndrome, in SAD people usually experience hypersomnia (struggling to waken in the morning), daytime somnolence, carbohydrate craving and weight gain. Since many of us experience these seasonal changes to some degree, the line between 'normality' and 'disorder' is necessarily somewhat arbitrary, but around 3 per cent of the UK population suffers from clinically significant SAD. It is most common among women of reproductive age. Since 'light deprivation' is the main cause, it is unsurprising that moving to live further away from the equator confers an increased risk.

Management of mild to moderate symptoms includes encouragement to continue exercise and daylight exposure during the winter months. Light therapy, most commonly with lightboxes or with dawn-simulating alarm clocks, is the usual first choice of treatment when moderate to severe symptoms are present. In SAD there is circadian phase delay and circadian rhythms can be advanced by bright light, usually of about 30 minutes' duration, around breakfast time. When patients prefer, or when light therapy is unavailable or only partially effective, non-sedative antidepressants (usually SSRIs) can be prescribed.

Childbirth and affective disorders

Mood changes in the postpartum period are common and well recognized. In order of increasing severity, these comprise maternity blues, postnatal depression and puerperal psychosis.

'**Maternity blues**' or 'postpartum blues' are so common as to be normal, and are reported by about two-thirds of women. Symptoms include weepiness, irritability and despondency. They peak on days 3–7 postpartum and are usually transient and self-limiting, although severe maternity blues sometimes merge with depression.

Postnatal depression is deemed to affect 10–15 per cent of women, although attention has recently been drawn to international differences in prevalence. Onset is usually within 6 weeks of delivery. The usual symptoms of depression occur, although mood can be more fluctuating, with irritability and impaired attention often being prominent. Aetiologically, the profound and rapid falls of circulating hormone levels (e.g. progesterone, oestrogen and prolactin) after delivery are considered important. Having a baby is also, of course, a significant and complex life event, giving rise to major family, relationship and occupational changes. Women very commonly experience postpartum physical complaints, including backache, fatigue and perineal pain (which may be with associated sexual difficulties). Coping with a new baby is not straightforward, yielding a mix of emotional and social disruption, often exacerbated by sleep deprivation. Despite all this, new mothers are expected to be happy; this expectation may contribute to the depression itself and to the unfortunate finding that the majority of postnatal depression goes undetected. Detection and treatment are important, not only for the woman herself, but because the children of untreated postnatally depressed mothers have been shown to experience developmental delay. Depressed mothers usually benefit from discussing their difficulties within a supportive therapeutic relationship, and more formal therapies such as CBT and interpersonal therapy are of established effectiveness. Antidepressants are prescribed for moderate to severe depression with due attention to possible breastfeeding; sertraline is one drug which is present in only minimal amounts in breast milk.

Puerperal psychosis occurs at a frequency of 1 or 2 per 1000 deliveries. The vast majority of these serious illnesses are affective psychoses, and women are about 20 times more likely to experience a manic illness in the first month postpartum than at any other time of their lives. Women with a history of bipolar affective disorder are at hugely increased risk, at around one in three, and there is a similar risk of recurrence after a previous puerperal psychosis. Early detection can be facilitated by acquiring this history. The onset is usually acute and within the first week after childbirth. Among the usual symptoms of affective psychosis, there is often also perplexity and confusion. Danger to the baby and to the mother (largely through suicide) must be closely assessed. If possible, admission should be to a psychiatric mother and baby unit so that both can be cared for while mother–infant bonding is facilitated.

Pregnancy was traditionally regarded as a time of emotional well-being for women. There is now convincing evidence that this is not the case. Around 10 per cent of women will experience depression during pregnancy and as many as 7 per cent will have an anxiety disorder. One study found that less than 6 per cent of women with an antenatal psychiatric disorder received treatment. This is particularly unfortunate since antenatal disorder can proceed untreated into the postnatal period. Furthermore, independent of postnatal maternal well-being, it is now known that the children of mothers who are depressed or anxious in pregnancy do less well than other children; they are at higher risk of emotional and behavioural difficulties and they are prone to developmental delay. Psychological interventions (CBT, interpersonal therapy, group therapy) are usually the first options, given the wish to avoid medication in pregnancy if possible. However, in view of the possible long-term sequelae, psychotropic medications are not uncommonly prescribed. Newer medications have not been prescribed in sufficient numbers of pregnancies to be certain about their safety, but while it may be associated with a slight risk of prematurity, fluoxetine is considered essentially safe during pregnancy.

Premenstrual depression

Changes in well-being across women's menstrual cycles have long been recognized, with cyclical physiological and emotional symptoms being referred to as premenstrual syndrome, and this may include some features similar to depressive illness. When more severe psychiatric symptoms prevail, premenstrual depression can be diagnosed. Typical symptoms comprise low mood, anxiety/tension, anger/irritability, lethargy, poor concentration, and changes in sleep and/or appetite. However, it is worth noting that this diagnostic category is not free of controversy with some rejecting the concept as they feel that a woman's biology is being construed as a psychiatric disorder. However, in some cases the quality of life can be markedly improved with treatment.

Summary

The key points relating to mood disorders can be summarized as follows:

- depressive disorders are very common;
- depression occurs with increased frequency in a wide range of medical conditions;
- the detection and management of depression are core medical skills;
- about 50 per cent of depression is not detected by doctors, often because patients present with somatic symptoms;
- depression usually responds to antidepressants and/or psychological therapies;
- very few other medical interventions rival the effects of treating depression on a patient's quality of life;
- bipolar affective disorders occur in about 2 per cent of the population;
- depressed patients should be asked routinely about manic/hypomanic episodes;
- especially in elderly people, mania can arise from other medical conditions or from prescribed medications;
- untreated mania can pose a significant risk to the patient's and/or others' safety;
- patients with bipolar disorders usually require long-term treatment with a mood stabilizer.

Further reading

Anderson IM, Ferrier IN, Baldwin RC, et al. (2008) Evidence-based guidelines for treating depressive disorders with antidepressants: a revision of the 2000 British Association for Psychopharmacology guidelines. Journal of Psychopharmacology 22: 343–396.

Brosse AL, Sheets ES, Lett HS, Blumenthal JA (2002) Exercise and the treatment of clinical depression in adults. Sports Medicine 32: 741–760.

Gellatly J, Bower P, Hennessy S, et al. (2007) What makes self-help interventions effective in the management of depressive symptoms? Meta-analysis and meta-regression. Psychological Medicine 37: 1217–1228.

Goodwin GM, Anderson I, Arango C, et al. (2007) Bipolar depression. ECNP consensus meeting. Nice, March 2007. European Neuropsychopharmacology 18: 535–549.

Halbreich U, Karkun S (2006) Cross-cultural and social diversity of prevalence of postpartum depression and depressive symptoms. Journal of Affective Disorders 91: 97–111.

National Institute for Health and Clinical Excellence (NICE) (2009) Depression: the treatment and management of depression in adults. National Clinical Practice Guideline 90. National Institute for Health and Clinical Excellence; available at www.nice.org.uk

Pilling S, Anderson I, Goldberg D, et al. (2009) Depression in adults, including those with a chronic physical health problem: a summary of NICE guidance. British Medical Journal 339: 1025–1027.

Ruo B, Rumsfeld JS, Hlatky MA, et al. (2003) Depressive symptoms and health-related quality of life: the Heart and Soul Study. Journal of the American Medical Association 290: 215–221.

Simon GE, VonKorff M, Piccinelli M, et al. (1999) An international study of the relation between somatic symptoms and depression. New England Journal of Medicine 341: 1329–1335.

Üstün TB, Ayuso-Mateos JL, Chatterji S, et al. (2004) Global burden of depressive disorders in the year 2000. British Journal of Psychiatry 184: 386–392.

Vesco KK, Haney EM, Humphrey L, et al. (2007) Influence of menopause on mood: a systematic review of cohort studies. Climacteric 10: 448–465.

Weissman MM, Bland RC, Canino GJ, et al. (1996). Cross-national epidemiology of major depression and bipolar disorder. Journal of the American Medical Association 276: 293–299.

CASE STUDY 1: SOMATIZED DEPRESSION

You are a general practitioner consulted by a 26-year-old man with dyspepsia. You notice that he is glum and he has felt low since splitting up with his partner 6 months ago.

What symptoms would you ask about in relation to a possible diagnosis of depression?

The first task is to establish his symptoms of dyspepsia, and to treat these if this is appropriate.

You want to know the timescale of his low mood, and whether this is improving or worsening.

The specific symptoms to check include diurnal variation of mood, loss of interest, anhedonia, sleep, appetite/weight change, energy/motivation, concentration and suicidal ideation.

You conclude that he has symptoms of moderate depression. Which factors might lead you to advise initial CBT rather than antidepressants?

No urgent need for treatment (e.g. low suicide risk) as CBT will take longer to commence.

Patient preference.

Negative thinking and behaviour patterns are prominent.

Intelligent and psychologically minded patient.

No previous good response to antidepressant.

CASE STUDY 2: POSSIBLE RECURRENCE OF MANIA

You are a general practitioner and a patient's wife has called to express anxiety that her husband is becoming hypomanic.

What would you ask her on the telephone to ascertain whether he is indeed manic/hypomanic?

If you did not know already, you would ask if he is prescribed prophylactic mood-stabilizing medication and whether he has continued taking this.

The symptoms you would ask about would include elevated mood/excessive cheerfulness, increased energy, reduced sleep requirement, irritability, impulsivity and grandiosity.

You see him and find him to be hypomanic, but he does not want to see a psychiatrist. Which factors would make you insist that he does?

These would include:

The severity of his symptoms.

Your assessment of risk, e.g. is he safe to drive (or willing to stop driving), is he able to make decisions rationally, is he excessively impulsive (e.g. financially), is he irritable/aggressive, can he care for children if this is an issue?

His willingness to accept treatment and your willingness to provide it – this will range from his complete refusal to his being willing to restart a medication which has previously been rapidly effective.

The home situation in terms of support from his wife (plus other relatives/friends) and the presence of young children.

ANXIETY DISORDERS

Ciaran Mulholland

KEY CHAPTER FEATURES

- Clinical presentation of anxiety and medically unexplained symptoms
- Important aspects of generalized anxiety disorder, panic disorder, obsessive compulsive disorder, stress-related disorders, somatization disorders and conversion disorders
- Treatment approaches for the above conditions

Introduction

This chapter describes psychiatric disorders in which anxiety is a key feature of the overall presentation, including the anxiety disorders themselves, stress-related disorders, such as post-traumatic stress disorder (PTSD), and obsessive compulsive disorder (OCD). Phobic anxiety disorders (agoraphobia, social phobia and specific phobias) are described in Chapter 8. This chapter also briefly describes two groups of disorders that present with medically unexplained symptoms: the somatoform disorders (somatization disorder, hypochondriacal disorder, somatoform autonomic dysfunction, persistent somatoform pain disorder) and a group of disorders

Exercise

Anxiety is probably easier to understand than some of the other conditions in this book as all of us have been anxious at some time. From your own experience of anxiety-provoking situations try to answer the following questions.

What are the physical and psychological symptoms of anxiety?

When do you think anxiety is appropriate and when is it inappropriate?

When you are anxious how do you try to manage the anxiety?

Can you think of inappropriate or unhelpful techniques that some people adopt to try to overcome anxiety?

The answers to this exercise are summarized later after some of the above issues have been addressed.

Box 7.1: Neurotic, stress-related and somatoform disorders (from ICD-10)

F40 Phobic anxiety disorder

F41 Other anxiety disorders

F42 Obsessive-compulsive disorder

F43 Reactions to severe stress and adjustment disorders

F44 Dissociative (conversion) disorders

F45 Somatoform disorders

F48 Other neurotic disorders

called the dissociative or conversion disorders. All of the disorders above are grouped together in the ICD-10 classification system as 'neurotic, stress-related and somatoform disorders' (Box 7.1) as they have historically been seen as inter-related and are often associated with psychological stress.

Why this is relevant to you

The anxiety disorders are very common. All doctors deal with patients with these conditions, especially GPs, and of course psychiatrists. A full understanding of the presenting symptoms and treatment of the anxiety disorders will help you in your future career.

Medically unexplained symptoms present frequently to GPs, physicians, surgeons, and all other doctors. These symptoms are often puzzling and are sometimes bizarre. There is a risk of over-investigation and overtreatment when patients present in this way and an awareness of the presentation of such symptoms and the treatment options available is thus necessary for all doctors.

What is anxiety and what is 'normal' anxiety?

Anxiety is a mental state that is characterized by physical and psychological symptoms as shown in Box 7.2. Most of us can quickly grasp the nature of the anxiety disorders as we have all felt anxious when faced with a stressful situation. Anxiety in such situations is normal and adaptive (if we aren't a little anxious prior to an important examination, for example, then we might not study hard enough). The symptoms of anxiety are outlined in Box 7.2 and are likely to be familiar to all readers. Anxiety is considered normal or appropriate if it is present in circumstances that warrant it as suggested by being anxious if undertaking an exam (and this may be exacerbated if there has been insufficient study). In summary, normal anxiety is a response to a known problem, usually a definable and external threat of short duration. Obvious examples of such threats include giving a speech or performing on a stage and others may be facing a new situation or meeting new people.

Box 7.2: Features of a state of anxiety

Affect	Feelings of fearfulness
	Apprehension
Thoughts	Themes of misfortune
	Belief of inability to cope with stress
	Unrealistic ideas of danger
Arousal	Increased arousal/alertness
	Hypervigilance
	Restlessness
	Poor sleep (especially initial/middle insomnia)
	Poor concentration
	Exaggerated startle response
Behaviour	Reduced purposeful activity
	Increased purposeless activity
	Avoidance of some situations
Somatic	Palpitations
	Hyperventilation
	Light-headedness
	Numbness or tingling
	Retrosternal constriction
	Muscle tension
	Nausea
	Diarrhoea
	Sweating
	Trembling
	Headaches
	Dry mouth
Associated symptoms	Depersonalization/derealization
	Irritability
	Low mood

When might anxiety be a problem?

Given that most of us experience some anxiety at some point, it can be easy to underestimate how those suffering from anxiety disorders might be compromised by their conditions. Anxiety is considered abnormal (or pathological or clinical anxiety) and a problem if it is extreme (that is, it overtakes the situation and prevents the individual getting on with the tasks of daily living or interferes with life in other ways) and/or misplaced (that is, it is not confined to recognized 'stressful' situations and/or begins to spill over into preventing effective everyday functioning). Some individuals have what is known as high-trait anxiety (or an anxious personality), that is they are more anxious than the average person but do not meet criteria for an anxiety disorder as such. Anxiety is present without any stressful context, that is it is almost the 'natural state of being' for an individual and they might have an anxious personality as discussed in Chapter 15.

Exercise

Summary of answers to exercise

The physical and psychological symptoms of anxiety are listed in Box 7.3.

Anxiety is appropriate in a stressful situation, so long as it is not more extreme than the stressful situation would normally provoke. Normal anxiety is a response to a known problem, usually a definable and external threat of short duration. Anxiety is inappropriate if it is extreme and/or misplaced (that is, it is not confined to recognized 'stressful' situations and/or begins to spill over into preventing effective everyday functioning).

Individuals vary but appropriate ways of managing anxiety include various relaxation techniques (for example, yoga) and taking exercise.

The most obvious examples of inappropriate or unhelpful techniques to overcome anxiety are smoking and the misuse of alcohol and benzodiazepines.

Box 7.3: Panic attacks are characterized by acute development of several of the following symptoms, reaching peak severity within 10 minutes

Escalating subjective tension

Sweating, chills

Chest pain/discomfort

Palpitations, tachycardia

Tremor

Nausea, 'butterflies'

Dizziness/feeling faint

Depersonalization/realization

Dread, i.e. fear of loss of control or dying

Parasthesiae

With pathological or clinical anxiety, there is a sense of fear which is not well defined. Any threat is not immediate (for example an examination that is many months away) or there may be no threat whatsoever. The threat may be 'internal' to the person and the situation is often chronic. Reassurance is rarely effective and can exacerbate the situation as it confirms the original misperception that there was reason to worry.

Pathological anxiety can occur as a secondary feature to other psychiatric illnesses, such as depression, dementia and psychotic disorders. Pathological anxiety can also occur secondarily to a range of physical conditions. Examples include a range of endocrine disorders including thyrotoxicosis, hypoparathyroidism, carcinoid syndrome, Cushing's disease, phaeochromocytoma, pituitary disorders and hypoglycaemia. Cardiovascular conditions (hypoxia, congestive heart failure, pulmonary embolism, hypertension, angina, myocardial infarction, arrhythmias, mitral valve prolapse), neurological conditions (seizures) and respiratory conditions (chronic obstructive pulmonary disease, asthma) can also present with anxiety.

Drug intoxication (for example cocaine, amphetamines), drug side-effects (theophylline, steroids, anticholinergics) or drug withdrawal (especially from benzodiazepines and alcohol) commonly cause anxiety-type symptoms. Another potential cause of anxiety symptoms is excess use of caffeine or 'caffeinism' (Box 7.4). Stopping caffeine suddenly is not a good idea as withdrawal effects are

---

Box 7.4: Caffeinism

Caffeinism occurs when an individual suffers side-effects from caffeine, takes larger amounts and needs to keep drinking caffeine to function properly (including a craving for caffeine)

250–500 mg of caffeine a day is OK (four cups tea or coffee). Caffeinism occurs if one has an intake of above 600–750 mg of caffeine per day. Drinking more than 1000 mg per day is well into the toxic range and likely to produce the symptoms of anxiety. The US Olympic Committee considers caffeine a stimulant

Suddenly stopping taking caffeine can produce problems. Withdrawal from even moderate amounts of caffeine can produce headaches (52%), anxiety (10%), rebound drowsiness, fatigue and lethargy

likely. The best plan is to gradually reduce caffeine intake, preferably over several weeks. Psychoeducation about the effects of caffeine may also be useful.

Finally, large numbers of individuals have primary anxiety disorders: generalized anxiety disorder and panic disorder (covered in this chapter), and agoraphobia (with or without panic disorder), social phobia and specific phobias (covered in Chapter 8). The other conditions dealt with in this chapter have prominent anxiety symptoms as part of their clinical presentation.

Neurosis

In the past, the term 'neurosis' was used to describe many of the conditions now classified in Box 7.1 and the term remains in the ICD-10 title of this group of conditions. The word was coined in 1784 by Cullen, a physician who recognized that some of his patients presented with what were at that time medically unexplained symptoms:

> In a certain view, almost the whole of the diseases of the human body might be called nervous … in this place I propose to comprehend the title neurosis to all those preternatural affections of sense and motion which are without pyrexia as part of the primary disease and which do not depend on a topical affection of the organs but upon a more general affectation of the nervous system.

In the eighteenth and nineteenth centuries the term neurosis was used for a wide range of conditions which are now known to have an underlying physical pathology (for example, diabetes, epilepsy, chorea) or which have since been classified more accurately as specific psychiatric conditions (for example, melancholia/depression).

Neuroses were traditionally seen as disorders characterized by unimpaired reality testing (that is, the person is in contact with reality compared with psychosis, where this contact is lost or impaired), with preservation of insight and an absence of any demonstrable organic basis. There was an implication that 'psychotics' were very ill but didn't recognize it, and that 'neurotics' were less ill but were very aware of it. (The term the 'worried well' has been applied to 'neurotics'.) This is not necessarily the case. The ICD-10 and DSM-IV classification systems have largely dropped the term neurosis, recognizing that the term has come to be used as a generalization for any situation in which anxiety or emotional symptoms are prominent and is often used pejoratively.

Aetiology of the anxiety disorders

Anxiety disorders are not homogeneous and do not have a single cause. Important aetiological factors include personality traits, psychosocial stress and the degree of social support available to an individual. Genetic factors are less important for the anxiety disorders than for some other psychiatric conditions but they are not unimportant. Older twin studies suggest that anxiety disorders in general terms show heritability. In more recent studies, panic disorder and agoraphobia demonstrate the greatest, most consistent genetic effects. In relatives of individuals with panic disorder there is a four to seven times increase in risk for panic disorder (PD). There is no increased risk for generalized anxiety disorder (GAD) in these individuals. Relatives of individuals with GAD have up to a five times increased risk of GAD and also an increased risk of alcoholism, but do not have an increased risk of PD or agoraphobia. These effects are generally reduced if milder cases are examined and are less marked in population studies than in hospital clinic studies.

Prevalence of the anxiety disorders

Anxiety disorders are very common. The National Comorbidity Survey (NCS), carried out in the USA, found that 25 per cent of the population will meet criteria for an anxiety disorder at some time in their lives. The lifetime prevalence of GAD was 5 per cent in this study. The Epidemiologic Catchment Area (ECA) study, also in the USA, demonstrated a prevalence of 3.8 per cent for GAD over a 6-month period and of 8.5 per cent over a lifetime. Panic disorder had a 6-month prevalence of 0.8 per cent and a lifetime prevalence of 1.6 per cent in the same study. In a UK study (OPCS General Household Survey – UK, 1995) a rate of GAD in females of 5 per cent, and in males of 4 per cent was demonstrated. The corresponding figures for panic disorder were 1 per cent for both sexes, and for a concept termed 'mixed anxiety and depression' 10 per cent for females and 5 per cent for males.

Clinical assessment

When assessing an individual who presents with anxiety symptoms it is of course necessary to take a full history and to complete a mental state examination in order to clarify the diagnosis. A physical health problem presenting with anxiety symptoms should be excluded (and physical tests may be necessary in order to fully exclude such a possibility). As anxiety symptoms may occur in other psychiatric conditions, such as depression and psychotic disorders, it is important to exclude these disorders. If a diagnosis of an anxiety disorder is indicated it is important to carefully differentiate between panic disorder, phobic anxiety disorders and generalized anxiety disorder (GAD).

One particular diagnostic conundrum is when symptoms of anxiety and depression are both present, but neither is clearly predominant, and neither type of symptom is present to the extent that it justifies a diagnosis if considered separately. In these circumstances a diagnosis of 'mixed anxiety and depression' is justified. However, when both anxiety and depressive symptoms are present and severe enough to justify individual diagnoses, both diagnoses should be recorded and the category of mixed anxiety and depression should not be used. Taking a careful history can help establish if anxiety followed low mood and poor self-confidence or whether the mood followed the frustrations of anxiety and being limited in daily life. In the latter situation the person may be someone who was predisposed to being anxious with minor triggers.

Generalized anxiety disorder

Diagnosis

GAD is defined as persistent (occurring more days than not for more than 6 months) 'free-floating' anxiety, with at least four associated features from the following list: palpitations, sweating, trembling, dry mouth, difficulty breathing, feelings of choking, chest pain, nausea, dizziness, derealization, depersonalization, fear of losing control, fear of dying, hot flushes or cold chills, numbness or tingling, feeling keyed up, difficulty swallowing, irritability, poor concentration, disturbed sleep (early/middle insomnia), muscle tension and restlessness.

'Free-floating' anxiety is generalized and persistent but not restricted to, or even strongly predominating in, any particular environmental circumstance. Fears that the patient or a relative will become seriously ill or have an accident are often expressed.

Onset is usually in early adulthood. In younger age groups it is twice as common in females, but there are only slightly more female patients in older age groups. For most sufferers GAD is mild but the illness course is often chronic and is often worse in females. GAD is distinct from panic disorder and is often comorbid with other psychiatric disorders (such as obsessive compulsive disorder, social phobia and dysthymia).

Management of GAD

The anxiety disorders often go unrecognized. Many individuals do not present themselves to their GP as they do not realize the meaning and significance of their symptoms. This is particularly true of men. When individuals do present the GP might not ascertain the meaning of symptoms such as breathlessness or chest or stomach pain. Misdiagnosis and inappropriate or inadequate treatment may result. The overall effect is that there are greater levels of social disability as a result of the anxiety disorders than is necessary, with a resulting high economic cost. Longstanding problems are often also more difficult to treat, as maladaptive coping strategies may have been employed over many years.

There are several other important issues when considering the assessment and treatment of patients with anxiety disorders. As a general rule you should be reluctant to make a new diagnosis of an anxiety disorder in an older patient: they may actually be troubled by an underlying medical condition. Be aware of the possibility of a patient 'self-medicating' with alcohol or benzodiazepines. Also, do not forget the importance of patient motivation if a successful treatment outcome is to be achieved.

Pharmacological interventions are rarely appropriate as the first-line intervention for mild forms of anxiety, which can usually be managed in primary care with basic psychological interventions. Psychological approaches range from simple reassurance, especially from the GP in person, through self-help, including guided self-help, counselling and problem solving carried out at the primary care level. More sophisticated approaches, applicable to those individuals who are referred to mental health services, include cognitive behavioural therapy (CBT) and 'anxiety management' (often carried out in a group setting).

If the disorder is more severe or chronic a referral to mental health services is indicated. Combined treatment, pharmacological and psychological together, is often best. The SSRI antidepressants are the first-line pharmacological approach, although they may cause exacerbation of symptoms initially (because of their activating effect) and patients should be warned about this. Tricyclic antidepressants are also effective, but they are used much less often because of their side-effect profile and their toxicity in overdose.

Benzodiazepines should in general be avoided (because of their addictive qualities and because they quickly induce increased tolerance) although they can occasionally have a short-term role. Buspirone, a non-benzodiazepine anxiolytic with negligible sedative side-effects, and which is a partial agonist at the 5-HT$_{1A}$ receptor, is probably less effective than the benzodiazepines but provides another therapeutic option. Beta-blockers, such as propranolol, are useful for somatic anxiety symptoms such as tachycardia, sweating and tremor but do not treat the core anxiety symptoms. They are, perhaps, more useful in social anxiety disorder.

Panic disorder

Diagnosis

The essential feature of panic disorder (also sometimes known as episodic paroxysmal anxiety) is recurrent attacks of severe anxiety (panic), which are not restricted to any particular situation or set of circumstances and are therefore unpredictable. As with other anxiety disorders, the dominant symptoms (Box 7.3) include sudden onset of palpitations, chest pain, choking sensations, dizziness and feelings of unreality (depersonalization or derealization). There is often also a secondary fear of dying, losing control or going mad. The patient fears further attacks (phobophobia) and often changes his or her behaviour in relation to attacks.

The onset of panic disorder is usually in adolescence or the mid-30s. New onsets after the age of 45 are rare. The illness course may be of varying severity. In younger age groups, there are twice as many female as male cases but this difference equalizes with age.

It has been established that there is an increased incidence (30–50 per cent) of mitral valve prolapse (MVP) in people with panic disorder (compared with perhaps 5–15 per cent in the general population). The reason for this association is not clear. There is not a simple relationship: MVP does not cause panic disorder and persists after panic disorder is treated. It is possible that MVP acts as an autonomic precipitant or that both MVP and panic disorder are part of a syndrome of autonomic dysfunction.

Assessment and treatment

Panic may occur as part of other psychiatric conditions. For example, panic disorder should not be given as the main diagnosis if a patient has a depressive disorder at the time the attacks start: in these circumstances the panic attacks are probably secondary to depression. It is also important to exclude epilepsy and intoxication with or withdrawal from drugs or alcohol when assessing a patient who presents in such a way.

In general, assessment is essentially the same as for GAD. Again, combined pharmacological and psychological treatment is usually best. The SSRI antidepressants are recommended as a first-line treatment, although the tricyclic antidepressants have also been shown to be effective. Fast-acting benzodiazepines, such as alprazolam, may be used in the short term, but in general it is best to avoid these medications in panic disorder. If a patient is seen when he or she is actually experiencing a panic attack a better strategy is to ask them to re-breathe their own air by the simple expedient of breathing into a paper bag. However, many patients (especially in such a state) may dislike the sensation of something over their mouth and should be encouraged to focus on emptying the lungs on expiration as hyperventilation syndrome is associated with rapid shallow breaths that do not allow adequate outbreaths.

Of the relevant psychological approaches CBT has the best evidence for sustained improvement. Exposure therapy, relaxation techniques and self-help are also effective.

Obsessive compulsive disorder

Diagnosis

The essential features of obsessive compulsive disorder (OCD) are recurrent obsessional thoughts or compulsive acts, or both together. Obsessional thoughts (or ruminations) are ideas, images or impulses that enter the patient's mind again and again in a stereotyped form. They are almost invariably distressing and the patient often tries, unsuccessfully, to resist them. They are recognized as his or her own thoughts, even though they are involuntary and often repugnant (common themes include fears of the person themselves acquiring disease or of coming to harm in some way, and of causing physical or sexual harm to others). Sometimes the ideas are an indecisive, endless consideration of alternatives, associated with an inability to make trivial but necessary decisions in day-to-day living. The result may be 'obsessional slowness'.

Compulsive acts or rituals are stereotyped behaviours that are repeated again and again. They are not inherently enjoyable and they do not result in the completion of inherently useful tasks. Their function is to prevent some objectively unlikely event, often involving harm to or caused by the patient, which he or she fears might otherwise occur. A patient might, for example, count up to a certain number repeatedly to ensure that his or her child is not involved in a car accident. Usually, compulsive acts are recognized by a patient as pointless or ineffectual and repeated attempts are made to resist them, but often to little avail. Family members can often become embroiled in the obsessional behaviour as initially this may appear to be helpful, but longer term this is rarely the case. Anxiety is almost invariably present. If compulsive acts are resisted the anxiety gets worse.

The majority of compulsive acts are concerned with cleaning (particularly hand washing), repeated checking to ensure that a potentially dangerous situation has not been allowed to develop, and orderliness and tidiness.

The presentation of OCD can vary considerably. Sometimes obsessional thoughts are to the fore, for example upsetting and violent sexual thoughts regarding family members. Sometimes compulsions are to the fore, for example endlessly checking the kitchen cupboards to ensure that the labels on every jar and tin face in the same direction.

Prevalence

At one time OCD was considered to be a relatively rare condition, but in recent years it has become apparent that it may affect between 1 per cent and 3 per cent of the population over a lifetime. Many individuals do not present to services, however, but just view the behaviours as an integral part of who they are. Perhaps half of those with OCD have a comorbid anxiety disorder. Rates in males and females differ in childhood with more males affected, but in adulthood rates are about equal. Age of onset is earlier in boys and is more often associated with tics. The course of OCD tends to be chronic. Males have a worse prognosis.

Aetiology

The aetiology of OCD is unclear, but it is clear that it is at least in part a genetic condition and there is increasing evidence for underlying brain abnormalities. First-degree relatives of individuals with OCD have higher rates of anankastic/obsessional personality (explained below), depression and OCD (the rate in first-degree relatives is 10 per cent) than the general population. The OCD concordance rate between monozygotic twins is 50–80 per cent, whereas between dizygotic twins it is 25 per cent.

Abnormalities of the serotoninergic system appear to play a role in OCD: studies have demonstrated hypersensitivity of postsynaptic serotonin receptors in some patients. OCD symptoms are particularly common in Gilles de la Tourette syndrome, a neuropsychiatric disorder characterized by multiple motor and vocal tics and sometimes coprolalia (the shouting out of swear words). Up to 80 per cent of individuals with Tourette's have obsessional symptoms. Abnormalities of the basal ganglia area may well play an important role in both OCD and Tourette syndrome: brain imaging has demonstrated abnormalities of brain circuits linking prefrontal cortex (especially the orbitofrontal region) and the striatum and thalamus. Overactivity of thalamocortical pathways may be the important mechanism.

Assessment

A thorough assessment is necessary to exclude various possible differential diagnoses. It should be remembered that obsessional symptoms often occur in both childhood and adulthood, especially the former, but do not mean that a person has OCD. (In studies, up to 14 per cent of the population have obsessions or compulsions.) Some obsessional behaviours start as a way of managing anxiety but then become habitual, so that by the time patients present to services the picture may be quite confused.

Obsessional symptoms may also occur in other psychiatric conditions, especially in schizophrenia and early dementia and other organic brain conditions. The relationship between obsessional ruminations and depression is particularly close and a diagnosis of OCD should be preferred only if ruminations arise or persist in the absence of a depressive episode.

Premorbid anankastic or obsessional traits (or personality disorder) are common. They are characterized by feelings of doubt, perfectionism, excessive conscientiousness, checking and preoccupation with details, stubbornness, caution and rigidity. There may be insistent and unwelcome thoughts or impulses that do not attain the severity of OCD.

A diagnosis of OCD is appropriate if an individual has obsessional thoughts or compulsive acts for most days over a period of 2 weeks. The obsessions and acts need to have a number of features: they are from the patient's own mind, they are repetitive and unpleasant, there has to be a degree of resistance to them, the thought or the act is not a pleasurable experience, the condition leads to some form of disability (with effects on relationships, work, family) and the symptoms are not related to a psychotic illness or mood disorder.

Management

Serotoninergic antidepressants – the SSRIs and clomipramine – have proven anti-obsessional effects. Dopamine blocking agents may also be useful. In very extreme cases neurosurgery (anterior capsulotomy or subcaudate tractotomy) may be useful. More recently, a new technique called deep brain stimulation has been subject to clinical trials.

Various psychological interventions have a clear role in the treatment of OCD, including response prevention and graded exposure (for rituals), thought stopping (for obsessional thoughts) and CBT. In exposure and response prevention a therapist asks the patient to expose themselves to a particular situation that brings on anxiety and/or a compulsive act. The patient is asked to resist from engaging in that act

for as long as possible and eventually the drive and resulting anxiety decreases.

Reactions to severe stress and adjustment disorders

These disorders are identified not just on the basis of certain symptoms and illness course, as are the majority of psychiatric disorders, but also by aetiology or cause. As the umbrella title indicates the presumed causes are either acute or chronic psychological stresses. Individual stressful events, or continuing unpleasant life circumstances, are considered to be the primary and overriding causal factor and the disorder would not have occurred without their impact. The disorders in this section can thus be regarded as maladaptive responses to severe or continued stress, in that they interfere with successful coping mechanisms and therefore lead to problems with social functioning (that is, the ability to cope with day-to-day life).

Acute stress reactions

Diagnosis

The first category in this section is the acute stress reactions. These are transient disorders that develop in an individual without any other apparent mental disorder in response to exceptional physical and mental stress, for example witnessing a murder, and usually subside within hours or days.

An individual's vulnerability to stress and ability to cope play very important roles in the occurrence and severity of acute stress reactions. The symptoms typically show a mixed and changing picture and include an initial state of 'daze' with some constriction of the field of consciousness and narrowing of attention, inability to comprehend stimuli and disorientation. This state may be followed either by further withdrawal from the surrounding situation (to the extent of a dissociative stupor, see below), or by agitation and overactivity (a flight reaction). Autonomic signs of anxiety (tachycardia, sweating, flushing) are commonly present.

The symptoms usually appear within minutes of the stressful event and disappear within 2–3 days (often within hours). Partial or complete amnesia for the episode may be present. If the symptoms persist a change in diagnosis should be considered.

Acute stress reactions have been shown to occur in

around 15 per cent of the population at some time in their lives. The rate for individuals who have suffered a severe traumatic event is approximately 30–40 per cent (that is, the majority of individuals who have been exposed to such trauma do not experience an acute stress reaction).

Management

It is important to explore the event that precipitated the acute stress reaction. Most often no intervention is required or indicated as the disorder is self-limiting. Simple explanation and support may be helpful. Brief CBT may help with an acute stress disorder that is characterized by dissociation and symptoms of PTSD. There was a trend to offer 'post-traumatic counselling' soon after an individual experienced trauma in the hope that this would prevent development of problems, but it has now been realized that this can be unhelpful. It is very important to allow individuals the time to make sense of the events for themselves.

Post-traumatic stress disorder

Diagnosis

The concept of post-traumatic stress disorder (PTSD) is a relatively recent one, but clearly the condition cannot be new. That some individuals develop longstanding symptoms after a traumatic incident became apparent over some decades.

In the nineteenth century 'railway spine' was diagnosed when passengers were involved in railway accidents. Physicians of the time thought that the symptoms were due to the 'excessive speeds' of the trains. In war after war it was apparent that soldiers were adversely affected in a psychological sense. In the American Civil War the preferred diagnosis was 'irritable heart', in the First World War 'shell shock', in the Second World War 'combat neurosis' and finally in the aftermath of the Vietnam War the diagnosis of PTSD was described.

PTSD arises as a delayed or protracted response to a stressful event or situation (of either brief or long duration) of an exceptionally threatening or catastrophic nature, which is likely to cause pervasive distress in almost anyone. Predisposing factors, such as personality traits or previous history of psychiatric illness, may lower the threshold for the development of the syndrome or aggravate its course, but they

are neither necessary nor sufficient to explain its occurrence.

Typical features include episodes of repeated reliving of the trauma in intrusive memories ('flashbacks'), dreams or nightmares occurring against a persisting background of a sense of 'numbness' and emotional blunting, detachment from other people, unresponsiveness to surroundings, anhedonia, and avoidance of activities and situations reminiscent of the trauma. There is usually a state of autonomic hyperarousal with hypervigilance, an enhanced startle reaction and insomnia.

Anxiety and depression are commonly associated with the above symptoms and signs, and suicidal ideation is common. The onset follows the trauma with a latency period that may range from a few weeks to months. The course is fluctuating but recovery can be expected in the majority of cases. In a small proportion of cases the condition may follow a chronic course over many years, with eventual transition to an enduring personality change.

The lifetime prevalence for PTSD has been estimated in various studies at a low of 1 per cent and a high of 10 per cent. For obvious reasons certain groups are more likely to develop PTSD: soldiers, those who have been exposed to natural and man-made disasters, assault and rape victims, and victims of torture. Between 30 per cent and 40 per cent of women who have been sexually assaulted will develop PTSD, as did 20 per cent of American Vietnam War veterans. Around one-third of individuals with PTSD suffer from a severe form of the condition.

Three factors that may predict the onset of PTSD are the scale of the trauma, the patient's previous experience of trauma and the level of social support available. There may also be some genetic predisposition. The hippocampus (responsible for memory) and the amygdala (the fear centre of the brain) may be oversensitive in people who develop PTSD. Magnetic resonance imaging scans have shown decreased hippocampal size in patients with PTSD.

Management

An initial period of engagement and the establishment of trust are important. Psychological treatment in the form of either trauma-focused CBT or what is known as 'eye movement desensitization and reprocessing' (EMDR) are recommended as the first-line treatments by the National Institute for Health and Clinical Excellence (NICE). EMDR is a somewhat controversial treatment, which involves generating rapid and rhythmical eye movements while holding traumatic images in the mind.

The key component of trauma-focused psychological therapies is to expose the patient to the traumatic event repeatedly. This is often accomplished by getting them to write a detailed account of the traumatic event and recording it (a 'testimony'). The idea is that repeating the trauma will reduce symptoms as an individual becomes used to the experience. Various non-specific psychological and social treatments such as stress management and family and support groups can be helpful, but it is probable that trauma-focused treatments are more effective.

Pharmacological treatment, using SSRI antidepressants, is the recognized second-line treatment. There is no role for routine prescription of benzodiazepines. Pharmacological treatments can of course be combined with psychological treatments, and often are.

Any comorbid conditions, including physical health problems, should be treated. Prognosis is good if the individual concerned had a healthy premorbid function, the trauma was brief and of limited severity, there is no past psychiatric history, no family history of psychiatric illness and the individual has good social support. Approximately 65 per cent of patients recover within 18 months.

Adjustment disorders

Adjustment disorders are states of subjective distress and emotional disturbance, usually interfering with social functioning and performance, arising in the period of adaptation to a significant life change or a stressful life event. The stressor may affect the integrity of an individual's social network (bereavement, separation experiences) or the wider system of social supports and values (migration, refugee status), or represent a major developmental transition or crisis (going to school, becoming a parent, failure to attain a cherished personal goal, retirement).

Individual predisposition plays an important role in the risk of occurrence and the shaping of the manifestations of adjustment disorders, but it is nevertheless assumed that the condition would not have arisen without the stressor.

The manifestations vary and include low mood, anxiety or worry (or a mixture of these), a feeling of inability to cope, plan ahead or continue in the present situation, as well as some degree of disability in the performance of daily routine. The predominant feature may be a brief or prolonged depressive reaction, or a disturbance of other emotions or conduct. The prevalence of adjustment disorder is not known although it is clearly a very common condition.

Management of adjustment disorders

There is generally no need to intervene. If an individual is very distressed or is thought to be at risk it is best to treat individuals for the predominant symptoms present, that is PTSD treatments for PTSD symptoms, or anxiety and depression treatments for individuals with predominant anxiety and depressive symptoms.

Dissociative (conversion) disorders

Individuals with dissociative disorders (previously termed 'conversion hysteria' or simply 'hysteria' – these older words are still in use) present with a wide array of physical symptoms that are presumed to be psychological in origin. These disorders are not seen very often, but when they are they are seldom forgotten as the patient's presentation may be very bizarre and dramatic indeed.

The dissociative disorders are presumed to be psychological in origin because of the frequently observed association between the symptoms and the timing of traumatic events, insoluble and intolerable problems, or disturbed relationships. There is often evidence that the loss of function experienced is an expression of emotional conflicts or needs. The symptoms often appear suddenly and represent the patient's concept of how a physical illness would present rather than the actuality of how such an illness would present. The patient can often be rather indifferent to the problem presented and appear disassociated from the presentation. Medical examination and investigation do not reveal the presence of any known physical or neurological disorder.

Some dissociative disorders remit after a few weeks or months, particularly if the onset is associated with a traumatic life event. More chronic disorders, particularly paralyses and anaesthesias, may develop if the onset is associated with insoluble problems or interpersonal difficulties.

Only disorders of physical functions normally under voluntary control and loss of sensations are included in the dissociative disorders category. Disorders involving pain and other complex physical sensations mediated by the autonomic nervous system are classified under somatization disorder. Some of the many varieties of dissociative disorder are outlined briefly in Box 7.5.

Prevalence

The exact prevalence of the dissociative disorders is not known. We do know that people with PTSD, substance misuse, eating disorders and who have been abused in childhood (either sexually, physically or emotionally) have a high frequency of dissociative experiences or symptoms and many will meet ICD-10 criteria for dissociative disorders.

Risk factors

The aetiology of the dissociative disorders is not clear but it presumably is due to a psychological mechanism. There is no evidence of any genetic contribution. There is clear evidence that psychological trauma precipitates dissociative states.

Management

Initially it is important to establish that there is in fact no underlying physical disorder that explains the patient's presentation. Sometimes this can be difficult although usually it is not. Patients will often arrive at the psychiatric clinic after months of thorough assessment at medical or surgical clinics, or indeed after months or years of pointless medical or surgical treatment, and by then any unusual physical illness will have been excluded. Long-term follow-up studies have demonstrated that even bizarre presentations may sometimes turn out to have an actual underlying pathology, however, and the possibility of the later appearance of serious physical or psychiatric disorders should always be kept in mind.

It is sometimes possible to ascertain the actual underlying psychological cause. If such a cause is identified, therapeutic efforts can be focused on this but even if no such direct cause can be pin-pointed,

---

Box 7.5: The main dissociative disorders and their presentation

F44.0 Dissociative amnesia

Loss of memory usually of important recent events, not due to organic condition. This is usually partial or selective and centred on traumatic events

F44.1 Dissociative fugue

This has all the features of dissociative amnesia plus purposeful travel beyond the usual everyday range. For example, a patient may turn up at a hospital many miles from where they came from, apparently unaware of their origin. The patient's behaviour during this time may appear completely normal to independent observers

F44.2 Dissociative stupor

Profound diminution or absence of voluntary movement and normal responsiveness to external stimuli such as light, noise and touch when examination and investigation reveal no evidence of a physical cause

F44.3 Trance and possession disorders

These are disorders in which there is a temporary loss of one's sense of personal identity and full awareness of one's surroundings. The diagnosis should only be made when such trance states are involuntary and should not be applied to trances which are religious or culturally appropriate

F44.4 Dissociative motor disorders

In the commonest varieties there is loss of ability to move the whole or a part of a limb or limbs. There may be close resemblance to almost any variety of ataxia, apraxia, akinesia, aphonia, dysarthria, dyskinesia, seizures or paralysis

F44.5 Dissociative convulsions

May mimic epileptic seizures very closely in terms of movements, but tongue-biting, bruising due to falling and incontinence of urine are rare, and consciousness is maintained or replaced by a state of stupor or trance

F44.6 Dissociative anaesthesia and sensory loss

Loss of sensation to an area of skin. The area of skin involved often has boundaries that make no anatomical sense and it is clear that they are associated with the patient's ideas about bodily functions. Loss of vision and hearing can also occur but are rarely total

F44.8 Dissociative identity disorder

Patients may complain of experiencing multiple different personalities – otherwise known as 'multiple personality disorder'. This is a somewhat controversial diagnosis though there is some evidence for its validity. There is a very strong association with childhood trauma

psychological therapy, usually in the form of long-term psychotherapy, often helps.

Somatoform disorders

Somatization refers to 'physical symptoms suggesting physical disorder for which there are no demonstrable organic findings or known physiological mechanism and for which there is positive evidence, or a strong presumption, that the symptoms are linked to psychological factors or conflicts'. Somatoform disorders are at the extreme end of the somatization spectrum.

The main feature of the somatoform disorders is repeated presentation of physical symptoms together with persistent requests for medical investigations, in spite of repeated negative findings and reassurance by doctors that the symptoms have no physical basis. If any physical disorders are present, they do not explain the nature and extent of the symptoms or the distress and preoccupation of the patient.

A differential diagnosis of these conditions and of the conversion disorders is that of simple malingering, where an individual is feigning symptoms to avoid an adverse consequence, for example loss of a relationship or criminal proceedings.

Somatization disorder

The main features of somatization disorder are multiple, recurrent and frequently changing physical symptoms of at least 2 years' duration. Most patients have a long and complicated history of contact with both primary and specialist medical care services, during which many negative investigations or fruitless exploratory operations may have been carried out. Symptoms may be referred to any part or system of the body. The course of the disorder is chronic and fluctuating, and is often associated with disruption of social, interpersonal and family behaviour.

Hypochondriacal disorder

The essential feature is a persistent preoccupation with the possibility of having one or more serious and progressive physical disorders. Patients manifest persistent somatic complaints or a persistent preoccupation with their physical appearance. Normal or commonplace sensations and appearances are often interpreted by patients as abnormal and distressing, and attention is usually focused upon only one or two organs or systems of the body. Marked depression and anxiety are often present, and may justify additional diagnoses.

Somatoform autonomic dysfunction

Symptoms are presented by the patient as if they were due to a physical disorder of a system or organ that is largely or completely under autonomic innervation and control, that is the cardiovascular, gastrointestinal, respiratory and urogenital systems.

The symptoms are usually of two types, neither of which indicates a physical disorder of the organ or system concerned. First, there are complaints based upon objective signs of autonomic arousal, such as palpitations, sweating, flushing, tremor, and expression of fear and distress about the possibility of a physical disorder. Second, there are subjective complaints of a non-specific or changing nature such as fleeting aches and pains, sensations of burning, heaviness, tightness, and feelings of being bloated or distended, which are referred by the patient to a specific organ or system.

Persistent somatoform pain disorder

The predominant complaint is of persistent, severe and distressing pain, which cannot be explained fully by a physiological process or a physical disorder, and which occurs in association with emotional conflict or psychosocial problems that are sufficient to allow the conclusion that they are the main causative influences. The result is usually a marked increase in support and attention, either personal or medical.

Prevalence

Somatization is common amongst the general population – in one study in the USA 4.4 per cent of a community sample complained of significant unexplained somatic symptoms. The prevalence of somatoform disorders however is much lower, perhaps as low as 0.03 per cent. In general, somatoform disorders are more common in women.

Risk factors

Genetic studies in this area have not provided any clear answers. Childhood experience does however appear to play an aetiological role. A number of studies suggest that adults who somatize have mothers who somatize, or have parents who in fact are or were ill. The process of continuously seeking medical reassurance may reinforce the associated behaviour and thus perpetuate the disorder. It is important to note that patients with depression may present with somatic symptoms as their primary and perhaps only symptom. This is not uncommon in patients from South Asia.

Assessment

Full assessment is vital in these conditions to exclude any physical problem but it is not helpful to continue investigation when such investigations are no longer clinically indicated.

Management

The starting point is making the link between physical symptoms and psychological distress. Treatment is then psychological rather than pharmacological. Psychological intervention is more likely to be successful if a patient accepts that psychosocial factors are making an important contribution to their clinical problem. Early treatment is also more likely to be successful (within 2 years of the onset of symptoms).

Summary

The anxiety disorders are very common – perhaps a quarter of us will suffer from such a disorder at some time in our lives. However, many of these conditions remain undiagnosed and untreated. Increased awareness among all medical practitioners will help to alleviate unnecessary suffering as the anxiety disorders are amenable to both pharmacological and psychological treatments.

The other disorders described in this chapter can broadly be categorized as disorders that present with unexplained medical symptoms, often with anxiety as a prominent clinical feature. Patients with these disorders usually present to GPs, physicians and surgeons before they present to psychiatrists, and when they do present to psychiatrists they may be reluctant to entertain the notion that their symptoms are psychological in origin. If a patient comes to accept that this may be the case then psychological intervention may well help to resolve their symptoms.

Further reading

Lader MH, Udhe T (2006) *Fast facts: Anxiety, Panic and Phobias*. Oxford: Health Press Limited.

Beck AT, Emory G, Greenberg RT (2005) *Anxiety Disorders and Phobias: A Cognitive Perspective*. New York: Basic Books.

Rosqvist J (2005) *Exposure Treatments for Anxiety Disorders (Practical Clinical Guidelines)*. Oxford: Routledge.

CASE STUDY I

A 30-year-old woman describes episodes of severe anxiety that occur unpredictably but frequently and regularly. During attacks she experiences acute breathlessness, chest pain and palpitations. She frequently attends casualty departments as she fears that she is having a heart attack.

What is the most likely diagnosis?

Would you carry out physical investigations?

What treatment would you initiate?

The most likely diagnosis is panic disorder. If the anxiety symptoms were suffered more or less continuously then the diagnosis would be generalized anxiety disorder.

While patients such as the one described here often fear a heart attack it is usually relatively easy to exclude such a possibility on clinical grounds. Often however some limited physical investigation (carrying out an ECG for example) may be helpful when a patient first presents, both to reassure the patient and to absolutely exclude physical pathology.

Simple explanation and reassurance are the starting point – such measures can have a dramatic and immediate effect for a patient who has come to casualty fearing the worst. Whether a referral is made to mental health services depends on the severity and chronicity of symptoms. An SSRI antidepressant is the most common pharmacological treatment, either given alone or combined with a psychological treatment. It is recommended that a psychological treatment, often CBT, is tried first in the majority of cases.

CASE STUDY 2

A 45-year-old man presents to mental health services stating that he cannot see. He has been extensively assessed by neurological specialists who state that there is no evidence of any underlying physical pathology. When questioned closely he reveals that he had been in some trouble over a sum of missing money at his workplace just before the onset of his difficulties.

What is the most likely diagnosis?

What is the most appropriate approach – an SSRI antidepressant or long-term psychotherapy?

This is a case of dissociative or conversion disorder. Some clinicians would still use older terminology and would call this 'hysterical blindness'. As in this case, patients with conversion disorders often spend many months, or even years, being investigated by various specialists before it becomes clear that there is no underlying physical pathology.

An antidepressant will not help with the underlying problem though it is possible that depression may develop in such an individual as a secondary feature and may require such treatment. Long-term psychotherapy is much more likely to prove fruitful. In psychotherapy the therapist explores the underlying causes of a patient's symptoms and hopes to resolve the symptoms by helping the patient to understand more about themselves.

PHOBIAS

Richard Day

KEY CHAPTER FEATURES

- Definition of phobic anxiety
- Phobic disorders: risk, epidemiology, assessment and management
- Useful questions to elicit phobic symptoms
- How to assess of severity of phobic symptoms
- How to differentiate phobias from other causes of anxiety

Introduction

There are times when it is very appropriate and useful to be anxious – if a hungry and angry tiger burst into the room as you are reading this chapter, it would not be helpful to your long-term survival to calmly place a bookmark in this page and then survey the room to consider your options for escape (perhaps you could offer to make it some tea?). Instead, you would feel fear; your sympathetic nervous system would be activated in the 'fight or flight' response and you would quickly respond to the dangerous situation with prompt activity (probably this would involve running away fast but that may depend on your previous experience of facing such threats!). We would consider this a normal response to a threatening situation.

What, however, if you repeatedly showed the same response, and the same degree of response, to the sight of a small, harmless spider on the other side of the desk? Or to travelling over a bridge (an entirely safe and structurally secure bridge)? Or to finding yourself in a busy supermarket? Or to eating in public? This situation, where a person experiences a degree of anxiety or panic that is predictable (i.e. happens in recognizable circumstances), is far in excess of what is necessary (i.e. disproportionate) and this causes a significant emotional distress to the individual is what is meant by the term phobia.

Exercise

Have you ever used the word 'phobia' or 'phobic' to describe yourself or have you heard others use the word? What did you (or they) mean by the word?

What behaviour or feeling was being described by the use of the word 'phobia'?

Aside from a description of an illness, can you think of other medical or non-medical uses of the suffix -phobic, e.g. xenophobic?

How does your own use and general use of the word 'phobia' relate to its use as a description of a particular mental health problem?

We can all be excessively anxious about different things and it can be difficult to distinguish between this 'normal' anxiety and phobic anxiety. Does this lack of clear-cut distinction bother you? Are you more comfortable with the definition of hypertension? In what ways do the definitions of hypertension or obesity have similar limitations to that of anxiety? It may be useful to revisit Chapter 1 in which we discussed the problems that may arise when the line between what is a disorder and what is not are unclear.

Types of phobias

Phobic situations are divided into three different types depending on the nature of the feared situation: agoraphobia, social phobia and specific phobia.

- In agoraphobia, the anxiety is caused by being in a busy situation or an open area where there is no immediate possibility of escape to a 'safe' area (the 'agora' in ancient Greece was an open area where crowds would gather together and was also used as the busy marketplace).

- For social phobia, the anxiety is a 'fear of scrutiny' by others, associated with being the focus of attention and being embarrassed or humiliated. It is typically relatively small social settings that are feared, such as eating with others, speaking in a small group setting, or even simply social interaction with another person who is not well known.

- Specific phobias are many and varied but all involve a very specific situation that is the cause of fear: a particular type of animal, the sight of blood or injury, darkness, flying, etc. Most specific phobias usually fall into one of the following six groups: fear of animals (usually relatively small animals and 'creepy-crawlies'), heights, water, enclosed spaces (claustrophobia), dental treatment and blood/injury/injection.

Prevalence

In terms of lifetime prevalence in the general population, agoraphobia as a primary diagnosis is less common (1–8 per cent) than social phobia and specific phobias which are the two commonest anxiety disorders in studies (both about 2–14 per cent).

Agoraphobia tends to present in young adults (50 per cent have presented by the age of 20 and 75 per cent by the early thirties). In contrast, social and specific phobias present in childhood or soon afterwards – 75 per cent by early adolescence and 90 per cent by the age of 23.

Risk factors

It is not very well understood how some people develop phobias and others do not. There is evidence for phobias having some genetic element in that rates are increased in family members of someone affected (a relative risk of about 2–3) and monozygotic twins (genetically identical) are more likely to be either both affected or both unaffected when compared to dizygotic twins (sharing only 50 per cent of genetic material).

Several social factors are associated with phobias – those who are married have lower rates of phobia than the unmarried, divorced or widowed; being unemployed, having a low income and low educational levels are associated with higher risk of phobia. It is not clear though which may be causing the other in that having a phobia may make an individual less able to form close and sustained relationships, less able to do 'normal social' things and adversely affect their education and employability.

Agoraphobia

Agoraphobia is often related to panic disorder in that a person can begin to experience unpredictable panic attacks and, as a result of this, subsequently develops agoraphobic symptoms whereby they fear having a panic attack while out, and therefore avoid going out. However, it is possible to develop agoraphobia without previously having panic attacks. It is not clear why some people with panic disorder develop agoraphobia and others do not – but those who do develop agoraphobia tend to have higher levels of premorbid anxiety as children, depression and have more dependent or avoidant personality traits. They also tend to have lower perceptions of self-efficacy and self-dependence. It is about three times as common in women as in men.

Social phobia

Social phobia has previously been an overlooked and underestimated diagnosis. In many people it goes unnoticed and untreated and they are merely thought of as being 'shy'. Although people who are very shy are more likely to have a social phobia than people who are not shy, very shy people may also not have a social phobia but instead have other psychiatric diagnoses. Also, people may develop a social phobia without the presence of shyness in their premorbid personality. People who are shy are unlikely to have the presence of symptoms of anxiety or panic about social contexts in general (although may be nervous about specific issues such as meeting new people or having to speak out) and less likely to have anticipatory anxiety. In shyness the degree of anxiety can vary as with any other personality traits. People with social phobias are also more likely to perceive other people as potentially negative and critical.

Previous prevalence rates of 2–3 per cent have now

been increased to 12–13 per cent as a result of more careful evaluation. It tends to present at a very early age (i.e. at school) with a slight female preponderance. It is a risk factor in children for poor school performance and school refusal and in adults for poor work performance, unemployment and low socioeconomic status. There is some evidence that there are higher rates in children who have experienced either parental rejection or overprotection but no clear relationship to overall childhood adversity.

More specifically, social phobia has been linked to a heritable personality trait known as behavioural inhibition. This is a tendency to react to novel situations by avoidance and withdrawal to safety (i.e. the caregiver) with the expression of distress (crying or fretting). It is evident early in childhood (toddlers and pre-school) and has been associated with the later development of anxiety disorders in general and social phobia in particular.

Functional neuroimaging indicates increased bilateral activation of the amygdala and increased regional cerebral blood flow to the amygdala and related limbic areas that normalizes on successful treatment (whether SSRI or cognitive behavioural therapy (CBT)).

Specific phobia

For specific phobias, explanations of aetiology now generally use learning theory or evolutionary explanations rather than assuming unconscious and traumatic psychodynamic factors related to early childhood.

It has been hypothesized that a person may develop a specific phobia after exposure to a particular stimulus or situation has been associated (by classical conditioning) with trauma and anxiety. This situation is then feared and avoided. If the person subsequently is exposed to the same feared situation they begin to feel anxious again and escape from the situation. This leads to a reduction in their level of anxiety, which thus serves to reinforce the fear of that specific situation. Similarly, if they are faced with the prospect of the feared situation they begin to feel anxious and if they manage to then avoid the situation they again experience a reduction in anxiety which reinforces their avoidance.

This may explain some specific phobias, but many people with a phobia cannot remember any earlier traumatic experiences and it does not explain why we tend to develop specific phobias to only a relatively small range of situations.

Evolutionary theories are based on the observation that most of the common specific phobias are focused on situations that could in the past hundreds of thousands of years have posed a significant threat and that therefore the phobia is some kind of evolutionary adaptation to increase survival. However, this theory is difficult to prove and does not explain why we have evolved a tendency to be phobic of small 'creepy-crawlies' such as spiders but not of larger predators that could be just as dangerous and threatening to personal survival (nor were there many dentists around 100 000 years ago).

There may well be multiple explanations for how people develop specific phobias and there is also some evidence that some people might be more prone to develop phobias by, for example, being more aware of bodily sensations and therefore more likely to link the somatic manifestations of anxiety with particular circumstances. Children's fears differ in nature across different ethnic groups. Culturally mediated beliefs, values and traditions may play a role in their expression and what is identified as a phobia or not.

Presentation

It is helpful to consider the effects of phobic anxiety in the three areas of cognitive (psychological) symptoms, behavioural responses and somatic (physical) symptoms. Phobias are associated with autonomic (sympathetic) nervous system activation with a large number of consequent physical symptoms (see Table 8.1).

Cognitive symptoms

The cognitive symptoms, as well as the experience of anxiety itself, often involve fear of losing control, fainting or even dying. The person may experience derealization or depersonalization. In derealization a person experiences their external environment as in some way unreal, for example people and objects may appear to be like 'cardboard cut outs' or like actors being watched on a TV screen. It is as though they have stepped out of their environment. In depersonalization it is the individual themselves who feels that they are in some way distanced or remote from everyone else around them, as if they were 'not

Table 8.1   Presentation of the somatic, behavioural and cognitive features of phobias

Somatic/physical	Behavioural
Dry mouth	Escape from the feared situation
Feeling of choking	Avoidance of the feared situation
Difficulty in breathing	
Chest pain/chest discomfort	**Cognitive**
Palpitations/pounding heart/accelerated heart rate	Feeling that objects are unreal (derealization) or that self is distant or 'not really here' (depersonalization)
Nausea/abdominal distress, e.g. churning	Fear of losing control, 'going crazy' or passing out
Sweating	Fear of dying
Trembling/shaking	
Hot flushes/cold chills	
Numbness/tingling sensations	
Feeling dizzy, unsteady, faint or lightheaded	

really there' or a passive observer of what is happening rather than actively involved in proceedings – they can still feel this even while, in reality, they are actively involved in what is happening. In this experience, it is as though they have stepped outside of themselves. It is important not to confuse these presentations with features of psychosis.

Behavioural symptoms

The major behavioural symptoms are either to hurriedly exit the feared situation (e.g. to rush out of a busy supermarket leaving the shopping trolley in an aisle with the shopping in it) or marked avoidance of the situation itself (so avoidance of the supermarket altogether). Thus a person with agoraphobia may get a relative or friend to do their shopping in busy places or else go themselves at very quiet times, often only if accompanied by a trusted other person; a person with a specific phobia of bridges may take a very convoluted route in order to avoid going over a bridge). The impact of the coping strategies, for example avoidance behaviour, may be what leads the patient and/or family to seek help.

In severe forms, agoraphobia can result in a person becoming virtually housebound, or a person with social phobia may avoid all contact with people beyond their immediate social circle. Avoidance of the feared situation can also lead to avoidance of

other things that might lead to exposure to the feared situation; thus, someone with a phobia of spiders may go to such great lengths to avoid spiders that they find themselves unable to search in the corner of a dark cupboard because there *might* be a spider there. The avoidance could also mean that they are unable to watch a video of a spider, look at a picture of a spider or even talk about spiders.

Typically, the fear and associated symptoms can also be felt even at the *thought* of being exposed to the phobic situation. This is called anticipatory anxiety. Thus a person with social phobia may become very anxious at the prospect of having to give a small group presentation in several weeks' time. Someone with agoraphobia becomes anxious even if they talk about perhaps going out sometime in the future.

A characteristic of phobic anxiety is that the person affected recognizes that their fear and the associated avoidance are excessive and unreasonable but is nevertheless unable to overcome them. Someone with a bridge phobia will be able to acknowledge that a bridge is safe and that there is minimal risk in walking over it; they will be able to agree that other people are perfectly correct to walk over it without giving it a thought; but still, if they approach the bridge themselves, they become so overwhelmed with anxiety that they are unable to cross over it.

Phobic anxiety is also characterized as being manifest only or mainly in the feared situation or when thinking about the feared situation. That is, there is not the more pervasive anxiety about lots of different things as in generalized anxiety disorder nor do the bouts of fear occur unpredictably, such as in panic disorder.

The emotional distress felt by the person can be directly as a result of the symptoms themselves, or a consequence of the avoidance of the feared situation. In fact, the consequences of phobic avoidance are often the biggest disruption to a person's life. They may place significant limitations on what someone is able to do because of what has to be avoided. If a person has a severe agoraphobia it will be almost impossible for them to work unless they have a job where they can virtually work from home. Think of yourself as a medical student – would it be easy for you to complete your studies if you had a social phobia such that you found it almost impossible to give group presentations, to perform an aspect of history taking or physical examination in front of a group of your peers?

Somatic symptoms

These are as for anxiety and shown in Table 8.1.

Agoraphobia

Agoraphobia is relatively rare on its own but much more commonly develops in association with panic disorder. Typically, agoraphobia develops as a result of repeated unpredictable panic attacks such that the affected person begins to avoid going outside for fear that they might have a panic attack in public. There is often focus on the physical symptoms experienced and their feared effects. The focus of anxiety is a fear that they will occur while the person is out in an area from which there is not easy escape rather than the fear being focused on a particular location or setting. There is typically fear or avoidance of crowds and public places, travelling alone or travelling away from home.

Comorbid rates of depression are very high, as are substance misuse (including alcohol and benzodiazepine dependence) and other anxiety disorders.

Social phobia

In social phobia, the fear is of being the focus of attention from other people and fear of behaving in such a way as to be socially embarrassed or humiliated. This is associated with avoidance of situations in which the person might be the focus of attention. Social phobia can be limited to specific forms of social scrutiny such as eating in public, speaking in public, meeting known people or entering small groups such as parties, meetings or classrooms. It can also be a more generalized fear of all or most of these different social situations.

Someone with social phobia will exhibit some of the somatic and cognitive symptoms of anxiety described earlier, including, at least one of, specifically:

- blushing or shaking
- fear of vomiting
- urgency or fear of micturition or defaecation.

Comorbidity with other psychiatric diagnoses is common with other phobic disorders and panic disorder being commonest but depression and alcohol misuse (about 20 per cent risk) also being recognized.

Specific phobias

A major consideration with specific phobias is that although a very large number of people (up to 60 per cent) may have a degree of phobia about a specific situation in that they exhibit an exaggerated fear that they recognize as such, the vast majority of these do not cause significant distress or disruption to ordinary life and so can be considered to be subclinical. It is the minority of phobias that do interfere with everyday life to such an extent that require treatment. This may be either because of the severity of the distress and avoidance or because of the frequency with which the feared situation would ordinarily be encountered. For example, a severe blood/needle phobia may be much more problematic (and therefore require treatment) for a medical student than a student studying accountancy.

In particular, exaggerated anxiety in certain situations is very common in children, but in the majority of cases this phobic anxiety spontaneously reduces with age and does not cause a problem in adulthood. It would be unusual though for a specific phobia to emerge in adulthood if it had not been present as a child or adolescent.

As with the other phobias, there is commonly comorbidity with other anxiety disorders in specific phobias but less commonly with depression or substance misuse.

Assessment

The key aspects of assessment in phobias are to establish whether phobic anxiety is present; if so, then to identify the nature of the feared situations; to look for any other associated psychiatric symptoms; and to consider the variety of treatment options (including beginning to identify the underlying beliefs and assumptions that may be targeted in any cognitive therapy).

To establish the phobic nature of the anxiety it is necessary to confirm that the anxiety is episodic and occurs relatively predictably upon exposure (or the thought of exposure) to a small number of situations. Or alternatively, that those situations are so well and habitually avoided that very little anxiety is actually experienced.

Enquiry about what situations are feared and avoided and what it is about those situations that is feared should help to distinguish between agoraphobia, social phobia and specific phobias. For example, three people might say that they are fearful of meeting their friend in the local shopping centre but for different reasons. When asked what it is they fear about going to the shopping centre, one will say that it is because it is very busy there and they fear that they will have a panic attack or faint (agoraphobia); another says that it is because they will have to go with their friend to one of the cafes for a coffee and they get very anxious eating or drinking when there are other people around (social phobia); the third says that it is because the only way to get into the shopping centre is to use one of the lifts and they always get very panicky in lifts (specific phobia).

Phobic anxiety may also present secondary to a number of other psychiatric diagnoses. Enquiry about the time course of the phobic anxiety in relation to other symptoms will help to clarify whether the phobia is a primary problem or merely a manifestation of the other diagnosis.

Assessment of comorbidity

A depressive illness can result in the development of phobic anxiety. This may happen without any history of previous phobic anxiety or it can occur when a relatively minor degree of phobic anxiety is exacerbated to the extent that it causes a significant amount of impairment. In this case there will be evidence of depressive symptoms that pre-date the phobic anxiety. There may be a history of previous episodes of phobic anxiety (associated with previous depressive episodes) but there should not be a lifelong history of clinically significant phobic anxiety. Alternatively, depression can occur in someone who has phobic anxiety and in this circumstance the long-term and early-onset nature of phobic symptoms should be evident together with more recent development of depressive symptoms.

It is also commonly comorbid with obsessive compulsive disorder and substance misuse problems. As with depression, it can be difficult to distinguish which has come first.

It is also important to avoid confusion with other disorders in which patients may demonstrate avoidant behaviour because of psychotic symptoms or longstanding personality traits, for example in patients with schizophrenia and paranoid delusions or in those with schizoid personalities.

Other key features to assess

One consideration in the assessment of phobias is the degree of distress and loss of function caused by the symptoms. Thus someone in Britain who has a specific phobia of spiders may experience much more distress and interference with everyday life than someone with a similarly severe (in terms of symptoms) specific phobia of scorpions.

Another consideration is how motivated a person is to engage with and persevere with the various treatment options. The degree of anxiety may be so great that a person is unable or reluctant to engage with treatment because they expect that the very nature of that treatment (which will involve thinking about and ultimately encountering the feared situation) will be unbearable and too stressful.

Careful questioning will help to identify some of the false assumptions that are operating in that person's thoughts. Asking questions such as 'What is it you most fear happening if you …?', 'What would that mean?' may help the person to verbalize their automatic thoughts that will need to be challenged in subsequent cognitive therapy. So, someone with a social phobia may describe that they fear embarrassing themselves socially, that they have an image of how they ought to perform but are convinced that they will fail to reach that degree of performance and that others are judging them in similarly negative ways.

General principles for the management of phobias

There are some general principles of treatment for phobias. For the reasons already stated, a person may be reluctant to engage with treatment if they are too fearful of confronting their feared situation. Careful assessment with empathy can be necessary to elicit these concerns, to discuss treatment options and highlight the options that may be least unacceptable, given a patient's concerns. If the overall assessment has identified other associated problems (such as depression), then this should be specifically treated as well and it may well be beneficial to treat depression before embarking on trying to treat the person's phobia.

Treatment for phobias can be psychological, pharmacological or a combination of both. The selection of treatment will depend on a combination of factors such as patient choice (an individual may have a strong preference for a particular treatment); availability of treatment (e.g. a 9-month waiting list for CBT); safety (there may be absolute or relative contraindications to particular drug treatments); psychological mindedness (some people struggle to make sense of what they are expected to do in psychological treatments and so are less able to make good use of them).

Psychological treatments

Useful psychological treatments are CBT and behavioural therapy. A number of behavioural techniques can be used and these generally involve the patient being exposed to the feared situations together with help to control their anxiety and relax.

The exposure can be in real life (actually going to a shop, eating under the scrutiny of others, crossing a bridge) or can use imagery (simply thinking about or visualizing the feared situation while sitting in the therapist's office). It can involve exposure to the most feared situation in the first instance or can use a hierarchy of increasingly feared things to build up gradually to the most feared situation. Table 8.2 shows the different psychological approaches to treating phobias.

Thus someone with agoraphobia may be exposed to a busy supermarket on a Saturday afternoon directly (an example of flooding) or may gradually gain confidence in less anxiety-provoking situations first: standing at the front door; going to the gate of their property; walking a short distance along the street; walking round the block; visiting the corner shop; going into town early on a quiet weekday morning, etc. (gradual exposure). Similarly, someone with a specific phobia of spiders may start with a small, simple drawing of a spider; then progress to a photograph; then to a video recording; then to a dead spider; then a very small live spider; then a larger one.

At each stage, the person continues in the situation until their anxieties have reduced. This can happen either as a natural process of extinction (i.e. fear tends to subside over time as no harm comes to the person by being in the feared situation) or by the use of relaxation techniques and anxiety management such as progressive muscular relaxation and breathing retraining. Cognitively based exposure techniques (cognitive remodelling) additionally involve getting the patient to enter the feared situation and test their feared predictions. Exposure can be done by the patient on their own, as 'homework', or accompanied by the therapist.

Pharmacological treatments

Pharmacological treatments include the three main groups of antidepressants – SSRIs (including the

Table 8.2   Cognitive and behavioural therapy approaches to treating phobias

Technique	Form of exposure	Rate of exposure	Relaxation management
Flooding	Real or imagined	Sudden	No
Graded exposure	Real	Gradual	Yes
Systematic desensitization	Imagery	Gradual	Yes
Cognitively delivered exposure	Real or imagery	Sudden or gradual	Yes

SNRI venlafaxine), tricyclics and MAOIs. There can be problems with initial exacerbation of anxiety with the start of drug treatment and also, given that drug treatment will need to be long term, adverse effects such as weight gain and sexual dysfunction can limit tolerability. Subsequent reduction or discontinuation of drugs may result in a relapse of the anxiety and so any reduction should be done gradually with careful monitoring of the re-emergence of symptoms.

If antidepressants are used, simple gradual self-exposure can be encouraged for whatever behaviours do not spontaneously improve. If psychological and pharmacological treatments are combined, then one way of doing this is to commence medications first of all to reduce intensity of the phobia and then use psychological treatments to further improve symptoms.

Agoraphobia

Pharmacological and psychological therapies are both reasonable options in agoraphobia and they can be used effectively together. SSRIs tend to be the medication of choice. Medication will be particularly appropriate if there is comorbid depression.

Psychological treatments may well use elements of graded exposure and systematic desensitization but would typically include a significant cognitive element that seeks to identify, challenge and remodel unhelpful, automatic thoughts.

Social phobia

As with agoraphobia, there is the option of using SSRI (or SNRI) antidepressants but pharmacological treatment usually needs to be long term (with relapse common if medicines are stopped). It can take 2–6 weeks for benefits to become apparent, with further improvement over 12–24 weeks. Again, antidepressants can be very helpful to treat any comorbid depression, or to improve symptoms to a level where psychological treatments are easier.

Psychological therapies are usually cognitively based rather than simply being behavioural and incorporate elements of progressive muscular relaxation, imagined and real-life exposure, cognitive restructuring and also social skills training. People with social phobia often display cognitive biases. They tend to interpret ambiguous information on their performance negatively, to focus their attention on finding and attending to negative information,

to be unable to recall positive information about their performance and react catastrophically to mild negative feedback.

People who have relatively mild social phobia can sometimes gain benefit from β-blockers (which reduce the somatic manifestations of anxiety without really affecting the cognitive feelings), which can be taken before feared situations on an 'as required' basis. Similarly, a benzodiazepine can be used as an anxiolytic on an occasional basis with minimal potential for tolerance and the development of dependence.

Specific phobia

The treatment of specific phobia is almost exclusively psychological with behavioural methods being well established as effective treatments. Depending on the severity of the phobia, behavioural methods can even be effective in a single session. It is also possible to use cognitive techniques to get patients to test out their erroneous and fearful beliefs in the avoided situation.

Summary

Phobias are relatively common but they usually only present for treatment when they interfere with a person's life. Phobias can have varying impacts on the lives of individuals and often individuals and their families have learnt to work around the phobia. Phobias may present with physical and/or psychological symptoms. Phobias, especially specific phobias, are amenable to treatment but require patients to be motivated sufficiently well to follow through treatment programmes.

Further reading

Baldwin DS, Anderson IM, Nutt DJ (2005) Evidence-based guidelines for the pharmacological treatment of anxiety disorders: recommendations from the British Association for Psychopharmacology. *Journal of Psychopharmacology* 19: 567–596.

Choy Y, Fyer AJ, Lipsitz JD (2007) Treatment of specific phobia in adults. *Clinical Psychology Review* 27: 266–286.

Perugi G, Frare F, Toni C (2007) Diagnosis and treatment of agoraphobia with panic disorder. *CNS Drugs.* 21: 741–764.

Stein MB, Stein DJ (2008) Social anxiety disorder. *Lancet* 371: 1115–1125.

CASE STUDY

Susan is a 24-year-old legal secretary. She presents with a 3-month history of variable low mood and tiredness. She is doing less in her evenings and weekends because she is too tired and 'can't be bothered'. Despite her tiredness her sleep has also deteriorated and she now has very unsettled nights.

She is very stressed at work because she is increasingly being expected to attend dinners and luncheons. She says that she just can't bear eating in front of other people and has so far always made excuses for not attending and once or twice has even stayed off 'sick' during the day in order to avoid going to the dinner at night. She is worried that her boss is dissatisfied with her performance because of this.

In the course of enquiry about other anxieties, she also mentions that she cannot bear the sight of spiders and if she sees one she has to catch it with a glass and throw it outside as soon as possible.

What would you include in the list of differential diagnoses for Susan?

Depressive episode: she describes a number of symptoms of depression with onset over the past 3 months.

Social phobia: the fear of and avoidance of eating in public together with the recognition that this is impacting her effectiveness at work raise the possibility of a social phobia diagnosis.

Specific phobia: the dread of spiders may indicate a specific spider phobia.

Generalized anxiety disorder needs to be considered.

Hypothyroidism: the tiredness and apathy warrants this in the list although is unlikely.

What questions would you ask to try to determine if she has a social phobia about eating in company?

Is the anxiety only specific to such situations?

Does she feel generally anxious at other times or get fearful at unexpected times?

When she eats on her own does she feel all right?

Can she attend meetings where she does not have to eat?

Does she avoid eating in public situations?

Ask what specific situations she is fearful of and what she fears will happen in these situations.

Does she recognize her fears as irrational?

continued ➤

CASE STUDY *continued*

Are her fears associated with any physical symptoms (e.g. blushing or shaking, fear of vomiting, urgency or fear of micturition or defaecation).

How long has she had these fears – have they developed in recent months or been present for years (e.g. since adolescence)?

She subsequently gives a 10-year history of social phobia for eating but has never had problems with depression before now. She says that she 'can't go on feeling like this' especially as she has an annual appraisal in 6 weeks' time. She had never realized that there was anything that could be done to help with her fears regarding eating but is keen to 'try anything' otherwise she thinks she may lose her job.

What information would you need to elicit in her history to work out how her apparent recent depressive illness relates to her probable social phobia?

What are the timelines of both sets of symptoms? Have her fears of eating in public been present for a long time and merely worsened since the development of depressive symptoms? Did they worsen first, lead to worsened social and occupational function or stress, prior to the development of depressive symptoms?

How would you decide if she also has a specific phobia of spiders?

There is clearly a fear of spiders but does it lead to avoidance or anticipatory fear? It sounds as though she is able to effectively deal with any spiders that she sees – is there significant distress or inability to function associated with her fears?

What will you tell her about treatment options?

Explain that there are both psychological treatments and medicines available to help; that psychological treatments require effort on her part, in between appointments, to put into practice what is discussed; that medications may be useful to help initially with her depressive symptoms but that there may be side-effects with them. She should know that it is important for her to be involved in the decisions made about what treatments to proceed with.

If you suggest that you can prescribe drugs, what will you tell her about possible side-effects and the time course?

She needs to know that the effect of any drugs used will have to be assessed over a matter of months rather than having a dramatic and sudden effect on her symptoms and that it is important to persevere with treatment over this time period. If you suggest an SSRI then she needs to know about the common side-effects, such as nausea and headaches, that she may experience

continued ➤

CASE STUDY *continued*

when starting the drug but which will often improve over the first 7–10 days. She should also know about other side-effects such as vivid nightmares and sexual dysfunction.

How would you explain the possible psychological treatments and what they involve?

Explain that her fears are related to how she views the threatening situations and that treatment aims to help her alter the way she thinks and the unhelpful, unrealistic expectations she has. It helps her see the situation in alternative ways that do not lead to the same fear. Treatment will involve her looking at the automatic assumptions that she makes and help her intentionally relax in threatening situations. She will then be encouraged to, probably gradually, enter progressively more threatening situations, using the new skills she has learnt.

SCHIZOPHRENIA

Brian Lunn

KEY CHAPTER FEATURES

- Introduction to schizophrenia
- Epidemiology and presentation
- Aetiology of schizophrenia
- Management and assessment of acute episodes and chronic disorder

Introduction

If a member of the general public was asked to describe their archetypal 'madman' the chances are that their reference point would be an individual with schizophrenia. Asking this archetypal layman for terms they associate with schizophrenia the odds are that 'split personality' and 'violence' are liable to be mentioned. Both terms are highly stigmatizing and in the case of the former, simply wrong, and in the case of the latter, inaccurate. In this chapter the aim is to introduce the reader to a more scientific understanding of the disorder starting with a historical perspective.

Schizophrenia is a major health problem both in the United Kingdom and worldwide. It is a relatively common condition in which the first acute symptoms usually occur in early adult life but it is often misrepresented and poorly understood by the general public. The acute illness is typically followed by a gradual deteriorating course. The symptoms and signs of the illness cause severe distress to patients and their relatives. Extensive resources are required for the management of the acute illness and long term support in the community. Across a patient's lifetime the costs add up to make it the most expensive individual illness treated in the NHS.

Why is this relevant to you?

Although only around 4 per cent of UK medical students will go on to become psychiatrists it is inevitable that doctors in every field of medicine will come across patients with schizophrenia. This complex disorder unfortunately is also associated with poorer physical health including higher rates of heart disease, cancer, diabetes, etc. An understanding of schizophrenia and psychosis in general is therefore essential for these patients to receive the care they need.

It is perhaps worthwhile first considering what 'psychosis' means.

Psychosis

Psychotic symptoms can occur in the context of a wide variety of different clinical situations. The presence of psychotic symptoms will frequently suggest that a patient may suffer from schizophrenia and this illness will be the main focus of this chapter. However, there are other so-called 'functional' psychoses, such as schizoaffective disorder and delusional disorder, that share some features with schizophrenia. (As discussed in Chapter 2, the term 'functional psychosis' was coined in the days when nothing was known about the evidence for biological factors in the cause of psychotic illness and was thus used to distinguish presentation of symptoms that clearly indicated disturbance of brain function but which were in the absence of what could, at that time, readily be perceived as organic brain disease, such as tertiary syphilis, a brain tumour or post-encephalitic state.) Psychotic symptoms may also present in the context of severe mood disorders, abuse of alcohol and a variety of other drugs, organic brain disease (e.g. Alzheimer's disease), poorly controlled complex partial seizures, in delirium, in conditions such as porphyria and occasionally as an adverse effect of usual doses of prescription drugs.

When we say a person is 'psychotic' we imply that they have to some degree lost touch with reality. Usually the person will have no insight or only limited insight into this. The most common and obvious features will be the presence of delusional ideas and/ or hallucinations, which are usually driving some significant disturbance of behaviour. It is often the behavioural disturbance that results in the person being presented to mental health services. These individuals are also usually said to be 'paranoid', and paranoid thinking is one of the most ubiquitous manifestations of psychosis. However, it is important to understand what we mean by the term 'paranoid'. Someone who is paranoid tends to see everything as relating to themselves in some way. This may be in the sense that they feel others are to harm them or that they feel others are taking about them. However, it does not just imply people or events relating to them in a potentially detrimental way, although this is often the way the term is used in more loose conversation. It may be that they see themselves as responsible for, or linked to, real events that they are not in reality connected to, leading perhaps to a grandiose view of themselves. Or they may believe another person is in love with them, for example, leading to delusional ideas about a romance.

Recognising psychosis is not a diagnosis in itself but the first step towards making a diagnosis. The ready availability of laboratory tests and brain imaging techniques usually makes it relatively easy to exclude obvious organic brain disease in the majority of cases where such may be suspected. However, it can often be extremely difficult in the early stages to distinguish between the other potential causes. For example, schizophrenia and schizoaffective disorder merge across a continuum of symptoms; some drug-induced psychoses can be slow to resolve and the related social dysfunction may create a presentation akin to schizophrenia. The final diagnosis often depends on the acute symptoms and also the response to treatment and/or evolution of the illness over a period of weeks or months.

What does schizophrenia mean?

A brief history of schizophrenia is presented to convey how our understanding of this has changed over time. The diagnosis of schizophrenia, as for the majority of psychiatric disorders, is not on the basis of pathology or one individual symptom but on the occurrence of clusters of symptoms, which allow consistency in the diagnosis of the disorder. Schizophrenia was first recognized as a discrete syndrome in the middle of the nineteenth century, although the term schizophrenia was not used until 1911, by Bleuler. There are, however, descriptions of what sound like similar psychotic disorders in Vedic and ancient Egyptian texts from several thousand years earlier as well as descriptions in Arabic medical writings from the Middle Ages.

The first modern phenomenological description of what we now term schizophrenia was proposed by Morel in 1853. He referred to *Demence Precoce* characterized by bizarre behaviour and mental function, withdrawal and self-neglect starting in adolescence. Fifteen years later Kahlbaum identified a cluster of symptoms, including stereotyped movements, outbursts of excitement and stupor that he called *Katatonie*. The description of *Hebephrenia* in 1871 by Hecker was very similar to Morel's *Demence Precoce*. The most important step forward in identifying a phenomenologically clear disorder was made by Kraepelin in 1893, when under the term *Dementia praecox* he grouped together all of the previously described disorders with the addition of what he called *dementia paranoides*. Kraepelin considered hallucinations, delusions, thought disorder, negativism and emotional blunting to be characteristic of *dementia praecox*. He also observed that the onset was usually in early adult life and often progressed to a 'demented' end stage. Kraepelin did however realize that the breakdown was not intellectual, the onset was not necessarily in adolescence and the prognosis was not always poor. He did not use the term dementia in the way that we currently do but rather to convey a deteriorating picture of global functioning that included psychotic symptoms.

When using the term 'the schizophrenias', Bleuler described four groups of symptoms that he thought were characteristic. These four 'As' were:

- **a**mbivalence
- **a**utism (Bleuler didn't use this term in the modern sense and meant an extreme withdrawal of oneself from the fabric of social life into a vivid internal fantasy life)
- flattened **a**ffect
- loosening of **a**ssociations.

From the description of *dementia praecox* by Kraepelin up until the 1950s the focus of interest in schizophrenia was on cognition. Schneider, in 1939, described his 'first rank symptoms' (Box 9.1), which he proposed were diagnostic of schizophrenia in the absence of overt brain disease. The discovery of chlorpromazine at the end of 1950 and its clinical use in the following years led to a shift from the focus on cognition to a therapeutically driven emphasis on tranquillization. As a result there needed to be clear diagnostic criteria to support therapeutic trials, with an inevitable focus on psychotic symptoms. Diagnosis began to be framed around Schneider's first rank symptoms.

Although the majority of patients with Schneider's symptoms will probably have schizophrenia, the symptoms are not specific for schizophrenia (8 per cent of psychotic patients with these symptoms do not have schizophrenia) and most typical of the acute phase of the illness. A minority of patients with first rank symptoms may be suffering from delusions or hallucinations in the context of a severe mood disorder or an organic disorder. Twenty per cent of patients with chronic schizophrenia never have a first rank symptom.

Psychiatrists tend to use one of two classification systems both in clinical work and in research: ICD and DSM (as outlined in Chapter 1). These classification systems allow the diagnosis of schizophrenia to be made in both acute and chronic phases of the illness and reduce the likelihood of the misdiagnosis of schizophrenia in those with other primary disorders such as mood disorders and organic syndromes such as toxic confusional states, drug-induced psychoses and epilepsy.

Box 9.1: Schneider's first rank symptoms

1. Auditory hallucinations of a specific type

Audible thoughts: a voice anticipating or repeating the patient's thoughts aloud

Two or more voices discussing the patient in the third person

Voices commenting on the patient's behaviour

2. Thought alienation

Thought insertion

Thought withdrawal

Thought broadcasting

3. Passivity phenomena

Experiences of bodily influence

Made acts/impulses/affects: experiences which are imposed on the individual or influenced by others

4. Delusional perceptions (a two-stage process)

First a normal object is perceived then second there is a sudden intense delusional insight into the object's meaning for the patient, e.g. 'The traffic light is green therefore I am the King'

Epidemiology

The usually cited figure of lifetime incidence of schizophrenia is 1 per cent. A 2002 systematic review stated that the figure might well be lower, suggesting a figure of 0.55 per cent. In the United Kingdom prevalence is roughly 200 per 100 000. The older literature suggested that there is no significant difference in the incidence of the disorder between males and females but onset is typically earlier in males. More recent first-episode studies have suggested that there may actually be a higher incidence in males. Peak onset for males is between the ages of 20 and 28 years, whereas for females the peak range is between 26 and 32 years. Schizophrenia can occur in childhood and in middle to old age but incidence in these age groups is much lower. In adolescents presentation of schizophrenia may be slightly different from the standard pattern seen in later life in that there may be vague, non-specific symptoms that are only recognized as the onset of the disorder in retrospect. Another interesting observation is that there is no difference in social class of parents. The clustering of patients in lower socioeconomic classes would therefore seem to be a result of the illness, suggesting downwards social drift.

A World Health Organization study originally seemed to suggest that there was little difference in prevalence between different countries. However, closer examination of this coupled with data from more recent studies suggest that there may be significant differences between countries. There are two important difficulties in trying to elucidate this issue: (a) it is often difficult to ascertain all cases as a proportion of people with psychosis (perhaps 20 per cent) will not present to doctors; (b) it can take some years of follow-up to determine a final diagnosis with reasonable certainty. There is clustering of cases in urban areas. One explanatory theory for this is 'urban drift' in that resources for managing patients with schizophrenia tend to be found more commonly in areas with higher population densities, but some studies have suggested that the urban environment itself may have a role to play in the aetiology of the disorder. So-called 'urban drift' was first demonstrated 60 years ago by Faris and Dunham, who showed that although the geographical distribution of residence of the parents of patients (between upper-class suburbs, intermediate areas and inner-city areas) was the same as the overall population the patients were much more likely to be found living in the inner-city areas. Patients also drift downwards in terms of socioeconomic status: the university student who drops out and becomes a part-time shop worker, the factory worker who loses motivation and becomes unemployed. However, there is also some evidence to support the proposition that some of the preponderance in lower socioeconomic groups is because of a slightly higher incidence of the illness in urban areas and among such groups.

Presentation

Symptoms of schizophrenia are typically divided into 'positive' and 'negative' subtypes. The former are typified by psychotic symptoms such as identified by Schneider (Box 9.1), i.e. delusions, hallucinations, thought disorder, etc. By contrast, negative symptoms can be characterized as losses of normal functioning, e.g. blunting of affect, social withdrawal, poverty of thought, etc. It is important to realize that not all such symptoms may be related to schizophrenia but may represent other disorders such as depression or be related to recreational substance use. A useful way to think about signs and symptoms might be to use the headings of a mental state examination as in Box 9.2.

Prior to the onset of acute symptoms (and not due to mood disturbance or substance abuse) and following an acute episode many patients exhibit less dramatic symptoms:

- marked social isolation and withdrawal
- impairment in social role, e.g. as a wage earner or student
- peculiar eccentric behaviour
- poor personal hygiene
- blunted or inappropriate affect
- vague speech
- odd beliefs
- unusual perceptual experiences
- lack of initiative or energy.

Subtypes of schizophrenia

A number of subtypes of schizophrenia have been described, based on particular patterns of clinical symptoms. However, these subtypes are not entirely distinct from each other and do not have clearly different aetiology from each other. Thus, they have a limited value in everyday clinical practice:

- simple schizophrenia: negative symptoms predominate
- hebephrenic schizophrenia: mood is inappropriate with giggling and shallowness, behaviour is irresponsible. Delusions and hallucinations are fragmented. Thoughts are disorganized. Onset typically age 15–25 years
- paranoid schizophrenia: complex delusions and hallucinations. Delusions may be persecutory, grandiose or religious
- catatonic schizophrenia: psychomotor disturbance varying from stupor to sudden outbursts of activity. Waxy flexibility, automatic obedience and negativism.

Aetiology

A number of probable aetiological factors have been identified. The contribution of any individual factor (e.g. obstetric complications) to the total incidence of schizophrenia in the population is usually modest, but may be important for an individual case. Overall, however, it would seem that aetiology at a population

Box 9.2: The features of mental state examination in possible schizophrenia

Appearance and behaviour

This can be completely normal but classical presentations include perplexity, social awkwardness, withdrawal and odd behaviours such as smiling in response to no apparent stimuli. Impulsivity along with over-aroused behaviours can occur as can aggression, but this is less common than a pattern of withdrawal

Speech

In the acutely ill patient this can be difficult to follow reflecting thought disorder. Just as common is poverty of speech, not just in relation to quantity but also poverty of ideas and vocabulary. Classically described are neologisms (made up words; sometimes a condensation of more than one word)

Mood

Mood changes are common in schizophrenia, something often forgotten by students. These changes can be divided into three main types. These are:

- blunting of affect where emotional responsiveness is flattened or absent leading to the patient appearing indifferent to events
- mood changes such as depression (relatively common in the acute phase) and euphoria/elation
- incongruous mood where the emotional response is not in keeping with the trigger e.g. smiling when describing sad or upsetting events

Thought form

Disorders of form of thought are already mentioned in the section on speech but it is worth emphasizing here. The train of a patient's thoughts may be difficult to follow, the ideas expressed may be 'concrete' reflecting impaired abstract thought or the links between ideas expressed may be tenuous or incomprehensible (loosening of associations). Other observed abnormalities may include thought block where the patient suddenly stops speaking mid-sentence and has the subjective experience of their thought coming to an abrupt halt

Thought content

Delusions are common. Although primary delusions are classical they are not common. Much more frequently seen are secondary delusions. These are commonly persecutory but may be grandiose, delusions of reference (where external events have a direct and special meaning for them), delusions of external control (may be called passivity phenomena) or delusions of thought alienation. The latter covers thought broadcasting, thought withdrawal and thought insertion. More detail is in Chapter 3 (mental state examination)

Perceptions

The most common hallucinations are auditory with those set out in Box 9.1 having particular significance. Hallucinations can occur in any sensory modality. Delusional interpretation of hallucinations is common

level is multifactorial and may also often be so for individual patients. Most often for individual cases it is impossible to identify a cause, although families will frequently ask this question.

Theories include the dopamine hypothesis, neurological dysfunction, and environmental and genetic theories.

Dopamine hypothesis

Abnormalities in dopamine pathways have been implicated in the causation of schizophrenia (see Chapter 2, Table 2.5). Dopamine became implicated initially following obervation that dopamine agonists such as amphetamines and L-dopa could cause schizophrenia-like symptoms in some people, and that all drugs effective for schizophrenia are dopamine receptor antagonists. In fact, drugs with geometric isomers are only effective when the isomer given is a dopamine receptor antagonist. It should be remembered however that the therapeutic effects of antipsychotic drugs on psychotic symptoms are not restricted to schizophrenia. Current evidence suggests it is likely that any abnormalities in dopamine neurotransmission are not the primary cause of schizophrenia but are secondary to some other abnormality, perhaps in the glutamatergic system. Nevertheless, the only currently available treatments for the 'positive' symptoms are drugs which are DA receptor antagonists. Disturbance of glutamatergic systems have been found and may be related to some of the underlying neuropathological changes seen. Research into the 5-HT system has not suggested this as primarily important, but manipulation of this may be relevant to certain symptoms, such as low mood, and to the presence of some of the effects of the second generation antipsychotic drugs. Accepting that neurotransmitters play a role in schizophrenia it is unclear whether the neurochemical findings in research are indicative of primary or secondary pathological processes, or are the result of compensatory mechanisms or environmental influences.

The role of recreational drug use in schizophrenia is complex. In clinical practice it is difficult to identify whether an individual's drug use has unmasked an underlying illness, has caused the illness in a vulnerable individual or may be the consequence of the illness in an individual with a subclinical picture. The answer like almost everything in psychiatry is liable to be complex. Cannabis use for example increases the risk of illness but this is most significant in individuals with an underlying genetic vulnerability and has a strong correlation with early (prior to the age of 15) cannabis use.

Neurological dysfunction

Symptoms similar to schizophrenia are seen in complex partial seizures where left temporal lobe limbic structures are involved, e.g. temporal lobe epilepsy. It has also been observed that birth complications are associated with an increased risk of schizophrenia. Along with the observations of structural brain abnormalities seen in brain imaging studies, an association with an increased prevalence of childhood developmental problems and the presence of soft neurological signs (e.g. minor abnormalities in coordination), these observations suggest neurological insults at an early age may play a role in the development of schizophrenia in some individuals.

It has also been suggested that schizophrenia is the price we pay for the evolutionary advantage gained from our development of language.

Environmental

The role of environmental factors remains unclear. As already mentioned there is an increased incidence of schizophrenia in urban populations, and it has been suggested that pollution may play a role. Other factors include obstetric complications and winter births (in males). Heavy cannabis use can contribute to the risk, although this may be mediated by genetic factors.

Environmental factors such as stressful life events can have a role in precipitating episodes of illness, and highly charged emotional environments (high expressed emotion) may well have a maintaining role and increase risk of relapse.

Speculation about particular styles of child rearing as an aetiological factor has not been supported by evidence and only serves to fuel feelings of guilt in some parents.

Genetic

The risk for individuals with an affected relative is significantly greater than for the general population and can be seen most strongly in twin studies where dizygotic twins have a risk not much different from non-twin siblings, but the risk for monozygotic twins is about four times higher. Further reinforcement has come from adoption studies where the risk for adopted children remains high. This has been covered in more detail in Chapter 2.

Management

Management of schizophrenia can be best thought of as assessment followed by management of the acute and then chronic stages.

Assessment

Although the initial assessment of the acute illness often takes place in hospital, depending on local services it may be carried out in community settings either by community mental health teams or crisis/home treatment teams. Where the assessment takes place will depend on how the individual presents (for example if acting upon delusions or hallucinations the police may be involved), severity, risk and/or level of support available. It is unusual for an individual to 'self-present', more typically it is the concerns of others that result in involvement of mental health services. An assessment should include:

- a full history and mental state examination, in particular identify delusions, hallucinations, thought disorder;
- a check for clouding of consciousness;
- an interview with third-party informants as relevant to that individual;
- a physical examination and appropriate investigations depending on age and mode of presentation, e.g. urine drug screen to exclude a drug-induced psychosis, EEG, brain imaging, neuropsychological assessment;
- a social assessment: housing, work, etc.

The aim is that by the end of the assessment:

- information supporting the diagnosis should have been collected;

- particular risks the patient may present to themselves and others should have been identified;
- vulnerability factors such as a family history of schizophrenia should have been considered;
- possible precipitants to the acute illness should have been identified (the 'Why now?' question);
- factors that may maintain the illness or make relapse more likely should have been explored, such as high critical expressed emotion within the family or stresses at work;
- whether the patient is prepared to accept treatment should have been decided;
- a differential or coexisting disorder should have been considered.

Management of the acute episode

In the acute stage of schizophrenia the focus is typically on management of acute psychotic symptoms and risk. The mainstay of treatment is pharmacotherapy with antipsychotic drugs combined with various types of social, practical, emotional and psychoeducational supports, as appropriate to the person's stage of illness. Second generation antipsychotic drugs should be tried first but it may sometimes be appropriate to try a first generation drug if one or two second generation drugs are not effective. The pharmacology of these drugs is described in Chapter 17.

As a first-line treatment oral medication is used, with some drugs giving the option of an 'oro-dispersable' preparation where compliance is in doubt. In more difficult cases depot preparations administered every 2–4 weeks allow monitoring of patient compliance, as they are administered intramuscularly. This can also address variability in first-pass metabolism and provide more predictable plasma levels in individuals who often have chaotic lives.

In the acute phase, antipsychotics provide sedation, which helps with excitement, irritability and insomnia. It is more usual for improvement in the psychotic symptoms such as hallucinations and delusions to take longer. Although antipsychotics help manage the acute psychotic positive symptoms such as hallucinations and delusions, they are less effective at managing the negative symptoms. Indeed many of the claimed benefits from the trials of newer drugs in this respect may only reflect differing side-effect profiles or issues with study design.

In patients with more extreme behavioural disturbance, rapid or acute tranquillization may be required, usually with short-acting benzodiazepines either on their own or in addition to an antipsychotic. This is covered in more detail in the Chapter 18. As many patients when acutely well lose insight and lack capacity as a direct result of their illness, mental health legislation is sometimes needed to ensure that they are treated. Compulsory treatment is dealt with in Chapter 5.

Prognosis following the first episode varies considerably. Patients whose first presentation is with an episode of acute psychosis, but in whom the nature of persistence of symptoms does not meet the diagnostic criteria for schizophrenia, can have a very good outcome with perhaps twenty per cent never experiencing a further episode of illness. However, the majority of those who meet the diagnostic criteria for schizophrenia will have some persistence of symptoms. This may range from a mild level of negative symptoms to persistent and distressing delusions and/or hallucinations accompanied by significant social disability. Age at onset and mode of onset of symptoms are the two most reliable prognostic indicators. Younger age of onset predicts poorer outcome. Males have earlier onset than females and thus, on average, also less good outcomes. More gradual, insidious onset also predicts poorer outcome. A sudden onset, over a few days, especially if prodromal features are absent (e.g. a prolonged period of social withdrawal) will usually have a good outcome. Patients whose illness appears (usually in retrospect) to have come on over many months do less well. Insidious mode of onset also predicts a longer duration of the period of untreated psychosis (i.e. before the condition is recognised) which itself predicts poor outcome. Heavy premorbid cannabis use may be another factor in poor outcome but persistent use after diagnosis is clearly detrimental.

Management of the chronic disorder

In patients who recover fully there is a need to consider strategies to prevent further episodes. The management involves pharmacological and psychosocial components. The more acute episodes a patient has in their life the worse the prognosis, so there is every reason to try and prevent relapses.

A common approach it to use long-term antipsychotics. This has to be balanced against the deleterious effects of possible side-effects on a patient's quality of life, not least because these side-effects may have a negative influence on compliance. Often clinicians will try and use lower medication doses in the maintenance phase in contrast to the treatment phase.

Consideration must be given to psychosocial interventions. It may be necessary to consider what levels of support activities of daily living require. Adequate housing and meaningful activities can also contribute. Family psychological interventions can target behaviours, such as high expressed emotion (see above), that can contribute to relapses.

Where a patient remains symptom free there will come a time when it is reasonable to attempt to stop antipsychotic medication. This needs to be preceded by a discussion regarding the possible risk of relapse balanced against the potential negative consequences of long-term antipsychotic use. The period before such a withdrawal is attempted is open for debate with no hard evidence, but in England and Wales NICE highlights the high risk if medication is discontinued in the first year or two and recommends close monitoring for at least 2 years following medication withdrawal.

Where there is incomplete response to treatment then treatment resistance, covered below, needs to be considered, but when the residual symptoms are predominantly negative medication change is unlikely to prove effective. In all these patients there is a recommendation for psychological interventions. Already mentioned are family interventions. Psychodynamic approaches may help in understanding the patient's problems and formulating responses. More recently there has been a shift in focus to cognitive behavioural therapy (CBT), which aims to aid the patient in challenging hallucinations and delusions and therefore allowing them to cope with greater ease.

In all cases ensuring that patients have adequate housing, are not in financial difficulty and are able to care for themselves or are supported in this is essential.

Treatment resistance

A proportion of patients with schizophrenia do not respond to standard treatment approaches. In all cases where patients do not appear to respond to treatment a reasoned, questioning approach needs to be followed. In the first case, adherence to treatment needs to be questioned. Failure to follow a medication regime may not be wilful but nonetheless needs to

be considered, and if suspected addressed. For cases where the negative symptoms and/or chaotic lifestyle of the patient lead to neglectful non-compliance, the use of a depot or other strategies to ensure medication is taken warrant consideration.

Other causes also need consideration, such as use of alcohol and/or other recreational drugs, comorbid illnesses such as depression or significant ongoing stresses, and then these managed appropriately.

Only when these issues have been addressed and adherence is assured with evidence that a patient has had an adequate trial of at least two antipsychotic drugs (one of which must have been a second-generation drug) at an adequate dose for a sufficient period of time (at least 6 weeks) can there be said to be treatment resistance.

In cases of treatment resistance the next approach should be a trial of dozapine. Owing to the risk of agranulocytosis, patients require regular haematological monitoring. This starts off as weekly but falls in time to monthly. In some cases there will be failure to respond to clozapine. Here, as covered above, psychological interventions may help, but there remains the option of augmentation with other antipsychotics (e.g. amisulpiride or aripiprazole).

Physical health

Patients with schizophrenia are at greater risk of physical health problems, such as cardiovascular disease, diabetes and cancers. The causes of this include lifestyle, side-effects of medication and what appears to be a higher inherent risk.

Ideally all patients starting on antipsychotics should be first assessed physically, including an assessment of cardiac risk. If the patient is too disturbed to enable a physical examination at initial presentation, this should be done once the patient settles. The assessment should include:

- a history of smoking, diet, exercise and alcohol and recreational drug use;
- calculation of body mass index and measures of truncal obesity such as waist-to-hip ratio;
- recording of blood pressure.

Investigations include ECG, FBC, U&Es, LFTs, glucose and lipid profiles. As several of the drugs used may cause hyperprolactinaemia, prolactin should be assessed and added to the list of measures that require regular review.

Active management of problems identified at baseline or subsequently on repeat measures is essential. Psychoeducation programmes looking at healthy lifestyles should augment this. It is worth remembering that a patient who is stable and has given up smoking may need their medication reviewed as cessation of smoking leads to an increase in drug bioavailability.

Schizoaffective disorder

This is not a subtype of schizophrenia but a separate disorder. It is common in differential diagnoses, particularly by students, but should only be used in very specific circumstances. It is important to realize that mood symptoms are quite common in schizophrenia, particularly following early acute episodes of illness. It is important therefore that the diagnosis of schizoaffective disorder should be limited to cases where diagnostic criteria for both schizophrenia and a mood disorder occur during the same episode. Otherwise the diagnosis is of the predominant syndrome.

Summary

Schizophrenia is a relatively common mental illness and can have significant impact on those who have the disorder and their families. It is often poorly understood by the general public and non-mental health professionals, which means that patients can experience discrimination. Early recognition and reduction of relapses improves prognosis. Most present with acute symptomatology, although a significant minority never develop Schneider's first rank symptoms. Antipsychotic medications are extremely effective for many but maintenance doses can present some challenges.

Further reading

NICE Guidance, 'Core interventions in the treatment and management of schizophrenia in primary and secondary care (update)': http//guidance.nice.org.uk/CG82

Oyebode F (2008) *Sims' Symptoms in the Mind: An Introduction to Descriptive Psychopathology* 4th edition. London: Saunders Ltd.

Stein G, Wilkinson G (eds) (2007) *Seminars in General Adult Psychiatry* 2nd edition. London: Royal College of Psychiatrists.

CASE STUDY

A 19-year-old man is brought into A&E by the police after he had been found wandering in the street in the small hours of the morning. They describe him as sitting mumbling to himself, and occasionally looking to the side and talking as though replying to someone sitting next to him.

When you go to see him, he is sitting looking relaxed with a distracted smile on his face. On trying to engage him in conversation, you find his train of thought impossible to follow. He appears distracted and will break off conversation or not attend to what you are saying to look to a point just behind your right shoulder when he will smile as though in response to something that has attracted his attention.

What actions would you take to assess this young man?

An assessment of his mental state; this should focus on:

observing his behaviour

assessment of his speech (particularly looking for breakdown of syntax and pointers to disorders of form of thought)

assessment of his mood

exploration of his thoughts with a view to identify any abnormally held ideas such as delusions and/or overvalued ideas, thought alienation (thought insertion, withdrawal or broadcasting)

assessment of whether there are abnormal perceptions (hallucinations or illusions/misperceptions)

cognitive assessment with particular reference to his conscious state.

Assessment of history. This is most likely to be of value when a corroborative history can be obtained e.g. from a family member or close friend. Looking for a pattern of change over time, a history of drug use etc. would be of particular value.

Investigations in the immediate period might include urine or blood screening for recreational drug use.

What differential diagnoses would you consider?

Schizophrenia

Other schizophreniform illnesses

Intoxication with psychoactive substances

Drug-induced psychosis

Complex partial seizures

CHAPTER 10

SUBSTANCE MISUSE

Ilana Crome

KEY CHAPTER FEATURES

- Frequency of substance misuse
- Drug and drug addiction
- Susceptibility to and impact of substance misuse
- Assessing and treating substance misuse

Introduction

There are many myths about addiction, such as patients do not get better, there are no treatments, treatments do not work, 'once an alcoholic always an alcoholic', older people cannot be drug users, addicted parents are bad parents. I hope that this chapter demonstrates that this is exactly what they are: myths. Substance use, misuse and dependence are commonplace in the community, as well as in clinical settings. There are many different psychological and pharmacological treatments available, patients can and *do* improve, substance misusing parents are not necessarily poor parents, and older people *are* at risk of developing substance problems. Medical students and young doctors are very important partners in raising the profile of substance misuse issues, as well as collaborating with multidisciplinary teams in its identification and treatment.

Why is this relevant to you?

No major specialty or subspecialty in the whole of medical practice can *avoid* substance misusers. Even if the patient presents with a substance problem, this may not be his or her major problem. Conversely, patients may present with numerous conditions resulting from substance use. Accident and emergency units and departments of cardiology, dermatology, gastroenterology, neurology, infectious diseases, oncology, respiratory medicine, obstetrics, geriatrics and surgery will generate their share of patients with substance-related problems, as will trauma and orthopaedic departments. This is because people may present acutely due to the effects of intoxication and withdrawal syndromes and as a consequence of the chronic use of substances. Convulsions, acute disturbance (psychosis, panic, confusion, accidents), cancer, and cardiovascular and respiratory conditions are some of the conditions with which patients may present. Psychiatric specialties such as adult, child and adolescent and old age, forensic and liaison psychiatry in hospital, community and criminal justice settings are increasingly contributing to the treatment of substance misusers. General practitioners too will regularly be managing the impact of substance misuse on the individual, family and community, because it is very common. In addition, medical services often have to work with social care services, e.g. education, housing, child protection, and the criminal justice system to manage this group of patients.

How common is substance misuse?

Alcohol

Alcohol problems make up 4 per cent of the global burden of disease. Around 25 per cent of the population drink above safe recommended limits and per capita alcohol consumption has doubled over the last 50 years and is still rising (Prime Minister's Strategy Unit, 2004). There are 7 million hazardous drinkers in the UK. Hospital admissions for conditions related to alcohol consumption have doubled in the last 10 years, as have death rates over the last 15 years. Alcohol misuse costs the country £20 billion per annum and there are about 22 000 premature deaths from alcohol misuse every year. The mortality associated with alcohol and drugs can be up to 16 times higher than in the general population. Twenty-five per cent of young people (16–24 years) drink over the recommended weekly limits for low-risk drinking in adults (21 units for men and 14 units for women) and 9 per cent of young males and 6 per cent of young females drink over 50 units per week, which would be high-risk drinking behaviour in adults.

Illicit drugs

Box 10.1 shows the different classes of illicit drugs. It is estimated that about 11 million people (35 per cent) aged 16–59 have used illicit drugs in their lifetime, and that 3.25 million (10 per cent) have used illicit drugs in the previous year and 2 million (6 per cent) in the previous month. Cannabis is the most likely drug to be used, with 8 per cent of 16–59 year olds reporting use in the previous year. Just over 1 million people aged 16–59 have used Class A drugs in the past year, and the use of Class A drugs increased between 1998

and 2006/7. Trends in drug use since 1998 indicate that drug misuse has stabilized or decreased; however, drug misuse costs the country £15 billion per annum at a conservative estimate (Table 10.1). There are 2000–3000 deaths from drug misuse every year.

Table 10.1   Class A drugs in the British Crime Survey 2007 (Murphy and Roe 2007)

Time period	Age group	Percentage
Lifetime	16–19	9.3
Lifetime	20–24	22.3
Last year	16–19	5.4
Last year	20–24	10.4
Last month	16–19	2.9
Last month	20–24	5.5

Smoking

Since the early 1990s the prevalence of cigarette smoking has been higher among 20- to 24-year-olds than in any other age group in Great Britain, despite a fall in overall prevalence from 45 per cent of the adult population in 1974 to 22 per cent in 2006. There are approximately 120 000 premature deaths from cigarette smoking each year.

What is a drug and what is drug addiction?

What is a drug or substance?

The term 'drug' covers licit (e.g. tobacco and alcohol) and illicit substances, e.g. central nervous system depressants such as opiates and opioids (e.g. heroin and methadone), stimulants (e.g. cocaine, crack, amphetamine and ecstasy), and LSD, khat and magic mushrooms. Street use and non-compliant use of prescription and over-the-counter drugs, such as benzodiazepines and codeine-based products (e.g. cough medicines, decongestants) are also included. People may use a combination of all these substances, which is known as polypharmacy or polydrug misuse. This is what makes this work challenging and stimulating! Patients may buy, borrow and share, and

Box 10.1: The classes of illicit drugs

Class A	Ecstasy, lysergic acid diethylamide (LSD), heroin, cocaine, crack, magic mushrooms and amphetamines (if prepared for injection)
Class B	Amphetamines, cannabis, methylphenidate, pholcodine
Class C	Tranquillizers, some painkillers, gamma-hydroxybutyrate (GHB), ketamine

may use out-of-date drugs. They may wittingly or unwittingly not report all use and they may forget or may not realize that a substance is psychoactive. They may be deliberately misleading, sometimes because they think that they will be denied treatment.

Concepts of harmful use and dependence (addiction)

There are specific criteria for the diagnosis of substance problems, outlined in Boxes 10.2 and 10.3, for both the *International Classification of Diseases* (ICD-10) and the *Diagnostic and Statistical Manual* of the American Psychiatric Association (DSM-IV). For the purposes of treatment management, it is essential to distinguish non-dependent substance misuse from dependent or addictive use. The more serious the substance problem, the more likely there are to be associated psychological, physical and social problems, which require a more intensive level of treatment intervention. A diagnosis of dependence can be made if three of the following criteria have been present during the preceding 12 months:

- compulsion or craving, i.e. a strong desire to take the substance;
- tolerance, i.e. needing more to get the same effect;
- difficulties in controlling the use of substances;
- a withdrawal syndrome when substance use is reduced or stopped;

- relief of withdrawal by substance use;
- persistent use, despite evidence of harmful consequences;
- neglect of interests and an increased amount of time taken to obtain the substance or to recover from its effects.

Every substance has its own withdrawal syndrome. For example, the withdrawal syndrome for alcohol consists of tremor, sweating, craving, agitation, nausea and vomiting, whereas for opiates the features are runny eyes and nose, muscle aches and pains, diarrhoea and nausea (Table 10.2).

Can people suffer from addiction at all ages?

Substance misuse problems may commence in adolescence and continue into old age. Childhood maltreatment contributes to the prevalence of comorbid personality disorder in addiction populations.

Substance misuse may result in miscarriage, stillbirth, fetal distress, placental abruption, eclampsia, early labour and sudden death. Babies born to pregnant substance-misusing women may suffer from the effects of withdrawal, and neonates and infants may experience delayed development, which can have an impact in adolescence and young adulthood.

Young people are using substances more frequently, mainly alcohol, cannabis and nicotine

---

Box 10.2: Criteria for substance abuse (DSM IV) and harmful use (ICD 10)

DSM-IV (American Psychiatric Association 1994)

A. A maladaptive pattern of substance use leading to clinically significant impairment or distress, as manifested by one (or more) of the following occurring within a 12-month period:

1 Recurrent substance use resulting in a failure to fulfil major role obligations at work, school, or home

2 Recurrent substance abuse in situations that are physically hazardous

3 Recurrent substance-abuse-related legal problems

4 Continued substance abuse despite having persistent or recurrent social or interpersonal problems caused or exacerbated by the effects of the substance

B. Has never met the criteria for substance dependence for this class of substance

ICD-10 (World Health Organization 1992)

A. A pattern of psychoactive substance use that is causing damage to health; the damage may be to physical or mental health

Box 10.3 Criteria for dependence syndrome in DSM IV and ICD 10

DSM-IV (American Psychiatric Association 1994)

A. Diagnosis of dependence should be made if three (or more) of the following have been experienced or exhibited at any time in the same 12-month period:

1 Tolerance defined by either need for markedly increased amount of substance to achieve intoxication or desired effect or markedly diminished effect with continued use of the same amount of the substance

2 Withdrawal as evidenced by either of the following: the characteristic withdrawal syndrome for the substance, or the same (or closely related) substance is taken to relieve or avoid withdrawal symptoms

3 The substance is often taken in larger amounts over a longer period of time than was intended

4 Persistent desire or repeated unsuccessful efforts to cut down or control substance use

5 A great deal of time is spent in activities necessary to obtain the substance, use the substance, or recover from its effects

6 Important social, occupational, or recreational activities given up or reduced because of substance use

7 Continued substance use despite knowledge of having had a persistent or recurrent physical or psychological problem that was likely to have been caused or exacerbated by the substance

ICD-10 (World Health Organization 1992)

A. Diagnosis of dependence should be made if three or more of the following have been experienced or exhibited at some time during the last year:

1 A strong desire or sense of compulsion to take the substance

2 Difficulties in controlling substance-taking behaviour in terms of its onset, termination, or levels of use

3 Physiological withdrawal state when substance use has ceased or been reduced, as evidenced by either of the following: the characteristic withdrawal syndrome for the substance, or use of the same (or closely related) substance with the intention of relieving or avoiding withdrawal symptoms

4 Evidence of tolerance, such that increased doses of the psychoactive substance are required in order to achieve effects originally produced by lower doses

5 Progressive neglect of alternative pleasures or interests because of psychoactive substance use and increased amount of time necessary to obtain or take the substance or to recover from its effects

6 Persisting with substance use despite clear evidence of overly harmful consequences (physical or mental)

and the age of use is earlier now than previously. Children as young as 10 years may present with substance misuse issues. However, most presentations are during adolescence. Many young people who present to treatment units have numerous associated psychosocial problems (for example, self-harm, unstable accommodation, poor education, involvement in criminal activity and difficult family relationships) as well as mental and physical health problems. Their coping and adaptive strategies may be poorly developed or absent. The overall mortality rate of adolescent addicts is 16 times that of the general adolescent population.

Women who use substances in particular are more likely than a control group to have been exposed to sexual, physical and emotional abuse as children and are more likely to experience emotional distress than a control group of female substance misusers who do not have that background.

Older people suffer from physical and psychiatric comorbidity. They may be taking prescribed and over-the-counter medications for their ailments, as well as licit and illicit drugs. They may start using substances at an early age or when they are older. The number of older people is projected to increase, so that people over the age of 65 will constitute 23 per cent of the population by 2020.

Older people are at risk of substance misuse for many reasons, including the development of multiple, chronic physical and psychiatric illnesses, for which they receive prescription medications that they may or may not take compliantly and that may interact with physical and psychological illness and illicit and licit substance use. Some users who began their substance misuse in the 1960s continue it into old age, whereas some initiate substance misuse in older age due to isolation, losses and illness and others use substances to cope with disability, pain, anxiety and insomnia.

Table 10.2   Symptoms of intoxication and withdrawal (Crome *et al.* 2004)

Substance	Intoxication	Withdrawal
Alcohol	Disinhibition Argumentativeness Aggression Interference with personal functioning Labile mood Impaired judgement and attention Unsteady gait and difficulty in standing Slurred speech Nystagmus Decreased level of consciousness Flushed face Conjunctival injection	Tremor (tongue, eyelids, hands) Agitation, insomnia, malaise Convulsions Visual, auditory, tactile illusions or hallucinations
Opiates	Apathy Sedation, drowsiness, slurred speech Disinhibition Psychomotor retardation Impaired attention and judgement Pupillary constriction Decreased level of consciousness Interference with personal functioning	Craving Sneezing, yawning, runny eyes Muscle aches, abdominal pains Nausea, vomiting, diarrhoea Pupillary dilatation Goose flesh, recurrent chills Restless sleep
Cannabis	Euphoria and disinhibition Anxiety and agitation Suspiciousness and paranoid ideation Impaired reaction time, judgement and attention Hallucinations with preserved orientation Depersonalisation and derealization Increased appetite Dry mouth Conjunctival injection Tachycardia	Anxiety Irritability Tremor Sweating Muscle aches
Nicotine	Craving Malaise or weakness Anxiety, irritability, moodiness Insomnia Increased appetite Increased cough and mouth ulceration Difficulty in concentrating Tachycardia and cardiac arrhythmias	Insomnia Bizarre dreams Fluctuating mood Derealization Interference with personal functioning Nausea Sweating
Stimulants	Euphoria and increased energy Hypervigilance Repetitive stereotyped behaviours Grandiose beliefs and actions Paranoid ideation Abusiveness, aggression and argumentativeness Auditory, tactile and visual hallucinations Sweats, chills, muscular weakness Nausea or vomiting, weight loss Pupillary dilatation, convulsions Tachycardia, arrhythmias, chest pain, hypertension Agitation	Lethargy Psychomotor retardation or agitation Craving Increased appetite Insomnia or hypersomnia Bizarre and unpleasant dreams

Thus, every single patient you come across requires a substance misuse assessment, because it may have a bearing on diagnosis and treatment. Age is no barrier to the development of substance-related problems, as Case study 2 at the end of the chapter demonstrates.

Who is susceptible?

People who have psychological (e.g. anxiety, depression and psychosis) and physical (e.g. pain) problems are particularly susceptible to substance use through many mechanisms:

- a primary psychiatric and/or physical illness may precipitate or lead to a substance problem;
- substance misuse may worsen or alter the course of a psychiatric and/or physical illness;
- intoxication and/or substance dependence may lead to psychological and physical symptoms;
- substance misuse and/or withdrawal may lead to psychiatric or physical symptoms or illnesses;
- primary psychiatric disorder may precipitate substance use, which may lead to psychiatric and/or physical symptoms or syndromes.

In studies that have examined the association between substance misuse and psychiatric illness, roughly 30–50 per cent of people with psychiatric disorder have been found to use substances. Between 30 per cent and 50 per cent of substance misusers have psychiatric illnesses. Substance misuse may be associated with psychotic illnesses, such as schizophrenia, bipolar disorder, schizoaffective disorder, anxiety, depression, post-traumatic stress disorder, eating disorders, attention deficit hyperactivity disorder, personality disorder and dementia.

In an extensive review of risk factors in young drug users, the most consistent evidence revolved around family interaction. Biological factors (i.e. those which cannot be changed) include genetic predisposition, gender, age, ethnicity and life events, while some traits such as self-esteem, early behavioural disorders, impulsive and sensation-seeking behaviour, antisocial behaviour and mental disorder (as described above) may be very difficult to change. Behavioural or attitudinal factors, which may be susceptible to change, include family attitudes to substance misuse, substance use by family members, religious affinity and attendance, conduct disorder, and educational

aspiration and attainment. *Interpersonal relationships* with family and friends are potentially open to modification, with regard to parental supervision and control, familial bonding and harmony and childhood trauma. *Environmental* and *economic factors* are outside the individual's control and include socioeconomic status, neighbourhood unrest and the availability of local amenities, which require political involvement.

A number of these factors may be operative at any one time and they may be mitigated by protective factors such as family support and monitoring, good relationships with parents, religious affiliation, later age of initiation and academic achievement. The age at which exposure to substances takes place and the setting also have an influence on later substance use. Social problems such as family problems can also be a result of the substance misuse.

What is the link between substance misuse and violent behaviour?

The pharmacological effect of the drug itself, especially (but not only) if taken in high doses, may be disinhibiting and lead to impulsivity, aggression, abusiveness and argumentativeness, agitation and grandiosity (e.g. amphetamine or cocaine). Substances may also exacerbate a psychotic episode. Chronic misuse of substances may lead to a dependence syndrome, so that withdrawal causes unpleasant symptomatology, including a confusional state (benzodiazepine withdrawal) during which paranoid ideation may occur. The distress and discomfort arising from cravings, including anxiety and depression, may lead to disturbed behaviour. Accidents, injuries and violent acts may occur during intoxication, in part as a result of the individual's decreased ability to make sound judgements due to impaired attention and concentration, paranoia and even the presence of delusions and hallucinations. The combination of a psychosis and comorbid use of drugs results in a higher rate and severity of violence than in a population with psychosis and no comorbid substance use. Non-adherence to medication for a psychiatric disorder may also lead to violent behaviour. If patients are substance misusers and non-compliant with medication, violence is twice as likely as in those with either problem alone. The prevalence of violent behaviour generally increases with the number of psychotic symptoms, except in those with the most psychotic symptoms where violence risk is relatively low. This can be explained in terms of social isolation and a degree of impairment so severe that it incapacitates the person from carrying out violent acts.

Thus, drug-related violent crime could be classified both as violence arising from the effects of substances and violence associated with the interaction of a psychiatric illness and drug use, and also as violence connected with acquisition of drugs and violence linked to disputes between drug users, drug dealers and drug gangs.

Sex-related crimes such as prostitution and 'date rape' sexual assault are examples of illegal activity. Driving under the influence of drugs and alcohol may lead to injury, as well as criminal convictions. Crime and violence are associated with victimization, social instability and marginalization, including homelessness and economic deprivation. These often stem from childhood and adolescent trauma and family problems, as well as educational and social skill deficits.

What is the impact of substance misuse on individuals, families and communities?

Substances do not have to be regularly used or even misused to have a significant impact on the lives of individuals and families. You do not have to be addicted to experience serious effects from a substance. For example, a person may be intoxicated from alcohol abuse, become involved in a road traffic accident and suffer severe injuries. The consequences of substance misuse may be related to the degree of dependence, the quantity and the quality (purity, adulterants) of the substance and the route of administration (e.g. smoking or injecting).

Serious physical illness is, of course, an additional 'comorbidity' and one that is, perhaps, overlooked, underrated and undertreated. Physical problems such as pain, infection, injury and cancer may lead to mental illness and may result from substance misuse. If not adequately treated, these conditions not only add to the suffering of individuals, but also undermine treatment provided for substance misuse.

Substance use may be life threatening: intoxication from alcohol is characterized by impaired judgement, reduced consciousness, lack of coordination and ataxia, disinhibition and slurred speech. Coma, associated with hypoglycaemia and hypothermia, and even death may ensue. Accidents, injuries, falls, burns and choking are other consequences, along with convulsions as a result of head injury. Stimulant intoxication may lead to increased aggression, and paranoia and anxiety or irritability due to craving. Volatile substances are dangerous, since not only does use result in unsteadiness and lack of coordination but also in cardiac arrhythmias, which may prove fatal. Drugs such as opiates may depress respiration to the extent that coma results.

Withdrawal from substances can also be a medical emergency necessitating rapid response. Alcohol withdrawal is unpleasant since tremulousness, nausea, vomiting, sweating, general malaise and insomnia result. Benzodiazepine withdrawal presents in a similar fashion. Severe alcohol withdrawal results in delirium tremens (discussed further in Chapter 12), which includes severe agitation, confusion, hypertension, hyperthermia, delusions and hallucinations. This condition can be fatal but, if intervention is early, recovery is good.

Withdrawal from opiates is not as risky, but it is very uncomfortable. General aches and pains, diarrhoea and vomiting, runny nose and eyes, and difficulty sleeping may be part of the withdrawal state. As combinations of substances may be used, withdrawal symptoms from several drugs may occur. Stimulant withdrawal may lead to inertia, depression, increased appetite and retardation: suicidal ideas may develop.

Chronicity of use is another factor in the extent to which substances may impact on health. Alcohol and nicotine contribute to the development of cardiovascular and respiratory disorders and are associated with heart disease and stroke. They may also cause cancer: tobacco use is associated with cancer of the lung, lips, tongue, throat, larynx, oesophagus, kidney, pancreas and bladder, and alcohol use causes cancer of the liver, bowel, throat, mouth, larynx, breast and oesophagus. In addition, fertility may be reduced.

Injecting drug use carries the risk of infection, e.g. blood-borne viruses such as HIV, hepatitis B and hepatitis C as a result of contamination from the blood or body fluids of infected users. Septicaemia, localized infections, such as abscesses in the heart, skin and central nervous system, and emboli may result. Repeated injecting may damage the veins, causing ulcers, abscesses and thrombophlebitis. Deep vein thrombosis from injecting large vessels in, for example, the groin is of special concern because of the possibility of emboli.

Substance misuse is a strong predictor of self-harm and suicide, and previous history of self-harm is a strong predictor of completed suicide. This too is a psychiatric emergency, since poisoning with substances is common among patients presenting to accident and emergency departments with self-harm. Craving for substances, specific adverse effects or distress may provoke an overdose. Whether accidental or deliberate, overdose with depressants such as alcohol, sedatives and opiates may lead to coma and death, whereas stimulant overdose may lead to cardiac arrest. Reduced tolerance may develop during a period of abstinence, for example if the patient has been in prison, which may lead to an unintentional overdose.

As a result of these complications, 'comorbid' patients present to primary care, secondary care and general medical, surgical and mental health services.

What are the components of a good assessment?

The key to appropriate management is a thorough history as discussed in Chapter 3. It is helpful to consider what specific information you need to elicit to ensure a comprehensive substance misuse history. An understanding of the current social circumstances, e.g. living arrangements, family constellation and education or employment activities, is important as these may be precipitating and perpetuating factors. They may also influence potential interventions and the likelihood of their success. Details about all current licit and illicit substance use, as well as prescribed and over-the-counter medication should follow. Information about the history of use, e.g. age at first use, onset of weekly and daily use, route of use (e.g. oral, injecting, smoking), and pattern of use are core parts of the assessment. Whether withdrawal symptoms for any substance have developed, the cost of use, the maximum ever used, periods of abstinence and triggers to relapse provide a picture of the extent of the problem. Previous treatment for substance misuse, mental and physical illness and the effectiveness of treatment is another strand. The nature of substance misuse and mental illness in the

patient and their family provides vital background information, as do details of physical illness associated with substance use. Life events, such as bereavement or divorce, as well as the nature of family relationships (e.g. conflict or separation) can provide some understanding regarding the historical precipitants of initiation, continuation or cessation of substance misuse. The history of criminal activity and resulting charges and convictions, including level of debt, is also valuable. The degree of social and community support and details of other agencies involved should be discussed so as to plan a comprehensive response. Special groups, e.g. teenagers, older people, homeless people, parents with young children and immigrants, have particular needs, in terms of both assessment (e.g. consent and confidentiality) and treatment (for further details please see Further reading and websites). Child protection may be an important issue to consider when assessing parents who have substance misuse problems. After these basic details have been completed, the information obtained can be utilized in the general protocol that follows. It is adapted from one developed for nicotine dependence and is a useful way to formulate the assessment process, because it translates into specific management plans. These are all things you as a medical student can and should consider with every patient you see.

Phase 1: ask

- Ask all patients about alcohol and other substance misuse, including prescribed and over-the-counter medications.
- Differentiate between substance use, harmful use and dependence.
- Assessment is ongoing and the information should be recorded.
- Be aware of, and sensitive to, the ambivalence substance misusing patients may feel.
- Be non-judgemental and act in a non-confrontational way, as this can be a powerful determinant of engagement with treatment.

Phase 2: assess

- Educate patients about the effects of substances, for example inform them about withdrawal symptoms.

- Assess the degree of dependence.
- Assess the level of motivation or 'stage of change'.
- In this context, aim to provide advice or suggestions as to what the 'goals' (e.g. abstinence or harm reduction) are.
- Negotiate appropriate treatment options (e.g. pharmacological interventions, the need for admission to specialist services).
- Clinical manifestations of the condition may impair the history-taking process (e.g. dementia, confusion, poor concentration).
- Follow an assessment schedule.

Phase 3: advise

- Continue the assessment within a brief 5- to 10-minute 'motivational interviewing' framework.
- Provide the patient with the opportunity to express their anxieties and concerns.
- Offer personalized feedback about clinical findings, including physical examination and biochemical and haematological tests.
- Discuss and outline the personal benefits and risks of continued substance misuse.
- Provide self-help materials (e.g. manuals).

Phase 4: assist

- Provide support and positive expectations of success.
- Acknowledge that loss of confidence and self-esteem might have resulted from failed previous attempts.
- Suggest that, if the goal is abstinence, a 'quit date' is set, so that the patient can plan accordingly (e.g. get rid of any alcohol in the house) and safely (is it safe to stop drinking abruptly or not?).
- Work through a range of alternative coping strategies, e.g. identification of cues that might help to distract the patient.

Phase 5: arrange

Be prepared to refer or organize admission to a specialist or appropriate unit if the patient

- is in, or is likely to develop, severe withdrawal, including delirium tremens
- is experiencing unstable social circumstances
- is severely dependent
- has a severe comorbid physical or psychiatric illness, including suicidal ideation
- is using multiple substances
- has a history of frequent relapse.

During all phases, close attention should be paid to the appropriateness of various options for the particular individual – 'tailor-made' where possible. The vignette illustrates some of these issues.

What treatments are available and do they work?

The National Institute for Health and Clinical Excellence (NICE) (Scotland has an equivalent in SIGN; the Scottish Intercollegiate Guidelines Network), has produced a series of reviews of the treatment of opiate dependence, smoking and alcohol (see www.nice.org.uk/ and www.sign.ac.uk/). There is no equivalent organization in Northern Ireland. Psychological treatments are an important part of the spectrum of available interventions. For 'treatment' to be successful, aftercare and long-term support with social issues, especially employment and accommodation, are essential components. It is also about treating the combination of substance misuse disorders, rather than treating them separately. We have become increasingly aware that addiction is not a 'stand alone' disorder – in fact comorbidity is the norm within the family and community, with local or regional and even national and international ramifications, since substances and substance misusers have a habit of crossing national boundaries.

Psychological approaches

Substance misusers vary in their suitability for psychological treatments and interventions may be more or less appropriate in individual cases due to age, cognitive ability or dysfunction, education, willingness and capability or capacity to view problems as psychological. However, psychological treatments are nonetheless perceived as being pivotal to treatment effectiveness, even when pharmacological treatments are administered. Standardization of approaches and outcome measures is complex. Treatment philosophies, environments and settings may differ greatly (e.g. primary care, accident and emergency, prisons). Additional resources for treatment (e.g. support from other agencies such as housing, education, probation) may vary. Some groups may be discriminated against across a variety of services because of general stigma around substance misuse, poorly trained staff and lack of resources, or because of old age, female sex or ethnic minority status. It has been noted that it is the emotional and socioeconomic issues that present the major challenge to recovery.

Stages of change

The process by which change occurs has been formulated as a series of stages: preconception, contemplation, preparation, action and maintenance. This theory has been influential in treatment and research. There is considerable evidence from other health and social care fields that provision of information in itself may be of some help. Information needs to be accurate and up to date and must provide advice not only on the negative effects of substance use, but also on any potential benefits. Responses to situations in which overdose might occur, physical consequences and psychological problems are a useful baseline from which to start.

Counselling may be appropriate. However, *behavioural therapies* have become the mainstay of treatment over the past decade and encompass social skills and self-control training, motivational counselling (which includes motivational interviewing and motivational enhancement therapies), marital therapy, stress management, contingency management, community reinforcement and cognitive therapies. Cognitive behavioural therapy, 12-step approaches and motivational approaches, as well as behavioural self-control training, coping skills and marital/family therapy, have been demonstrated to be beneficial for drinkers in a variety of studies.

Brief interventions have become extremely popular and are especially useful in primary care, but are also helpful in medical and psychiatric care and, to some extent, in accident and emergency departments. Most work has been undertaken in drinkers and smokers. The key components are that treatment is delivered by a non-specialist, such as a general practitioner, opportunistically, in a non-confrontational style with a focus on the individual's preferences. Brief interventions provide the opportunity for all health and even allied professionals to raise and manage the initial intervention for people with substance problems.

The key characteristics of brief interventions are best described by the acronym FRAMES:

- Personalized **f**eedback or assessment results detailing the target behaviour and associated effects and consequences on the individual.
- Emphasizing the individual's personal **r**esponsibility for change.
- Giving **a**dvice on how to change.
- Providing a **m**enu of options for change.
- Expressing **e**mpathy through behaviours conveying caring, understanding and warmth.
- Emphasizing **s**elf-efficacy for change and instilling hope that change is not only possible, but also within reach.

Pharmacotherapies are available to treat a variety of situations, such as:

- emergencies, e.g. overdose, fits, dehydration, hypothermia and acute confusional state, including delirium tremens;
- detoxification and withdrawal syndromes, e.g. lofexidine, methadone, buprenorphine, chlordiazepoxide;
- substitution, e.g. methadone, buprenorphine, nicotine replacement therapy;
- relapse prevention, e.g. naltrexone, acamprosate, disulfiram;
- treatment of vitamin deficiency;
- comorbid psychiatric disorders, e.g. depression, anxiety and psychosis;
- comorbid physical disorders, e.g. HIV, hepatitis C, diabetes and hypertension.

More and more evidence is accumulating about the effectiveness of treatment. Several major studies have been undertaken in the UK and others in the USA, Australia and Scandinavia.

Who has responsibility for treating patients with substance problems? What are the challenges?

Given that any doctor may come across individuals with substance misuse in their work, we all have a responsibility in ensuring that they are properly assessed and managed. There may be a need to work closely with other doctors and health care staff. In Case study 6, a general practitioner, addiction psychiatrist, physiotherapist and pain specialist were involved in the patient's care.

There is an evolving diversity of models and guidance for best practice and best treatment and there are many pointers to what the components of a less risky and more comprehensive approach should be. This has to take into account the following needs of some patients.

- A holistic approach is required.
- Complexity: this sometimes involves the 'long haul' and practitioners need to be aware that it is not a 'quick fix'.
- Continuity: continuity and constant review and reappraisal of the changing situation are both reassuring and beneficial.
- Unpredictability: patients may present in crisis suddenly.
- Particular people have particular risks and vulnerabilities, e.g. the homeless, teenagers, older people.
- Need for support and knowledge about how to access available services.
- Need for supervision by experienced practitioners.
- Severity: the severe nature of medical, psychological, psychiatric and substance misuse problems with which patients, who are sometimes very young, present and the need for trained medical staff. It is not just a matter of prescribing, which must be undertaken by trained, experienced staff in the context of many other medical and social problems.
- Multidisciplinary team working within a service and good interagency working.
- Relationships between inpatient statutory services and how they are used regularly yet are very difficult to access.

- The dilemmas of disengagement in this vulnerable group.

The vignettes demonstrate that, in order to provide the best care for patients with addiction problems, colleagues in general medicine and general practice, general surgery, pain clinics, and accident and emergency and psychiatry departments must be involved. However, the Royal College of Psychiatrists is the only royal medical college to have an accredited recognized training curriculum for those who wish to practise in the addictions, although this is still a subspecialty of general psychiatry. The Royal College of General Practitioners (RCGP) has developed short courses for primary care and other professionals and general practitioners can take on a substantial role in shared care with addiction psychiatrists. It is vitally important that doctors in all specialities have access to regular relevant training in substance misuse. This reduces stigma and increases confidence in management by improved identification and intervention. Treatment has been shown to be cost-effective in that every pound spent saves many more.

Summary

I hope that while this chapter has dispelled some of the myths and highlighted developments over the last two decades, it has also faced the realities. Substance use, misuse and dependence are as predictable in clinical settings as they are unsurprising in our communities. There are many different treatments available and patients *do* get better, as long as the treatments are made accessible. Addicted parents are not necessarily poor parents, although they may need considerable support. Older people, like everyone else, are at risk of developing substance problems. However, they too can be treated and will improve substantially if offered the opportunity. Practitioners and services, patients and carers, policy-makers and communities need to work together to erase the impact of the socioeconomic challenges that undermine the potential for treatment to work. The treatment provided may be suboptimal because of resource constraints. Small, gradual improvements or prevention of further harm are also important steps in the route to achieving abstinence and should not be denigrated. It is sometimes very difficult for people to achieve a drug-free condition on the first occasion they attempt to reduce or stop substance use.

Medical students and young doctors are essential allies in this quest to support the individual, families and communities. At the present time a national undergraduate addiction curriculum is being rolled out, so that all medical schools can train students in the basic management of addiction patients.

Further reading

Crome I (2009) Commentary: new impetus to aim 'higher, faster, stronger'. *Addiction* 104: 173–178.

Crome IB (2010) Addiction psychiatry. In B Puri and I Treasaden (eds), *Psychiatry – An Evidence-Based Text for the MRCPsych*. London: Hodder Arnold.

Crome I, Bloor R (2009) Alcohol problems. In R Murray, KS Kendler, P McGuffin, *et al.* (eds) *Essential Psychiatry*. Cambridge: Cambridge University Press, 198–229.

Crome I, Bloor R (2010) Substance misuse and offending. In J Gunn and P Taylor (eds) *Forensic Psychiatry*, 2nd edition. London: Hodder Arnold.

Crome IB, Shaikh N (2004) Undergraduate medical school substance misuse training in the UK: Can medical students drive change? *Drugs: Education, Prevention and Policy* 11: 483–503.

Crome I, Ghodse H, Gilvarry E, McArdle P (2004) *Young People and Substance Misuse*. London: Gaskell.

Department of Health and the Devolved Administrations (2007) *Drug Misuse and Dependence: Guidelines on Clinical Management 2007*. London: National Treatment Agency for Substance Misuse.

Edwards G (2000) *Alcohol: The Ambiguous Molecule*. London: Penguin Books.

Edwards G, Marshall EJ, Cook CCH (eds) (2003) *The Treatment of Drinking Problems: A Guide for the Helping Professions*, 4th edition. Cambridge: Cambridge University Press.

Frisher M, Crome I, Macleod J, *et al.* (2007) *Predictive Factors for Illicit Drug Use Among Young People: A Literature Review*. Home Office Online Report 05/07. London: Home Office.

Latt N, Conigrave K, Marshall J, *et al.* (eds) (2009) *Addiction Medicine*. Oxford: Oxford University Press.

Miller WR, Sanchez VC (1993) Motivating young adults for treatment and lifestyle changes. In G Howard (ed.) *Issues in Alcohol Use and Misuse in Young Adults*. Notre Dame, IN: University of Notre Dame Press, 55–82.

Murphy R, Roe S (2007) *Drug Misuse Declared: Findings from the 2006/07 British Crime Survey*. Home Office Statistical Bulletin 18/07. London: Home Office.

Office for National Statistics and The Information Centre (2006) *Statistics on Young People and Drug Misuse: England*.

Prime Minister's Strategy Unit (2004) *Alcohol Harm Reduction Strategy for England*. London: Cabinet Office.

Prochaska JO, DiClemente CC (1984) Self change processes, self efficacy and decisional balance across five stages of smoking cessation. *Progress in Clinical and Biological Research* 156: 131–140.

Raw M, McNeill A, West R (1998) Smoking cessation guidelines for health professionals: A guide to effective smoking cessation interventions for the health care system. *Thorax* 53, Supplement 5.

Scivewright N, Parry M (2009) *Community Treatment of Drug Misuse: More than Methadone,* 2nd edition. Cambridge: Cambridge University Press.

Useful websites

Alcohol and Drug Abuse Institute: http://depts.washington.edu/adai/

Alcohol Concern: www.alcoholconcern.org.uk/

Australian Drug Information Network: http://www.adin.com.au/

Daily Dose: www.dailydose.net/

Department of Health publications: www.dh.gov.uk/en/Publicationsandstatistics/index.htm

DrinkandDrugs.net: www.drinkanddrugs.net/

Home Office: www.homeoffice.gov.uk/

National Institute for Health and Clinical Excellence: www.nice.org.uk/

National Institute on Drug Abuse (USA): www.nida.nih.gov/

National Treatment Agency for Substance Misuse: www.nta.nhs.uk/

NHS Information Centre: www.ic.nhs.uk/

National Institute on Alcohol Abuse and Alcoholism (NIAAA) (USA): www.niaaa.nih.gov/

Royal College of General Practitioners: www.rcgp.org.uk/

Royal College of Psychiatrists: www.rcpsych.ac.uk/

Scottish Intercollegiate Guidelines Network: www.sign.ac.uk/

Substance Abuse and Mental Health Services Administration (USA): www.samhsa.gov/

CASE STUDY 1

A 13-year-old girl was referred from school due to alcohol use affecting her school work and attendance. She was assessed by a substance misuse worker at school, as this was felt to be the most appropriate environment due to her age and she could be supported by people she knew. It also ensured minimal disruption to her education. The alcohol use was affecting all aspects of her life and was a result of home dynamics as well as an older boyfriend who was causing concerns. The worker continued to see her at a regular time in her timetable and brought in the support of the family therapist, who explored her relationships with others and accessed extra support for her education, as she had fallen behind. This work aimed to prevent exclusion from school and explore the reasons for her substance misuse to be able to address the underlying issues.

CASE STUDY 2

A 60-year-old man was found wandering around his local area picking up cigarette stubs and begging for money to buy alcohol. He was very dishevelled. Neighbours said that he had lost his job several months previously, because he had been drinking heavily. He had had chest pains and asthma and had been noted to have hypertension. He had not taken the treatment for his cardiovascular problems for several months. He was not eating properly and was neglecting himself. He had had a period of heavy drinking years ago, but had managed to cut down. His wife died suddenly and his social network seemed to have contracted to such an extent that he was isolated and bored, especially at the weekends. He had therefore taken to drinking regularly. On admission to a geriatric unit, he was diagnosed as having alcohol-induced dementia.

CASE STUDY 3

A 42-year-old man presented to the outpatient clinic for detoxification. He had a longstanding history of substance misuse. He had first tasted alcohol at the age of 8 years and started drinking regularly at 13 years. He had tried almost every substance, including solvents, amphetamines, ecstasy, magic mushrooms and heroin. He had been in custody for three periods because of theft, burglary and shoplifting offences, which were committed to fund the purchase of drugs or to maintain basic living needs. He had lost an eye as a result of an unprovoked attack. At the time of presentation, he was drinking alcohol, using benzodiazepines and topping up his methadone prescription with street opiates. He lived with his partner and two young children, in whose care he had a central role.

CASE STUDY 4

A specialist registrar was called to see a 49-year-old man in the surgical ward who was extremely agitated and distressed. He was attending for assessment for inpatient admission. Although he had drunk 7 pints of cheap cider that morning, he was tremulous, sweaty and confused. He did not know the date and had difficulty walking. He was depressed and said that he wanted to die. He complained of failure and guilt in relation to his children and felt hopeless about the future. He was unemployed and living alone. His blood pressure was 168/102 and his pulse rate was 100. After several hours, it became clearer that he was in severe alcohol withdrawal and so he was admitted immediately for detoxification and assessment of his mental state.

CASE STUDY 5

A 25-year-old woman presented to the accident and emergency department with cocaine misuse. Her parents, who were proud and respectable people, attended with her, having just recently found out about her habit. They were devastated, especially as her older brother had had a drug problem years ago, from which he had recovered. She complained of 'paras', i.e. thinking that people were staring at her. Her appetite and sleep were poor. She was a talented singer who had started a college course, but had had to drop out temporarily because of her drug use, though the college were prepared to keep her place. Her parents virtually placed her under house arrest so that she could not use. For 3 weeks it appeared that she was managing without drugs, but then she started to use cannabis, followed by alcohol. She then developed a full-blown amphetamine dependence, injecting several times a day and requesting needles daily. Her appearance deteriorated badly. She did not communicate well – she looked at the floor, replied in a monosyllabic manner and appeared gaunt, pale and unhappy. She said that she did not mind if she 'went over' after a binge of amphetamines. She appeared to have an insatiable desire to continue to use. She was referred to the specialist addiction service and continued to attend. Her parents thought that they could manage without any support and refused family therapy, saying 'we can manage without'. She usually attended when arranged and continued to make good progress.

CASE STUDY 6

A 16-year-old pregnant user was referred by her general practitioner, who had begun prescribing her buprenorphine. She appeared to be a nice friendly girl, who presented no particular problems. She lived with her boyfriend, who was an older, established drug user. Her supportive family did not know about her drug use. Her baby was born blind and had endocrinological problems. The client had been attending the service for 18 months and, while she appeared relatively stable on methadone, in fact she never produced a negative urine screen and her methadone gradually crept up. About 6 months later she was involved in a car accident and she continued to increase her use of heroin as well as being prescribed tramadol because of back pain resulting from the accident. She did not inform the specialist at the pain clinic that she was a drug user for fear of prejudice. She slept poorly because of the back pain, took little exercise, took comfort in eating chocolate but managed to go to physiotherapy. She attended the clinic fairly reliably and used some support for her child as well. Since her partner was a user, she was tempted to 'use on top' just a little each day and was always on the verge of feeling that she might need an increased dose of methadone. Her partner was fast-tracked for assessment and treatment and, once he was treated with a high dose of methadone, she improved.

EATING DISORDERS

John Eagles

KEY CHAPTER FEATURES

- Anorexia nervosa: prevalence, risk factors, assessment and management
- Comorbidity of anorexia
- Anorexia nervosas in children and males
- Bulimia nervosa: prevalence, risk factors, assessment and management
- Binge eating disorders

Introduction

Eating disorders have become more common during the last 50 years and they are among the most interesting illnesses encountered in clinical medicine. Their aetiology comprises a complex mix of biological, psychological and social factors, and their management is eclectic and challenging. Broadly eating disorders comprise restricting intake or binging and purging type disorders. Although there are some commonalities, they have different presentations, prognosis and management. However, both are more common in females and this may be linked to societal expectations of the ideal female body shape.

Why is this relevant for you?

General practitioners, other doctors and dentists need to be well informed and vigilant regarding the possibility of eating disorders, as their early detection is associated with a better prognosis. The physical symptoms and signs that may be present are discussed later, and sensitive exploration of these may lead to a diagnosis. Women may present with amenorrhoea and/or infertility to obstetricians and endocrinologists, and eating disorders need to be considered by these specialists. All young females are a high-risk group, and athletes, dancers and models are at very high risk. Although screening of high-risk groups may be helpful with instruments such as the SCOFF questionnaire, there is no substitute for a clinical consultation in reaching the diagnosis (see Box 11.1).

Doctors may also have a role to play in prevention which can be viewed from broad political and

Box 11.1: SCOFF screening questions

1 Do you make yourself **s**ick because you feel uncomfortably full?

2 Do you worry you have lost **c**ontrol over how much you eat?

3 Have you recently lost more than **o**ne stone in a 3-month period?

4 Do you believe yourself to be **f**at when others say you are too thin?

5 Would you say that **f**ood dominates your life?

educational perspectives, focusing on widely held dysfunctional attitudes arising from society's preoccupation with a thin body ideal. More general public education in healthy nutrition would be helpful. Educational programmes have been used to promote realism with regard to body shape ideals, to normalize peripubertal physical changes, to address low self-esteem and to inform about healthy eating patterns.

Classification and definition

The two common eating disorders are anorexia nervosa and bulimia nervosa. The typical features of both conditions will be described below and for the sake of clarity they will be regarded as neatly definable and separate illnesses. In practice, there may be considerable overlap and management will be tailored accordingly.

Other less common eating disorders will not be discussed in this chapter. Although obesity is clearly exceedingly common, and often has psychological consequences such as low self-esteem and depression, it is not regarded as a primary psychiatric disorder and will not be covered.

Anorexia nervosa

History and prevalence

William Gull is credited with the first description of anorexia nervosa in 1868. Even though Gull had described a psychogenic aetiology, psychiatrists seldom saw the condition in the nineteenth century. It is probable that the symptoms of emaciation and amenorrhoea were interpreted as reflecting somatic illnesses, and therefore patients were seen by physicians. However, notwithstanding its underdiagnosis, anorexia nervosa probably remained relatively uncommon in the first half of the twentieth century before its prevalence in Western societies began to rise in the 1960s and 1970s in tandem with increasing emphasis on the importance of a slim female body shape. The death from anorexia nervosa in 1983 of the celebrated American singer Karen Carpenter is often credited with raising awareness of eating disorders. Others in the public eye (for example Diana, Princess of Wales) subsequently acknowledged their own eating disorders, and the fact that these

illnesses were thus admitted to and detected more readily complicated studies of changing rates across time. It seems likely that anorexia nervosa continued to become more common into the 1980s, with no further increase in incidence over more recent decades.

Given the tendency of sufferers to conceal their symptoms, true prevalence rates are difficult to quote and are likely to be underestimates. In Western societies, the current prevalence rate of anorexia nervosa is estimated to be 0.3 per cent among young females. Rates among adolescents may be as high as 1 per cent.

Risk factors

Sociodemographic factors

Gender is an important risk factor, with females being around 10 times more likely than males to develop an eating disorder. The reasons for this are unclear and links have been made with evolutionary, biological, psychological and social theories of aetiology. One hypothesis was that the illness might constitute a way of avoiding adolescent changes, especially as it may prevent development of secondary sexual characteristics.

It was thought that eating disorders occurred more commonly among Caucasian girls in higher socioeconomic groups, and this was linked to the alleged causal factor of 'striving middle class parents'. These apparent ethnic and social class effects probably reflected detection biases and publications based on selected cohorts who were referred to specialist treatment centres. Ethnic and socioeconomic factors have not been confirmed by recent studies as important aetiological factors.

Theories of family pathology as causes of anorexia nervosa achieved prominence in the 1970s and 1980s. These included the ideas that anorexics were 'enmeshed' in inappropriately close relationships with parents and that they were 'triangulated' between parents who had a poor relationship, the conflicts of which were expressed in their child's illness. In these family pathology models, the child is seen as stuck and unable to exercise appropriate autonomy. However, it is problematic to regard these clinical observations of 'abnormal' families as straightforward aetiological factors, since patterns of family interactions may be results of, rather than causes of, illness in a child.

Biological factors

There is a sizeable genetic contribution to the risk of anorexia nervosa, in that a girl who has a first-degree relative with the condition is nearly 16 times more likely to develop it than a girl who does not. The genetics of bulimia nervosa appear to be rather less specific, with links to the heritability of impulsivity, mood variability and substance misuse. Genes that relate to serotonin function currently seem most likely to be implicated in the aetiology of eating disorders, and this is logical considering the close involvement of serotonergic activity in the physiology of eating and satiety.

There is some evidence for two very early biological risk factors, both similar to findings for schizophrenia, in the aetiology of anorexia nervosa. Future sufferers have experienced increased rates of pregnancy and perinatal complications and are more likely to be born in the spring and early summer, suggesting a contribution from seasonal intrauterine factors.

Despite above-average academic achievements, girls with anorexia nervosa often exhibit impaired visual memory and visuospatial skills, these deficits being independent of malnutrition. Brain imaging studies have detected abnormalities in the cingulate, frontal and temporal areas. These findings are currently inconsistent but it is possible that imaging and neuropsychological studies will elucidate specific areas of brain dysfunction in the future.

Psychological/psychiatric/medical factors

Sexual, emotional or physical abuse in childhood increases the risk of eating disorders in later life, and subsequent traumatic life events may link closely with the onset of illness. Early childhood feeding and digestive problems are predisposing factors, possibly for both psychological and biological reasons.

Excessive concerns about weight and shape, often linked to a more general negative self-evaluation, are common premorbid features. The personality factors that have been found to be the most important and consistent predisposing traits are neuroticism and obsessionality. General psychiatric morbidity, most commonly depression and anxiety, can both predispose and impact negatively upon prognosis.

Sociocultural factors

Evidence for the importance of sociocultural risk factors is more circumstantial, but striking. Although eating disorders are not unknown in developing countries, they are only common in areas of the world that have plentiful food supplies. As in the Chinese proverb 'to be fat is to be lucky', in many non-Western societies it is deemed positively desirable to be overweight. The modern 'epidemic' of eating disorders in developed countries has coincided with the emphasis upon the attractiveness of thinness in females. The increased incidence of eating disorders among models, athletes and ballerinas lends weight to social models of causality.

There has been controversy as to whether dieting itself may lead to eating disorders. However, clinical experience rather suggests that it is the reasons for dieting that are important rather than the dieting.

Presentation and assessment of anorexia

This section will focus on the typical young female patient, dealing much more briefly with the presentations seen in children and in males.

First health service contact

The first health service contact people with anorexia nervosa have is usually in primary care. This makes the role of the general practitioner pivotal in the assessment and diagnosis of eating disorders, especially since improved prognosis is associated with early detection and treatment.

Diagnosis of anorexia nervosa, and of other eating disorders, is challenging in primary care. When patients are identified by screening, research suggests that 50 per cent of such patients have gone unrecognized. A study in Glasgow found that, prior to diagnosis, females with eating disorders had consulted at an increased rate over the preceding 5 years. Presentations varied, but these women consulted particularly with gynaecological, gastrointestinal and psychological complaints. The highly differing rates at which different general practitioners refer patients with eating disorders to specialist services suggests very different levels of awareness; complaints such as menstrual abnormalities and constipation, especially when associated with weight loss or weight fluctuations, should lead to a high level of suspicion of an eating disorder.

Patients are generally ashamed and secretive, and thus may not readily disclose their symptoms. Despite this, the vast majority will divulge their symptoms, indeed they may be hugely relieved to do so, if a health professional inquires in an appropriately informed and sensitive manner.

Specialist referral

General practitioners may feel comfortable to adopt a supportive 'wait and see' approach with milder eating disorders, especially if there are adverse life circumstance that may have precipitated the problem and if they know the patient and their family. When the initial symptoms are severe, if the patient minimizes weight loss, or if symptoms are persistent, referral to specialist services is usually required, as primary care teams are unlikely to have the requisite skills for effective management of eating disorders.

Psychiatric assessment

In psychiatric practice, the assessment process frequently blurs into the start of therapy. This is particularly true of eating disorders, when the first interview usually has the purpose of assessment and of attempting to engage a (often resistant) patient in therapy. Given the patient's probable ambivalence about the issues, it is necessary for the interviewer to be sensitive, supportive and uncritical. To set the patient more at ease, it may also be helpful to make

'normalizing' statements before questions such as: 'You'll know that a lot of young people have concerns about their weight or body shape. Do you have any concerns like that?' A broad summary of a structure for the first assessment is shown in Table 11.1.

Premorbid/prodromal features

Early childhood feeding and digestive problems are often described, although these may be over-reported by way of retrospective explanation and may in part reflect difficulties in the mother–child relationship. Abuse in childhood, be it sexual, physical, emotional or a combination of these, may be elicited.

Traits of obsessionality and perfectionism are common, which may explain the finding that girls with anorexia nervosa are overachievers academically. Other symptoms of illness may also give rise to a focus on schoolwork while peers are expending more of their time and energy on relationships and other areas of normal adolescent development. Girls with anorexia nervosa frequently have low self-esteem, are overcautious and anxious, and perceive themselves as ineffective. Symptoms of anorexia can be seen as an attempt to gain control when a girl perceives her life (personally and interpersonally) as being outside her control; limiting and controlling her calorie intake and expenditure can be the one area of her life in which she feels a sense of control and effectiveness.

Table 11.1   Assessment of possible anorexia nervosa

History	Details of weight and diet history Typical current daily food and calorie intake Exercise patterns Purging activities Possible precipitating events Developmental and personal history Family history Psychiatric and medical history
Mental state examination	Note especially: attitude to food, weight and shape; mood; obsessive compulsive symptoms
Physical examination	Weight, height and body mass index (BMI) Pulse, blood pressure (sitting and standing), peripheral circulation Skin (including lanugo hair) Muscle strength
Investigations	Full blood count Urea and electrolytes, glucose, thyroid function, liver function tests ECG (if severely underweight or if hypokalaemic)

Premorbid obesity may occur in as many as one in five girls who develop anorexia nervosa. Teasing about overweight can be a precipitant, especially in the early years after puberty. Stressful life events, such as parental conflict or bereavement, may exert a particularly powerful effect.

Central features

The symptoms and signs listed in ICD-10 for the diagnosis of anorexia nervosa are summarized in Box 11.2.

Box 11.2: Summary of ICD-10 criteria for anorexia nervosa

(a) Body weight is at least 15 per cent below that expected (or failure to gain expected weight in prepubertal patients)

(b) Weight loss is self-induced by avoidance of fattening foods which may be accompanied by self-induced vomiting, purging, excessive exercise, use of appetite suppressants

(c) Body image distortion with a dread of fatness

(d) A widespread endocrine disorder manifested as amenorrhoea in females or loss of libido in males

(e) Delayed or arrested puberty occurs with prepubertal onset

---

Observable behaviour

The onset is often fairly gradual and insidious, and may be difficult to differentiate from a 'normal' diet or the desire to achieve a 'healthy lifestyle', which becomes progressively faddish. Although other measures to reduce weight are also frequently deployed (see below), reduction of food intake is almost always a core feature. Higher calorie foods are the first to be reduced or excluded from the diet, with progressive stages of dietary restrictions ensuing that may lead to vegetarianism or veganism. For example, there may be avoidance of 'fat', as fat in food is equated with bodily fat and a fear of becoming fat. Calories will usually be counted with a daily limit of less than 1000. As anorexia nervosa develops, sufferers generally become more secretive and seek to hide their problems and weight loss from family and friends. Sufferers will often try to avoid eating in company and may change their style of dress to obscure their diminishing size. These clandestine aspects of anorexia nervosa can often contribute to a delay in identification and intervention for the disorder. Eating frequently provokes obvious anxiety, the process slows significantly and watching someone with anorexia nervosa consume a meal can feel like an interminable experience.

Restricting and bingeing/purging subtype

In the restricting subtype of anorexia nervosa, weight loss derives predominantly from restriction of calorie intake. Those with the bingeing/purging subtype will have episodes of binge eating and engage in other behaviours such as self-induced vomiting and laxative misuse to help weight loss. These features occur in bulimia nervosa and will be discussed further below. Management approaches may differ according to the subtype of anorexia nervosa.

Exercise/overactivity

There is some evidence that young people who develop anorexia nervosa are not only more active than their peers during the disorder but have also engaged in more physical activity prior to its onset. The parents of children who develop anorexia nervosa also seem to be more physically active than the parents of children who do not.

Like restricted eating, exercising can be a secretive activity. Compulsive exercise appears to occur more enduringly in people with eating disorders who also have obsessional personality traits and is associated with higher levels of stress, anxiety and depression. Exercise can increase in frequency from the normal range to the point where it becomes a compulsive behaviour: the exercise schedule becomes rigid (often with detailed records), exercise takes priority over other activities and there is distress and guilt if exercise is postponed or interrupted. Unlike other exercisers, control of weight and shape is seen as a primary goal, and the degree of emotional distress experienced if exercise cannot occur is entirely disproportionate.

Psychological and social features

In more severe cases, it is often difficult to disentangle the primary psychiatric symptoms of anorexia from the secondary effects of the starvation induced by the anorexia. It may thus be helpful to consider briefly the psychological sequelae of starvation.

The psychological effect of starvation itself can be studied in such situations as famines, prisoners of war and hunger strikers. Starving people think, talk and dream progressively more about food the longer that starvation continues. This preoccupation has similarities to obsessional ruminations. Eating tends to slow in pace and people become emotionally unstable and irritable. Sex drive and social activity reduce. Sleep disturbance is common, and these symptoms can also be difficult to distinguish from those of a primary depressive disorder; the level of depressed mood has been found to correlate with the degree of weight loss in anorexia nervosa. Cognitive deficits develop, with impairment of concentration, attention and memory, factors that can complicate attempts at psychological therapies.

Early successful attempts at dieting will often elicit positive reinforcement from others and give rise to temporary feelings of achievement with improved mood and well-being. As preoccupations with food, weight and shape intensify, the 'success' with which weight loss equates battles against the 'failure' associated with weight gain. Sufferers develop a morbid fear of fatness, whereby they anticipate with dread the likelihood (as they see it) that even a small amount of high-calorie food, or an interruption to other methods of weight reduction, will render them significantly obese. This is coupled with body image distortion, so that cachectic patients can observe their starving frame in a mirror and pronounce themselves to be overweight. Although this misperception can seem to be of delusional intensity it is usually more accurately regarded as an overvalued idea. This failure to appropriately evaluate one's physique, which is not uncommon at lesser levels in 'normal' people, seems not to derive from deficits in perception but from distorted cognitive processes.

Physical symptoms and investigations

The physical symptoms and signs of restricting anorexia nervosa are discussed here. The physical complications of bingeing and purging that may occur in the bingeing/purging subtypes of anorexia nervosa are discussed later. Patients are often apprehensive and resistant about physical examination. so extra sensitivity may be required. Weight and height should be measured and body mass index (BMI, the weight in kilograms divided by the square of the height in metres) calculated. BMI can then be compared against standard values for gender and age, which can be found on widely available charts. Anorexia nervosa is characterized by a BMI of 17.5 or less; normal BMIs are in the range of 20 to 25. For younger patients growth charts are often more informative than BMIs. Other important components of a physical examination are shown in Table 11.1.

The physical consequences of restricting anorexia nervosa are summarized in Table 11.2, with the possible abnormalities that may be identified when further investigations are undertaken summarized in Table 11.3. Emaciation is a universal sign. Several of the symptoms and signs can be viewed as bodily responses to chronic low calorie intake, in effect a 'partial shutdown', notably bradycardia, hypotension, acrocyanosis, delayed gastric emptying, constipation and amenorrhoea. Patients may also complain of cold intolerance and may develop mild hypothermia. Lanugo hair is soft and downy and is seen predominantly over the face, trunk and arms. Its aetiology is unknown and one possibility is that it arises as an (ineffective) attempt at heat conservation. The mechanism whereby oedema ensues is ill

Table 11.2   Physical symptoms and signs of anorexia nervosa

System	Symptoms/signs
Skin/hair	Alopecia, lanugo hair, dry skin, acrocyanosis
Musculoskeletal	Myopathy, osteoporosis, pathological fractures
Endocrine/reproductive	Amenorrhoea, reduced fertility
Gastrointestinal	Delayed gastric emptying, constipation
Cardiovascular	Hypotension (postural and non-postural), bradycardia, palpitations, syncope
Renal	Renal calculi, oedema
Neurological	Peripheral neuropathies, seizures

Table 11.3   Abnormal investigation results in anorexia nervosa

Investigation	Findings
Electrocardiogram	Sinus bradycardia, arrhythmias, reduced voltage tracing
Haematology	Anaemia, leucopenia, bone marrow suppression
Metabolic/endocrine	Hypocalcaemia, hypokalaemia, hypoglycaemia, raised cortisol, low LH and FSH, raised growth hormone

understood and may relate to hypoproteinaemia. When women have been underweight for a protracted period, a dual-energy X-ray absorptionmetry scan of bone is usually indicated to investigate possible osteoporosis. This may help motivate therapy. For amenorrhoeic women who are concerned about their fertility, pelvic ultrasonography can be undertaken.

Psychiatric comorbidity

It can be problematic to differentiate associated symptoms of anorexia nervosa from the secondary effects of starvation. During the acute phase of anorexia nervosa, the majority of patients will also have symptoms of depression and there is an increased risk of suicide. Obsessional symptoms, often related to calorie counting or exercise, are common. When anxiety disorders occur, these are often related to situations that involve eating or loss of control over weight-reducing activities.

Anorexia nervosa in children

Rather like depression, the marked female preponderance in anorexia nervosa emerges only post-pubertally. Before puberty, girls are more often affected but boys may constitute as many as a quarter of cases. Eating disorders seem to be becoming more common in children. Although earlier menarche may contribute to younger age at onset, a larger part is probably played by concerns about weight and shape developing at a progressively early age.

Children (and early adolescents) may not present with actual weight loss but with a failure to attain expected weight gain. Puberty is usually delayed when anorexia nervosa develops at a young age, and growth retardation is common. Aetiologically, acute physical illnesses and teasing (most commonly about obesity) appear to be more important factors in young children who develop eating disorders. Symptomatically, children often describe their findings differently, depending on their stage of cognitive development, and may not be able to clearly formulate their food-related concerns. When weight loss or failure to gain weight appropriately occurs in prepubertal children, indications for concern include:

1 continued dieting after initial goals have been achieved

2 dieting and eating behaviour that gives rise to reduced social contact with friends

3 excessive exercising

4 increased unhappiness about body shape or weight as dieting continues

5 any purging activity.

Unusual 'faddy' eating is common among young children and is discussed in Chapter 14.

Anorexia nervosa in males

Without resorting to gender stereotypes, in general whereas females will express a wish to be slimmer than they are, males would prefer to be more muscular. Indeed, although males may be rather less affected by societal aspirations towards attractive body shapes (male magazines contain much less about body shape than the female equivalents, but this is changing), in adolescent boys there are clear parallels between disordered eating and the pursuit of muscularity. In terms of body image, puberty is a rather different experience for boys and girls. Girls experience an increase in body fat (distancing them from the modern 'female ideal') whereas boys become more muscular, thus bringing them closer to the 'male ideal' in body shape. There may be other factors (e.g. genetic or hormonal) that contribute to the marked sex difference between males and females, but most aetiological credence attaches to these psychosocial differences.

The presentations of males and females with

anorexia nervosa have many more similarities than differences, and only the differences will be highlighted here. Premorbidly, it is more common for males to have been athletic and the drive towards athletic excellence, through weight and shape modification, is more prevalent. Reduction in sexual drive is the symptomatic male equivalent of female amenorrhoea and this may complicate assessments of male sexuality. However, in one fairly large study over 50 per cent of males with anorexia nervosa were considered to be 'asexual'. This contrasted with bulimia nervosa in which 42 per cent of males were identified as either homosexual or bisexual. It is possible that sexual orientation is linked to differing body image aspirations. Males collectively present after a lengthier history than do females. This may reflect the traditional male reluctance to seek health care, but perhaps also suggests shame and doubt about having developed a 'female' disorder, giving an added motive for secrecy in an already clandestine disorder. Psychiatric comorbidity (notably depression, substance misuse and personality disorders) appears to be slightly commoner than among females with anorexia nervosa.

Given the relative rarity, it is difficult to know whether recent suspicions of an increase in prevalence of male eating disorders are well founded. However, given the current blurring and overlap of gender roles and the increased emphasis on physical appearance for both sexes, it would not be too surprising if there were to be a closing of the gap in prevalence between males and females in the years ahead.

Differential diagnosis

The main differential diagnoses are severe depression, obsessive compulsive disorder and atypical psychosis. Physically, other causes of weight loss in a young person – inflammatory bowel disease, chronic cardiac failure, coeliac disease, carcinoma (brain tumours can also cause disordered eating), diabetes, hyperthyroidism – should be considered. In none of these disorders will the characteristic psychopathology (the fear of becoming fat) of anorexia nervosa be present.

Sharing the diagnosis

Once diagnosis is reached, patients should be told and encouraged to become as well informed as possible about the condition. Without unnecessary scaremongering, it is helpful for women to know the current and longer term risks of unresolved anorexia nervosa, since hopefully this will help to motivate change and engagement in therapy. The relatively high mortality rates and long-term sequelae can also help to engage reluctant parents.

Management

General considerations

Most patients will initially be at best ambivalent, and often openly resistant, to changes in their eating and weight. These changes are generally not rapid and patients and relatives should know this; patients may find it reassuring and families will not expect too much progress too rapidly. Developing a collaborative and supportive ongoing relationship with a knowledgeable health professional is the first and most important step in the recovery process.

Education/dietary counselling

Management is best conducted within a multidisciplinary team and a specialist dietician will often be involved. If no dietician is available, it is important that a patient has access to appropriate, informed advice about food and nutrition to counteract possible misconceptions. It is helpful from the beginning for a patient to know what she will have to eat to gain weight steadily and to feel reassured that this will proceed at a reasonable rate but without the goal of making her 'fat'. It is usually helpful to set a target weight which would be at least 90 per cent of that expected for her age and height.

Gaining weight

Regular charting of weight is required to monitor progress, and it should be remembered that patients may 'cheat', for example by drinking water before being weighed – a pint of water weighs over a pound (approximately 500 g). Particularly with more significantly emaciated patients, there is a consensus that weight gain is required before patients have the cognitive and emotional capacity to make use of psychological approaches. A slow and steady weight gain of between 0.5 and 1.0 pounds (0.25 and 0.5 kg) per week would be a usual goal for an outpatient, whereas inpatients may be expected to gain weight a little more quickly. The medical management of the most severely malnourished patients is a specialist enterprise that is beyond the scope of this book. The main danger of unskilled management is 're-feeding syndrome' in which rapid re-feeding, especially with carbohydrates, gives rise to cardiac arrhythmias, cardiac failure and confusion, mediated principally by hypophosphataemia and hypokalaemia.

Family therapy

In the therapy of anorexia nervosa, as the 2004 National Institute for Health and Clinical Excellence guidelines on eating disorders say: 'it is now widely agreed that family interventions are best viewed as treatments that mobilise family resources rather than treating family dysfunction'. For younger patients, there is evidence that family approaches are effective and preferable to individual therapy, although the latter has use as an adjunct therapy. In the context of a supportive and educational approach, parents will be encouraged to take a joint, firm and consistent approach with their child's eating. It will usually be helpful to promote open communication within the family, and to help the parents to acquire control over their daughter's health.

Individual therapies

An individual approach is usually adopted with older patients. Common elements of this treatment will include support, education and nutritional advice. There is minimal evidence for the effectiveness of any particular approach. Therapy needs to be tailored to the individual's needs. For example, a patient's distorted perceptions of herself and her shape might be tackled with cognitive behavioural therapy (CBT), whereas emotional and relationship difficulties might be approached with techniques relating to interpersonal therapy.

Medication

Medication, such as an SSRI antidepressant, will quite often be used for psychiatric comorbidity such as depression or anxiety. There is little evidence of efficacy of medication for the treatment of anorexia itself.

Admission to hospital

The large majority of patients with anorexia nervosa will be treated as outpatients, especially since admission will separate patients from family and friends and interrupt their work or studies. The following factors, however, may indicate the need for admission:

1 severe weight loss (<75 per cent of expected BMI)
2 suicidal acts or plan
3 rapid worsening during outpatient treatment
4 poor motivation and insight
5 significant medical complications (e.g. hypokalaemia, dehydration, hypotension).

Day patient treatment ('partial hospitalization') may constitute a compromise between the benefits of admission and remaining at home.

Compulsory treatment

The need for compulsory treatment is rare, but may be necessary if the alternative is that the patient is likely to die. Resistance to treatment is common. To enforce the Mental Health Act, it needs to be clear that the patient is absolutely refusing treatment or is so ill that consent is not feasible. Patients in this category may be so severely physically ill that they are initially managed on a general medical ward and may require nasogastric feeding.

Outcome in anorexia nervosa

Among psychiatric disorders, anorexia nervosa has the highest mortality and one of the poorest prognoses. The risk of premature death in women with anorexia nervosa is increased by a factor of about 6 in patients who are severe enough to require inpatient care with an equivalent figure of 3 for all patients presenting to secondary care services. In the acute stages, the highest risk of death is from cardiovascular causes, notably when there is a bingeing/purging pattern. Increased mortality rates endure for at least 20 years after diagnosis from causes related to chronic malnutrition. Suicide rates are elevated throughout this period.

Just less than half of patients make a full recovery, about one-third improve but remain symptomatic to some degree while 20 per cent remain chronically ill. Poorer prognosis has been associated with comorbid psychiatric problems (depression, anxiety and obsessive compulsive personality features) and with specific symptoms (bulimia, vomiting and laxative abuse). Good prognostic factors include early detection and treatment and, for hospitalized patients, initial length of admission; this may attest to engagement in treatment, however, rather than to the efficacy of inpatient treatment *per se*. Patients who have recovered describe the importance of supportive non-familial relationships, therapy and maturation.

Bulimia nervosa

Bulimia nervosa shares many features with anorexia nervosa that have been described above. It is also a less serious condition in terms of physical health.

History and prevalence

The term 'bulimia' derives from the Greek and means the hunger of an ox. Although the practice of eating large amounts of food and vomiting thereafter dates back for thousands of years, and there were a few isolated cases described previously in the medical literature, the syndrome of bulimia nervosa was first described by Gerald Russell in 1979. During the last three decades, prevalence appears to have increased in Western societies but this may be related to improved awareness and willingness to present for treatment. The estimated prevalence is 1 per cent among young females but this may be a significant underestimate.

Risk factors

The risk factors for bulimia nervosa are very similar to those for anorexia nervosa, and the few differences will be mentioned below. Around 40 per cent of people with bulimia nervosa have experienced a previous episode of anorexia nervosa, which may have been brief or subclinical. A history of weight loss prior to the onset of bulimia is extremely common and dieting is an important aetiological factor. The huge increase in prevalence since the 1970s points strongly to the important causal factor of cultural pressures to be slim and to control eating and weight.

In childhood, traumatic events and abuse (sexual, emotional or physical) occur with increased frequency. Parental obesity is common, and this seems to be at least partly a genetic predisposition. Families of bulimic patients have increased rates not only of eating disorders, but also of depression, alcohol dependence and drug misuse. Serotonin dysregulation seems to play an aetiological role in that even after recovery from bulimia there is reduced serotonin receptor binding and diminished platelet–paroxetine binding.

Presentation, assessment and diagnosis

As with anorexia nervosa, females are about 10 times more likely than males to develop bulimia. It is exceedingly rare in childhood and the average age at onset is around 19 years, rather later than that for anorexia nervosa. The majority of patients with bulimia nervosa will be assessed and managed in primary care settings. As most are of normal weight, relevant questions may not be asked and the disorder remains undiagnosed. Given the high prevalence of bulimia nervosa, the condition should be suspected for younger women who present with any of the physical complaints/signs listed in Table 11.4 or with any of the psychiatric comorbidities mentioned below.

Psychiatric comorbidity

Depression of mood and anxiety occur with marked frequency, and not only as consequences of the bulimia itself. Of the specific anxiety disorders,

Table 11.4   Physical symptoms and signs in bulimia nervosa resulting from bingeing, vomiting and purging

System	Symptoms/signs
Gastrointestinal	Dental erosion, salivary gland hypertrophy, oesophageal tears/bleeding, abdominal distension, constipation, raised serum amylase
Renal	Oedema, electrolyte abnormalities (hypokalaemia, hyponatraemia), dehydration
Cardiovascular	Arrhythmias, sudden death
Neurological	Seizures, peripheral neuropathies, tetany

social phobia and obsessive compulsive disorder are the most common. Alcohol misuse is common, significantly more so than in anorexia nervosa. In bulimia nervosa, impulsivity is a common personality trait and is associated with raised rates of overdoses, other self-harming behaviours and promiscuity. There is an association with 'impulsive' personality disorders, notably with emotionally unstable/borderline personality.

Clinical features

The symptoms and signs of bulimia nervosa can occur as part of the clinical picture in the bingeing/purging subtype of anorexia nervosa. The major difference between these diagnostic groups is that patients with bulimia nervosa do not have a significantly low BMI or stunted growth.

ICD-10 criteria for the diagnosis of bulimia nervosa are summarized in Box 11.3. DSM-IV criteria also list exercise as a 'compensatory behaviour' and specify that both binge eating and the compensatory behaviours must occur on average at least twice per week over a period of at least 3 months.

Binge eating entails the consumption of an excessive quantity of food, usually over a period of less than 2 hours, coupled with a subjective feeling of loss of control. Foods consumed are usually high in calorie content, notably carbohydrates and chocolate. Several thousand calories may be consumed in a typical binge, and these will occur more days than not for the majority of people with bulimia nervosa.

Binges may, initially and transiently, provide relief from feelings of tension, anxiety and low mood. However, this quickly gives way to feelings of disgust and guilt. Sufferers, therefore, do their best to keep their behaviour secret; many will do this successfully,

---

Box 11.3: Summary of ICD-10 criteria for bulimia nervosa

A preoccupation with eating and a craving for food gives rise to episodes of binge eating

Patients attempt to counteract the fattening effects of food by self-induced vomiting and/or laxative abuse and/or alternating periods of starvation and/or medication (e.g. appetite suppressants, thyroid preparations, diuretics)

There is a morbid dread of fatness and a strong desire to be unhealthily thin

---

leading to underestimates of prevalence and often lengthy delays in receiving treatment, if indeed treatment is ever received at all.

Of the compensating behaviours to attempt to avoid weight gain, self-induced vomiting is the most common (induced by putting their fingers down their throats). Laxative misuse is the next most common strategy. Especially in tandem, vomiting and laxative misuse can give rise to dangerous hypokalaemia. Measures of the severity of an eating disorder correlate quite highly with the number of different compensatory behaviours that a patient deploys.

The characteristic psychopathology is very similar to that in anorexia nervosa. Patients are preoccupied with shape and weight and are usually aspiring to a low (usually inappropriately low) target weight. Unlike anorexics, patients with bulimia nervosa repeatedly 'fail' in their attempts to 'over-diet', lowering mood and self-esteem further and often forming something of a vicious circle with the bingeing/purging behaviour, which has the same effects.

Physical symptoms, signs and complications

The symptoms and signs specific to bulimia nervosa are those of bingeing and purging, and these are summarized in Table 11.4. Screening for electrolyte abnormalities (notably hypokalaemia) is the most important investigation.

Erosion of dental enamel from the repeated flow of gastric acid over the teeth can be striking, and dentists can assist in the diagnosis of eating disorders when they observe this sign. Painless swelling of the salivary glands, notably the parotids, can give rise to a characteristic 'hamster'-like appearance, and again this can be a helpful diagnostic clue.

People with bulimia nervosa eat more and recognize satiety less readily than control subjects and this may at least partly be a gastrointestinal effect. It has been found in bulimia that there is an enlarged gastric capacity, delayed gastric emptying and a low postprandial release of cholecystokinin.

Differential diagnosis

When depression co-exists, it may be necessary to unravel which disorder was primary, since this will guide treatment. Upper gastrointestinal disorders can give rise to recurrent vomiting, and pathology in the brain's frontal lobes can cause disordered, disinhibited eating, but neither is associated with the characteristic psychopathology of bulimia nervosa.

Management

Management starts by attempting to engage the patient in motivation to change during the assessment interview. There may be major concerns about losing control over weight and shape, but these are generally less than for patients with anorexia nervosa. In part, this has made it easier to engage bulimia nervosa patients in controlled trials and the evidence for the efficacy of treatment is significantly stronger.

Patients frequently present with mixed features of anorexia and bulimia nervosa, without being strictly classifiable into either category (diagnosed as 'Eating Disorder Not Otherwise Specified' – EDNOS in the US classification system). Patients with EDNOS with BMIs above 17.5 tend to respond well to approaches used for bulimia.

Psychological approaches

There is strong evidence for the effectiveness of CBT in reducing both bingeing and purging behaviours. Irrational feelings and beliefs about shape, weight and eating are elicited and challenged, in tandem with an educational approach. Behaviours such as vomiting and laxative misuse are addressed, for example by encouraging patients to eat gradually larger amounts of food without vomiting. Fifteen to 20 sessions, individually or in groups, are usually required.

Self-help approaches are often used for milder cases, and sometimes as the first step in a tiered treatment approach. These can be delivered either by books or online, and have a strong educational component. This will include highlighting the ineffectiveness of both vomiting and laxatives as weight control measures, and the way in which vicious circles are generated by bingeing and purging, both physiologically and psychologically. Self-help programmes have been shown to afford greater benefit for people with bulimia nervosa than remaining on a waiting list.

Pharmacological treatment

Although CBT is regarded as the treatment of choice, antidepressants are often prescribed as a first line of treatment, particularly at the time of first diagnosis in primary care. Fluoxetine has the best evidence of efficacy, and is effective in reducing binge frequency irrespective of whether the patient is also depressed. Higher doses are usually needed than for the treatment of depression. While CBT has been shown to improve long-term outcome, the effect of fluoxetine has only been demonstrated in the shorter term. In more severe cases, the two are often used together.

Outcome in bulimia nervosa

In 1997 Keel and Mitchell reviewed studies that aggregated more than 2000 women with bulimia nervosa. There was no increase in premature mortality. At 5–10 years' follow-up, 50 per cent had fully recovered, 30 per cent had recovered partially and 20 per cent were little changed. Severe symptoms, psychiatric comorbidity and impulsivity appear to be associated with a poorer prognosis.

Binge eating disorder

Binge eating disorder can be viewed as a milder form of bulimia nervosa. The symptoms comprise bulimia nervosa without purging or other compensatory behaviours. Binge eating disorder is relatively more common in males, with a female preponderance of only about 2 to 1. It often has an onset at a later age, and the onset is more likely to be stress induced. Sufferers are often overweight, and perhaps the main reason for attempting to differentiate it from 'ordinary' obesity relates to its treatability. Binge eating disorder has been found to respond to self-help interventions (as described for bulimia nervosa), to antidepressants (certainly in short-term trials) and to CBT. Management will usually be in primary care where a staged approach is appropriate, starting with self-help, moving on to SSRI antidepressants and then to CBT if necessary.

Summary

Some of the key points about eating disorders can be summarized as follows:

- anorexia nervosa is often a life-threatening condition;
- eating disorders are common, underdetected and undertreated;
- early treatment is associated with a better prognosis;
- there are significant and wide-ranging physical complications;

- the diagnosis hinges on a sensitive interview and a good mental state examination;
- the management of anorexia nervosa is essentially psychotherapeutic and eclectic;
- the management of choice in bulimia nervosa is cognitive behavioural therapy;
- much more could be done in the early detection and prevention of eating disorders.

Further reading

Berger U, Sowa M, Bormann B, *et al*. (2008) Primary prevention of eating disorders: characteristics of effective programmes and how to bring them to broader dissemination. *European Eating Disorders* 16: 173–183.

Carlat DJ, Camargo CA, Herzog DB (1997) Eating disorders in males: a report on 135 patients. *American Journal of Psychiatry* 154: 1127–1132.

Gorwood P, Kipman A, Foulon C (2003) The human genetics of anorexia nervosa. *European Journal of Pharmacology* 480: 163–170.

Hoek HW (2006) Incidence, prevalence and mortality of anorexia nervosa and other eating disorders. *Current Opinion in Psychiatry* 19: 389–394.

Keel PK, Mitchell JE (1997) Outcome in bulimia nervosa. *American Journal of Psychiatry* 154: 313–321.

Millar HR, Wardell F, Vyvyan JP, *et al*. (2005). Anorexia nervosa mortality in Northeast Scotland, 1965-1999. *American Journal of Psychiatry* 162: 753–757.

National Institute for Clinical Excellence (2004) Eating disorders: core interventions in the treatment and management of anorexia nervosa, bulimia nervosa and related eating disorders. www.nice.org.uk/nicemedia/pdf/cg009niceguidance.pdf.

Ogg EC, Millar HR, Pusztai EE, Thom AS (1997) General practice consultation patterns preceding diagnosis of eating disorders. *International Journal of Eating Disorders* 22: 89–93.

Papadopoulos FC, Ekbom A, Brandt L, Ekselius L (2009) Excess mortality, causes of death and prognostic factors in anorexia nervosa. *British Journal of Psychiatry* 194: 10–17.

Ricciardelli LA, McCabe MP (2004) A biopsychosocial model of disordered eating and the pursuit of muscularity in adolescent boys. *Psychological Bulletin* 130: 179–205.

Tozzi F, Sullivan PF, Fear JL, *et al*. (2003) Causes and recovery in anorexia nervosa: the patient's perspective. *International Journal of Eating Disorders* 33: 143–154.

CASE STUDY 1

Adeline had been a shy young child who was lacking in confidence. At primary school she started to become overweight, and on going to secondary school at the age of 11 she was teased about her weight. After her periods started at the age of 13 years she began to become especially conscious of her body shape. She decided to eat a bit less and surprised herself when she took up running to find that she was good at this, getting into the school cross country team. Gradually, she became more preoccupied with restricting calories and she told her family she had become a vegetarian. By the age of 16 she continued to diet and to exercise excessively, her mother noticed that she was pathologically thin, and took her to their general practitioner.

As the family general practitioner, on which areas of her history and mental state would you focus?

You would inquire sensitively about: timescale and degree of weight loss, feelings about her weight and shape, what she eats at present, current exercise and activity, her menstrual history, whether she binges and/or vomits, whether she takes laxatives and whether there is associated psychopathology such as depression/anxiety.

Would you conduct any investigations at this stage?

It is very important to establish weight and height and thus to get a baseline BMI.

The necessity for other investigations (see Tables) will depend on severity, but if she gives a history of vomiting it is advisable to screen for hypokalaemia.

How would you decide whether you would refer her to psychiatric services?

Since Adeline has a 3-year history and she is currently very thin, it is highly likely that you would refer her. In general, milder and less enduring cases would be those that might not be referred to psychiatry.

CASE STUDY

Sally was an outgoing but unhappy child. As a teenager, she was particularly moody and volatile, these traits being exacerbated by her parents' divorce. On going away to university, she felt low and lonely. After a spell of comfort eating and weight gain, she dieted and lost weight rapidly. She could not sustain the diet and started to binge eat (usually on bread and biscuits) with self-induced vomiting thereafter. After 6 months her bingeing and vomiting was occurring daily, it became apparent to her flatmates and they persuaded her to visit her general practitioner. When she sees you (her general practitioner) she tends to minimize the importance of her symptoms.

How would you explore the impact of her bulimia on her quality of life?

The areas you cover would probably comprise: the frequency of her bingeing and vomiting, the degree of preoccupation with issues relating to body shape/weight and eating, the effect of symptoms upon her social life, her relationships, her self-esteem, her studies and her finances.

She agrees that her symptoms are having a huge effect on her life. How might you discuss the management options with her?

It will be helpful to emphasize that the medium term prognosis is positive with appropriate treatment.

You would discuss the possibility of prescribing fluoxetine as a measure, which may provide some symptom control.

You would tell her that psychological therapy (CBT) is the usual first choice; given the severity of her symptoms, specialist referral would be preferable to self-help approaches.

ORGANIC DISORDERS

Simon Budd

KEY CHAPTER FEATURES

- Definition of organic disorders
- Dementia and delirium
- Assessment, diagnosis and management of organic disorders

Introduction

Organic disorders are those disorders that have an underlying physical or pathological cause. This commonly means medical, neurodegenerative or drug-related disorders (excluding those related to substance misuse). Disorders where there is no currently understood pathophysiological cause are often called functional disorders. A wide range of physical conditions can present with or cause psychiatric symptoms or syndromes. Details of some of these are given in Table 12.1. This is not exhaustive and only describes psychiatric presentations.

Exercise

What do you understand as the differences between dementia and delirium?

Why is this relevant to you?

The two commonest organic disorders and the focus of this chapter are dementia and delirium. These are the conditions you are most likely to come across in

both general medicine and psychiatry, as well as in the general hospital setting, where you are likely to spend time as a foundation level doctor. They are mainly disorders of older people, but both are well recognized in younger age groups, especially delirium which is common in children. Dementia and delirium significantly affect outcomes, increase mortality both in hospital and after, and increase associated morbidity, independent of other risk factors (Fig. 12.1). Given the increasing ageing population and especially the ageing hospital population, all doctors need to have a basic understanding of these disorders and their management. This is particularly relevant when one considers the comorbidity that elderly patients may have and their increased vulnerability to delirium.

Classification of organic disorders

Organic disorders can be classified using the World Health Organization *International Classification of Disease*, 10th Edition (ICD-10) (Box 12.1). It is important to remember that there may be an organic or underlying biological cause for a patient's psychiatric symptoms. Although it may appear as though psychiatrists do not manage most organic disorders,

Table 12.1   Organic conditions and their psychiatric presentations

Condition	Psychiatric symptoms	Further details
Cerebral lesions		
Stroke	Depression, emotional liability, personality changes, behavioural problems, dementia	High incidence of depression in first year, atypical presentations, affects rehabilitation
Cerebral tumours	Local effects may depend upon site of lesion, e.g. occipital may give rise to visual hallucinations, frontal to behavioural changes, hypomania, depression. Distant effects include depression	Also adjustment disorder and depression linked to the diagnosis
Epilepsy	Auras, hallucinations and other disorders of perception, *déjà/jamais vu* experiences, psychosis, neurotic disorders	Temporal lobe epilepsy: schizophrenia-like psychosis. Increased risk of suicide
Head injury	Amnesia, behavioural disturbances, cognitive impairment	Outcome dependent on extent of trauma, loss of consciousness and length of post-traumatic anterograde and retrograde amnesia
Metabolic		
Porphyria	Emotional disturbance and lability, delirium, depression, panic or anxiety episodes, psychotic episodes	Acute intermittent type
Hypercalcaemia	Depression fatigue and low energy, irritability, cognitive slowing	
Uraemia/renal failure	Depression, memory problems, delirium (~33 per cent), psychosis	
Endocrine		
Cushing's disease	Weight gain, depression, psychosis, insomnia, loss of libido	
Addison's disease	Depression, apathy, tiredness, weight loss, anorexia, mild cognitive impairment	
Hypothyroidism	Depression, mania, schizophrenic-like psychosis, cognitive slowing, dementia, ataxia, anorexia, weight gain, depressed mood or psychotic symptoms, loss of libido, poor memory	'Myxoedema madness'
Hyperthyroidism	Weight loss, increased appetite, anxiety, psychosis, irritability, loss of libido, restlessness, weakness	
Hypokalaemia	Depression, sleep disturbances	
Hypoparathyroid	Delirium, agitation, anxiety, depression, cognitive impairment, irritability, emotional lability, psychosis (rare)	
Hyperparathyroid	Depression, fatigue and low energy, irritability, cognitive slowing, dementia	
Phaeochromocytoma	Anxiety or panic	Episodic, associated with hypertension

Box 12.1: ICD-10 Categories of organic disorder (WHO, 2009)

F00 Dementia in Alzheimer's disease

F00.0 Dementia in Alzheimer's disease with early onset

F00.1 Dementia in Alzheimer's disease with late onset

F00.2 Dementia in Alzheimer's disease, atypical or mixed type

F00.9 Dementia in Alzheimer's disease, unspecified

F01 Vascular dementia

F01.0 Vascular dementia of acute onset

F01.1 Multi-infarct dementia

F01.2 Sub-cortical vascular dementia

F01.3 Mixed cortical and sub-cortical vascular dementia

F01.8 Other vascular dementia

F01.9 Vascular dementia, unspecified

F02 Dementia in other diseases classified elsewhere

F02.0 Dementia in Pick's disease

F02.1 Dementia in Creutzfeldt–Jakob disease

F02.2 Dementia in Huntington's disease

F02.3 Dementia in Parkinson's disease

F02.4 Dementia in human immunodeficiency virus [HIV] disease

F02.8 Dementia in other specified diseases classified elsewhere

F03 Unspecified dementia

F04 Organic amnesic syndrome, not induced by alcohol and other psychoactive substances

F05 Delirium, not induced by alcohol and other psychoactive substances

F05.0 Delirium not superimposed on dementia, so described

F05.1 Delirium superimposed on dementia

F05.8 Other delirium

F05.9 Delirium, unspecified

F06 Other mental disorders due to brain damage and dysfunction and to physical disease

F06.0 Organic hallucinosis

F06.1 Organic catatonic disorder

Box 12.1 – continued

F06.2 Organic delusional [schizophrenia-like] disorder

F06.3 Organic mood [affective] disorders

F06.4 Organic anxiety disorder

F06.5 Organic dissociative disorder

F06.6 Organic emotionally labile [asthenic] disorder

F06.7 Mild cognitive disorder

F06.8 Other specified mental disorders due to brain damage and dysfunction and to physical disease

F06.9 Unspecified mental disorder due to brain damage and dysfunction and to physical disease

F07 Personality and behavioural disorders due to brain disease, damage and dysfunction

F07.0 Organic personality disorder

F07.1 Post-encephalitic syndrome

F07.2 Post-concussional syndrome

F07.8 Other organic personality and behavioural disorders due to brain disease, damage and dysfunction

F07.9 Unspecified organic personality and behavioural disorder due to brain disease, damage and dysfunction

F09 Unspecified organic or symptomatic mental disorder

these are always important to consider as part of the differential diagnoses. All patients presenting with psychiatric symptoms should be screened for physical disorders, using physical examination and appropriate blood tests. This is particularly the case in older people where comorbid physical disorders may cause existing psychiatric conditions to deteriorate or lead to a psychiatric condition. For example, the chronic pain of arthritis may exacerbate or lead to depression and even attempted suicide; hypertension and hypercholesterolaemia need treatment to reduce the risk of stroke disease, which is linked to depression and vascular dementia. In younger patients psychotic symptoms may be related to space occupying lesions in the brain or metabolic disorders, e.g. porphyria (as in the case of King George III).

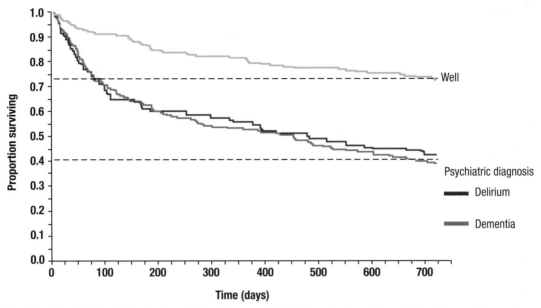

Fig. 12.1 Survival after hip fracture in patients with no psychiatric diagnosis, dementia or delirium. Those with organic disorders have a significantly reduced two year survival rate when corrected for other confounding factors (after Nightingale *et al.*, Psychiatric illness and mortality after hip fracture. *Lancet.* 2001; 357: 1264–5).

Dementia

Dementia is defined as a syndrome due to disease of the brain that is chronic or progressive in nature, and involves disturbances in multiple higher cortical functions in the absence of clouding of consciousness. It may be accompanied by deterioration in emotional control, social behaviour or motivation. Although it often presents with memory loss, it also impairs cognitive functioning, leading to dysfunction in daily living for over 6 months. It is a common disorder, with an estimated current number of sufferers at about 820 000 in the UK, a number projected to increase to 1 000 000 by 2012. This number will continue to increase as the proportion of the population over 65 years old continues to expand. The prevalence of dementia increases with age. Different studies have found varying levels of prevalence, and prevalence doubles every 5 years. The rates at 65–70 years are about 1 per cent, increasing to about 10 per cent in those aged 80–85 years and then to 25 per cent in those aged 85–90 years. In the over-nineties, the rates are 30–40 per cent (Fig. 12.2).

There are many causes of dementia, some common and some rare (Table 12.2). The actual prevalence of specific causes is difficult to determine, as, despite international criteria, the prevalence varies from study to study depending upon the techniques used to determine cases and the populations studied. It is generally accepted that Alzheimer's disease is the most common type, affecting more than 50 per cent of patients with dementia . Patients may also present with symptoms and/or signs typical of dementia but investigation reveals that they are suffering from severe depression or other treatable disorder. Such "treatable causes of dementia" are discussed further later.

Classification

Dementias can be divided into two main groups, the primary degenerative dementias (including Alzheimer's disease, Lewy body dementia and fronto-temporal dementia) and secondary (including vascular dementia).

Another division sometimes used is between cortical and subcortical dementias, referring to the primary area of the brain affected by the pathology. However, because of the multiplicity of intracerebral connections this should not be considered the only region affected. Cortical dementias include Alzheimer's disease, and are characterized by amnesia, dysphasia, apraxia and agnosia. Subcortical

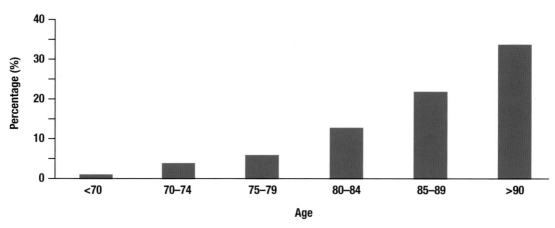

Fig. 12.2   Prevalence of dementia with age.

Table 12.2   Causes of dementia

Primary/ degenerative	Alzheimer's disease (50 per cent), vascular dementia (20–25 per cent with some regional variations, e.g. up to 50 per cent in Japan), Lewy body dementia (10–15 per cent) Frontotemporal dementia (about 5 per cent), Huntington's disease, Parkinson's disease, progressive supranuclear palsy
Tumours	Cerebral tumours, remote effects of carcinoma, lymphomas
Trauma	Infection, subdural haematoma, dementia pugilistica, post severe head injury
Infection	Neurosyphilis (including general paresis), Creutzfeldt–Jakob disease, other prion diseases (e.g. kuru), HIV-associated dementia, chronic infection with tuberculosis or fungi, post severe meningitis, progressive multifocal leucoencephalopathy, chronic rubella encephalitis
Neurological	Communicating and non-communicating hydrocephalus, progressive myoclonic epilepsy, neuroacanthocytosis, cranial arteritis, subacute sclerosing panencephalitis, motor neurone disease, multiple sclerosis, cerebellar ataxias, limbic encephalomyelitis, 'epileptic dementia', Steele–Richardson–Olszewski syndrome
Metabolic	Renal failure, dialysis dementia, hepatic encephalopathy, inborn errors of metabolism, Wilson's disease, lysosomal storage diseases
Endocrine	Myxoedema, Addison's disease, hypo/hyperthyroidism, hyper/hypoparathyroidism, Cushing's syndrome, hypopituitarism, hypoglycaemia
Toxins	Alcoholic dementia (including Korsakoff's syndrome), chronic drug usage, heavy metal poisoning, industrial agents (e.g. toluene), carbon monoxide
Anoxic	Anaemia, congestive cardiac failure, chronic pulmonary disease, post cardiac arrest
Systemic	Vitamin deficiency (B12, thiamine, nicotinic acid), folic acid deficiency, porphyria, Whipple's disease, systemic lupus erythematosus, sarcoidosis, xeroderma pigmentosum

dementias, including Huntington's disease, dementia due to Parkinson's disease, vitamin deficiencies, infections and metabolic states, are characterized by slowed cognition, slowed motor symptoms, memory impairments and changes in personality and mood. It should, however, be stressed that the most common form of dementia in the elderly is a mixed type with features of Alzheimer's and other types.

Alzheimer's disease

Risk factors

The biggest risk factor for Alzheimer's disease (AD) is age. The risk to first-degree relatives of patients with AD who developed the disorder at any time up to the age of 85 years is increased some threefold to fourfold relative to the risk in controls with no family history. People with Down syndrome will develop Alzheimer changes in the brain by the age of 40 years. A history of cardiovascular disease, Parkinson's disease, hypothyroidism or significant head injury also increases the risk. AD is equally common in males and females. In the vast majority of cases, even when there is a family history of AD, the risk to other family members cannot be accurately determined.

A known genetic risk factor is inheritance of the E4 allele of the apolipoprotein E gene. Among patients with AD, around 40–80% have at least one APOE4 allele. Heterozygosity for this allele increases the risk of AD by a factor of three and homozygosity increases it by a factor of fifteen. Around 0.1% of cases arise as an autosomal dominant familial AD due to inheritance of mutations in genes relating to amyloid precursor protein (APP) and presenilins 1 and 2.

Pathology

The principal pathology found at microscopic level has been known for many years. Senile plaques (SPs) are found extracellularly in cerebral cortical grey matter, hippocampus and certain subcortical nuclei. Neurofibrillary tangles (NFT) are found intracellularly, particularly in the hippocampus and cerebral cortex. Amyloid deposits may be found in leptomeningeal and cortical blood vessel walls. These findings are associated with cell loss, often of 30% or more, and reduced synapses. The extent of cell loss, SP counts and NFT counts correlates with the degree of dementia. Macroscopically, there is reduced brain volume and weight and generalized atrophy (greater than that expected for normal ageing), often more prominent in the medial temporal lobe and parietal lobes, along with enlarged ventricles, all of which may be evident on computed tomography (CT) or magnetic resonance imaging (MRI) scans as well as at post-mortem (Fig. 12.3).

The underlying biochemical pathology is complex and not yet fully understood. The SPs are made up of deposits of beta amyloid (Aβ). Aβ comes from amyloid precursor protein (APP) which seems to be metabolized differently in patients with AD. The aggregation of Aβ appears to damage the neurones though the final SP itself is relatively inert and acts only as a marker of the disease process. Abnormal phosphorylation of tau protein results in damage to the intracellular microtubules that are essential to intracellular transport. This results in formation of the NFTs.

The synaptic damage resulting from the above pathology results in deficits in function of a number of neurotransmitter systems, including acetylcholine,

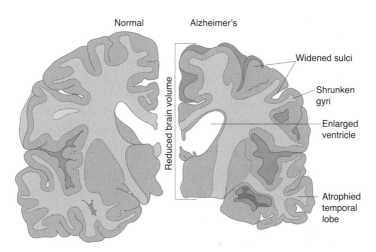

Fig. 12.3   Diagram showing differences between normal brain (left) and Alzheimer's disease affected brain, with atrophy, wide sulci, narrow gyri and enlarged ventricles (right).

noradrenalin, serotonin and dopamine. The cholinergic deficits, particularly those arising from the basal forebrain nuclei, are important in relation to the cognitive deficits as these nuclei project widely to the cerebral cortex and to the hippocampus, which is important in memory processes. Cholinergic neurones are lost, there is depletion of acetylcholine, nicotinic receptors are depleted and, late on, muscarinic receptors become depleted. This provides the theoretical basis for the only available pharmacological treatments, the cholinesterase inhibitors. These drugs principally inhibit the enzyme that inactivates acetylcholine in the synapse.

Presentation

Most commonly, this is seen in community settings and characteristically is slow and gradual. Memory problems and changes in behaviour are most often noted by carers or family rather than the patient. This will often initially be explained as normal ageing. In Alzheimer's disease, the onset is insidious, so that the disease process is well established and the problems can be significant by the time of presentation to health care services. Deterioration in self-care and repetitive phone calls, episodes of wandering, missed appointments, dangerous lapses of memory, getting lost and failure to learn new routines or other important information can also lead to presentation to services. Some patients will present themselves, especially those of higher premorbid intellectual abilities who may notice that their memory or other cognitive skills are deteriorating. Even in the early stages, patients often have little insight into their difficulties, minimize their difficulties or attribute the changes to ageing.

There is a slow intellectual decline in the early stages of the disease, with behaviour and general functioning within normal limits. The initial stages can last from 2 to 5 years, and patients may develop coping strategies to cover their deficits.

In Alzheimer's the main symptoms can be divided into five symptom areas or 'the five As of Alzheimer's':

- Amnesia
- Agnosia
- Aphasia
- Apraxia
- Associated behaviours.

Amnesia

The amnesia or memory decline in Alzheimer's is typically slow but progressive, with forgetfulness and the failure to retain newly learned information. Short-term memory is affected at first, and relatives will often report that patients ask the same question repeatedly, or need to be told the same piece of information repeatedly. Recent events or important dates are forgotten and items, such as bank cards or keys, can be misplaced. They find they cannot retrace their steps to relocate the misplaced object or recall information at all, even with prompts.

Patients have difficulties laying down new memories and retrieving older ones. They will adopt strategies to aid memory function, such as writing things down, or getting family members to help out with tasks that they could manage previously. As the dementia progresses, the misplacing of items can lead to the patient accusing people of stealing their belongings.

Initially distant memories are preserved, so they can give full details about their early life, but as the disorder progresses their long-term memories become fewer and confused, e.g. they may mix up children and grandchildren. They may begin to live in the past and may believe that their parents are still alive (occasionally this may be true, hence the importance of informant histories!). The patient may learn to confabulate to fill the gaps, but some of the confabulations may be true memories. They may try to go to work, despite having retired many years previously, or set the table for deceased family members.

The patient becomes disorientated, usually initially in time, losing track of dates and days, progressing to the season and years. They may even lose day–night awareness. The disorientation progresses to disorientation in place, so they may not recognize clinics or hospitals. They can lose awareness of their surroundings and this may progress to a state where patients no longer recognize their own home (although they may recognize where they used to live) or local environment, which can lead to wandering. If they go out, they may need to be helped home, as they lose track of where they are and what they are doing. Disorientation in person tends to deteriorate later than in time. Orientation in age tends to be lost early on.

Agnosia

Agnosia is the inability to recognize external sensory stimuli in any modality correctly, with relatively intact sensory pathways, which is displayed as the inability to recognize objects and people. Initially, this may be an inability to be able to put names to faces, but may deteriorate to not recognizing family members, or even spouses. They may believe that the other person is an intruder and this can occasionally lead to the patient attacking the carer. Patients may not even recognize themselves, which can lead to 'the mirror sign', where sufferers see their reflection in a mirror and will talk to it as if it is another real person. They may not recognize everyday objects, which can lead to abnormal behaviour, such as urinating in a waste paper basket, believing it to be a toilet bowl. This is exacerbated by the general decline with age of the senses, especially vision and hearing.

Apraxia

Apraxia is the decreasing ability to perform coordinated motor tasks, with an intact peripheral neuromuscular system, which begins to develop as the dementia becomes moderately severe. This causes problems with activities of daily living, such as difficulties with dressing, and may result in problems with writing and other tasks (usually in neuropsychological tests) as ideational apraxia develops (this is the loss of ability to conceptualize, plan and execute the complex sequence of motor actions involving the use of tools or objects in everyday life). Significant problems arise when the patient can no longer perform important tasks, such as using cutlery or providing themselves with food or drink.

Aphasia

Strictly speaking, aphasia does not occur until late in the dementia, and rather patients have dysphasias. In the early stages, they may have difficulty in participating in conversations because they have difficulty following the thread, or may find that they get stuck and do not know how to continue. The patient's vocabulary becomes contracted, and the ability to express themselves becomes reduced, as does the ability to use metaphors and analogies. They will have increasing difficulty word finding over and above the normal levels, to the extent it becomes noticeable to

others. The ability to name objects diminishes so that they describe objects or use alternative descriptions, e.g. a pen may be called 'that thing you write with' or 'a word scribbler'. Perseveration, characteristic of organic problems, may occur, often repeating the same segments of thought or stories repeatedly at interview. Speech abnormalities and semantic errors increase in frequency and marked dysphasia, both expressive and receptive, can occur (related to effects of the pathological processes in Broca's area and Wernicke's area, respectively). Patients, even in later stages, can get very frustrated by expressive dysphasia, as they are aware of what they are trying to say but cannot get the right words out.

Associated behaviours

These can be divided into three areas, the psychiatric symptoms, the behavioural symptoms and personality changes. It is usually these that produce the most stress for carers and lead to alternative care.

Psychiatric symptoms

A full range of psychiatric symptoms may occur in dementia. Depression is common in dementia (~20–25 per cent of patients), possibly related to the preservation of insight and less to cognitive impairment. It tends to present early, and symptoms of irritability, apathy, retardation and agitation may be present as well as typical symptoms of depression.

Psychotic features are relatively common, particularly delusions (in about 15 per cent), which are often persecutory (often of theft or persecution by neighbours or carers). Delusions, often linked to agnosia, of infidelity, misidentification (including the patient's own reflection), believing intruders are (or have been) in the house, and not believing that one's own house is one's own home may occur. These can be distressing to carers or relatives, especially spouses, and may develop into delusional misidentification or the non-recognition may even lead to aggression, e.g. believing that a spouse is a burglar or intruder. Hallucinations are common, are usually visual or auditory and occur in 10–15 per cent of patients.

Personality changes

These occur as the disease progresses, with the patient frequently displaying accentuated features of their premorbid personality and become more egocentric.

They may also display behaviour out of their character, such as sexual disinhibition or antisocial behaviour. They will become much more fixed and rigid in their routines and will have difficulty coping if these change. They gradually stop their usual interests and as the dementia progresses are able to spend the day doing very little. This apathy tends to be more distressing to carers than the patient. Emotional responsiveness and emotional control become reduced, the latter to the point where they can have 'catastrophic reactions', where there is a disproportionate outburst of anger or even aggression when they are pushed beyond their abilities (occasionally seen during cognitive assessment).

Behavioural symptoms

These are important to elicit as they are the most likely cause of admission to 24-hour care. They cause carer distress and may pose significant risk to the patient and others. They include wandering, aggression, incontinence, disinhibition (both social and sexual), sleep disturbance and marked apathy. Patients' behaviours may deteriorate around teatime (known as sun downing), which may make care more difficult at this time. Aggression may range from irritability to verbal hostility and aggression, but physical violence is uncommon. In later stages, the aggression may be related to resistance to carer interventions (or other residents in 24-hour care settings) with swearing or lashing out, but direct violence is rare. Any underlying reasons for the behaviour should be examined, such as pain or delirium.

Wandering is a common symptom and occurs in a majority of patients. It ranges from restlessness and pacing about their residence to leaving the house and getting lost, needing help to get home or to be located by police searches. There may be intent in the wandering, as some believe they are trying to get home or go to work.

Appetite may be reduced with significant weight loss, with patients eating very little, forgetting to eat or only eating when food is provided. Supplements may be needed, but other causes of weight loss should be considered before attributing it to the dementia.

Disinhibition is not common and may range from disinhibited conversation to sexual acts such as exposing genitals or soliciting intercourse.

Incontinence may be due to several factors and can be difficult to cope with. Patients may not recall where the toilet is or not be able to reach it in time or there may be agnosias. Comorbid conditions need to be considered, for example constipation and urinary tract infections. Careful toileting and management of fluids is helpful, as well as treating other pathologies.

Sleep disturbance may be problematic as patients wander around at night, keeping their carers awake. Older adults require less sleep generally but disturbed sleep can be exhausting for carers. Nocturnal wakefulness can lead to daytime sleepiness and the sleep–wake cycle, initially normal in the early stages, may become reversed.

Progression and prognosis

The abilities and cognitive functions of the patient gradually deteriorate. They gradually become inefficient or confused with activities of daily living, including washing, dressing, feeding, taking medication, and so on. Superficially, the patient may appear intact, but testing reveals impairments of judgement and reasoning, and abstract thinking also becomes impaired. They may have poor judgement over money matters and have difficulty managing their affairs. They may withdraw large amounts from the bank, carry it around with them, storing it at home (often misplacing or losing it) or spending it and not knowing how it has been spent. They may forget to pay bills, or sign up for services they do not need. They become vulnerable to exploitation from unscrupulous people, which may include their family or carers.

Patients eventually lose all ability to self-care and become difficult to engage with, inhabiting a world of their own; they resist interventions and require full nursing care as the link between body and brain is broken. The disease shortens the expected lifespan, with the average time from onset to death about 7–8 years, often due to other illnesses such as pneumonia.

Vascular dementia

Vascular dementia is the second most common cause of dementia, and is more common in males. It is related to arteriosclerosis, with the underlying pathology being strokes, usually multiple and small. Risk factors are as for other vascular or ischaemic diseases: smoking, hypertension, hyperlipidaemia, ischaemic heart disease, peripheral vascular disease, valvular heart disease, atrial fibrillation, diabetes. A family history of stroke and/or vascular dementia is also a risk. Unsurprisingly those ethnic groups at high risk of cardiovascular disorders (such as Indian, Bangladeshi, Pakistani and Sri Lankan) are also at increased risk of vascular dementia. There are essentially three main types of vascular dementia – the first caused by stroke, the second by small vessel disease and the third is a combination of the two. Dementia from strokes may develop after a single event (such as a single stroke), or may be secondary to multiple smaller ones (often called multi-infarct dementia), and onset can be relatively quick. Dementia caused by small vessel disease is also known as subcortical vascular dementia and in a severe form known as Binswanger's disease which as the name implies is caused by damage to small blood vessels in the brain. The damage is the result of the thickening and narrowing (atherosclerosis) of arteries that feed the subcortical areas of the brain. The symptoms develop more gradually than those of stroke and are often accompanied by walking problems. Symptoms are similar to Alzheimer's, but due to the nature of strokes, the presentations may be variable. Affective symptoms may present earlier

and classically there are sudden deteriorations in the cognitive functions linked to further cerebrovascular events, classically with a stepwise progression (Fig. 12.4). On examination there may be physical signs, such as focal neurology. Informant history is important as patients may present well, have little insight and on cognitive assessment may score highly on screening tests but have marked deficits on day-to-day functioning. Any underlying vascular risk factors should be screened for and actively managed, as this reduces the risk of further cerebrovascular events. It is also worth educating those at risk to minimize the frequency of ongoing transient ischaemic attacks because although these in themselves may not cause any ongoing or permanent damage, they are a strong signal that all is not well.

Lewy body dementia

This accounts for about 15 per cent of dementias and is more common in males. The age of onset is slightly earlier than Alzheimer's, typically in the sixth or seventh decade. Diagnosis is made clinically but pathologically there is generalized atrophy and

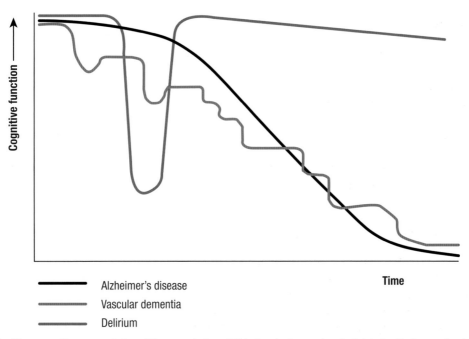

Fig. 12.4   Diagrammatic representation of the progression of Alzheimer's disease (gradual deterioration), vascular dementia (stepwise progression) and delirium (sudden crisis with resolution).

microscopically Lewy bodies are seen intracellularly, although there is no correlation between the number present and the degree of dementia (and they can also be found in Parkinson's and Alzheimer's diseases).

Presentations vary, but clinically there is a cortical dementia. Cognition may be fluctuant with pronounced variations in orientation and alertness (which may even mimic delirium). Performance on cognitive tests of attention, visuospatial function and the frontal lobe may show marked impairment, but memory impairment is not great in the early stages. About 40–50 per cent have depressive episodes. There may be recurrent detailed visual hallucinations (auditory hallucinations also occur frequently) and delusions (in about 70 per cent of patients). Patients develop spontaneous motor features of Parkinsonism including bradykinesia, tremor, rigidity and mask-like features. There will be recurrent falls or episodes of syncope. Care must be taken in treating the psychotic symptoms as there is marked neuroleptic sensitivity, and reactions may be severe or even fatal.

Frontotemporal dementia

This is a group of dementias with prominent changes in personality and social conduct that includes Pick's disease. The onset is insidious with slow progression, and the age of onset tends to be younger (50–60 years), affecting females more than males. It is uncommon but is probably underdiagnosed, with prevalence rates of 5–15 per cent. Aetiology is unclear but there is a familial history of dementia in about 50 per cent of cases.

Striking personality and emotional changes occur early in the illness, and lead to the patients rapidly having difficulties in managing their lives, with poor insight and judgement. Cognitive testing shows frontal lobe dysfunction (reduced verbal fluency, difficulty with abstraction, set-shifting and trail-making tests) but there is relative sparing of memory, orientation and visuospatial abilities. Behavioural features are prominent, including early losses of personal awareness (neglect of personal hygiene and grooming) and social awareness (lack of social tact and misdemeanours). Other recognized features include disinhibition (such as aggression, inappropriate jocularity and sexual disinhibition), mental rigidity and inflexibility, hyperorality (including Kluver–Bucy syndrome), stereotyped and perseverative behaviour (including wandering or mannerisms such as singing, dancing or hoarding), distractibility, and impulsivity and unrestrained exploration of objects in the patient's environment. Affective symptoms including depression, anxiety, hypochondriasis and bizarre somatic preoccupations are recognized, as are emotional unconcern (a lack of empathy and sympathy), apathy and lack of spontaneity. Language becomes increasingly impaired with empty speech, word-finding difficulties and poor verbal fluency. Stereotypy occurs with repetition of a limited vocabulary and themes, with echolalia and perseveration, and the patient eventually becomes mute. Patients develop neurological signs such as akinesia and rigidity late in the disease, but incontinence may present early.

Less common causes of dementia

Dementia in Creutzfeldt–Jakob disease

This disorder is rare, with incidence rates of about one per million people per year, with equal rates in males and females, and a peak age of onset at 40–60 years. However, it is thought to have a long incubation period and so symptoms might not appear until 40–50 years after transmission. There are three subtypes: familial (autosomal dominant inherited), variant and sporadic.

The symptoms are a mixture of psychiatric and neurological symptoms that are rapidly progressive. Symptoms suggestive of CJD include a severe dementia, pyramidal and extrapyramidal neurological disease, and a characteristic EEG (diffuse slowing, a characteristic triphasic pattern and periodic sharp wave complexes).

In variant CJD, there is a different clinical picture and the aetiological factor implicated in its emergence is the entry of infected central nervous system material into the food chain. In the late 1980s and 1990s, this was linked to a large increase in the occurrence of BSE. Sufferers are usually in their twenties, presenting with a progressive neuropsychiatric disorder, including a dementia. This is associated with peripheral sensory disturbance, particularly paraesthesia and painful burning feet, and cerebellar ataxia. The EEG does not show the typical patterns of CJD, and magnetic resonance imaging (MRI) scans frequently show a positive Pulvinar sign (high signal levels in the posterior thalamus). The duration of the disease is longer, with death ensuing 12–14 months after onset rather than in the usual 4-6 months with the other CJ dementias.

Dementia in Huntington's disease

Huntington's disease is an autosomal dominant inherited disorder, with the gene linked to the disorder located on the proximal arm of chromosome 4. It usually presents in the fourth decade of life, but there is a wide variation in the age of onset. It is uncommon, with prevalence rates varying from 4 to 7 per 100 000 of the population, although there are regional variations. There will be family history with males and females affected equally.

Psychiatric symptoms tend to precede motor symptoms and dementia symptoms occur early in the disease, with a subcortical picture, including non-specific memory disturbances, slowed cognition and apathy. Frontal lobe and executive functions are affected early but there is a lack of language disorder. Patients are easily distractible and exhibit poor visuospatial functioning. Depressive symptoms are common and insight is retained, with suicide accounting for 5–10 per cent of deaths. Prognosis is poor and the disease is inevitably fatal but progression is slow with the average duration of the disorder being around 14–15 years.

Dementia in Parkinson's disease

Unfortunately, dementia is an integral part of this illness, with increased incidence and prevalence with advanced disease. In total, 20–40 per cent of patients develop a dementia later in the illness. There is a subcortical pattern as discussed under 'Classification', with slowing of cognition, apathy, decreased intellectual function and memory disturbance. Frontal and executive symptoms are common and motor symptoms may make the confusion appear worse. The dementia worsens the delirium-producing effects of L-dopa medication.

There is a degree of overlap in symptoms and histopathological changes both of Alzheimer's disease and of Lewy body dementia, with evidence of both being present. It is most likely that there is a continuum and overlap between these disorders.

There may be psychotic symptoms, including hallucinations and persecutory delusions.

Dementia in HIV disease

With the increase in HIV infection worldwide, the prevalence of HIV-related brain disease and dementia is likely to rise, but may be mitigated by effective treatment regimes, as dementia related to HIV is usually accompanied by the onset of AIDS itself. It is variously known as 'HIV dementia', 'AIDS dementia complex', 'HIV encephalopathy' and 'HIV-associated dementia complex'. It is defined as dementia developing in the course of HIV disease, in the absence of any other explanation for the clinical features, and is due to direct neurotoxic effects in the brain tissues of viral infection. It causes widespread inflammatory changes and neuronal loss, particularly in the frontal lobes, though CT scans generally show mild cerebral atrophy and ventricular enlargement. Prevalence ranges from 5 per cent to 15 per cent, with lower rates in patients treated with antiretroviral agents. Another 20–30 per cent are likely to develop some mild neurocognitive symptoms. Dementia is rarely the presenting feature, but early cognitive impairments include psychomotor slowing, memory impairments and reduced concentration. Insight is frequently maintained for some time. Patients also may have motor symptoms, including reduced fine motor control, clumsiness and tremors, with early symptoms suggesting a subcortical picture. Behavioural symptoms such as apathy, social withdrawal and irritability or emotional lability occur, but marked affective symptoms or psychosis can occur. Prognosis is poor, as the dementia is associated with the HIV virus in the brain and the development of full AIDS.

Potentially reversible dementias

Vitamin deficiency

Although psychiatric manifestations of vitamin B12 or folic acid deficiency are rare, these deficiencies may present as dementias. Patients with dementia have poor nutrition so it may be difficult to determine cause and effect. Treatment of both deficiencies reverses the dementia, although improvement can be slow.

Depression

This is an important differential diagnosis to consider especially in the elderly. It is worth reiterating that depression especially in elderly people may present with cognitive impairment so that dementia is erroneously diagnosed. Depression may be a comorbid disorder in patients with dementia, in up to 20 per cent of sufferers, and makes cognitive deficits worse. Given that the patient with dementia may not be able to give a coherent account of their mood, patients should be monitored for symptoms such as depressed appearance, psychomotor slowing, apathy, agitation, loss of interest, reduced appetite and early-morning wakening. It is important to undertake a thorough assessment before diagnosing dementia as the management of the two disorders is different and depression is treatable. It may be useful to refer back to Chapter 6 and review depression in the elderly. Depression may also occur more frequently in physically ill elderly patients so doctors working in hospitals need to ensure they do not merely dismiss cognitive changes in the elderly as dementia without appropriate assessment.

Thyroid deficiency

Thyroid dysfunction can cause psychiatric symptoms, and in hypothyroid states a dementia can develop which clinically is not distinguishable from Alzheimer's disease. Other signs and symptoms of hypothyroidism may aid diagnosis, as will thyroid function blood tests, and the patient's response to the treatment. Hypothyroidism is a risk factor for Alzheimer's disease, with an increased relative risk of about 2.3.

Normal pressure hydrocephalus

This is rare but usually presents with the classic triad of symptoms of ataxia, urinary incontinence and dementia. The cognitive problems are often the first symptoms, and are associated with a general slowing and apathy that may resemble depression or frontotemporal dementia. There may be a history of significant head injury, subarachnoid haemorrhage or cerebral infection. CT scan is the main investigation and can show enlarged ventricles, but not the widening of sulci associated with Alzheimer's. Treatment is the insertion of a shunt, but the benefits may be small and need to be balanced against the risks and complications of surgery.

Subdural haematoma

This usually occurs after a head injury, although in older people, where this is most common, the actual injury may be minor or even not recalled. Physical signs are often minimal, but there is frequently an associated apathy or psychomotor slowing. Headache is not a common symptom and a confirmed diagnosis may only become apparent on CT scan because of the varied presentations.

Alcohol and other drugs

Chronic alcohol abuse can lead to the development of a dementia, as well as an increase in the risk of Wernicke's encephalopathy, Korsakoff's syndrome and vitamin B12 deficiency-related cognitive problems. This is probably due to the direct toxic effects of alcohol on brain cells, and up to 50 per cent of heavy drinkers over 65 years have some cognitive impairment.

Many drugs, particularly anticonvulsants and possibly lithium, may occasionally cause cognitive impairment to a degree that mimics dementia. Withdrawal of the offending drug may cause a reversal of symptoms, although improvements may be slow.

Wilson's disease

Also known as hepatolenticular degeneration, this is an inherited autosomal recessive disorder of copper metabolism that affects the liver and nervous system. It usually presents with hepatic or movement disorders, often early in life, although a significant number present with psychiatric symptoms, including dementia.

Syphilis

The psychiatric symptoms emerge in the tertiary stages of syphilis, and constitute neurosyphilis, or general paresis of the insane (GPI) which is linked to spirochaetes (*Treponema pallidum*) in the brain tissue. Although now rare in the developed world, as syphilis is generally treated before this stage is reached, the psychiatric sequelae are notable and may increase in the future because of the increasing rates of syphilis across the world, particularly associated with HIV infection.

About half of the cases present with uncharacteristic behaviour such as crimes, violence, or reckless behaviour with associated personality changes. Classically, general paresis can be subdivided into five categories, relating to the clinical presentation: grandiose, simple dementing, depressive, taboparetic and others.

In grandiose (~5–20 per cent of presentations), the patient expresses delusions of power and grandeur, frequently with delusions of being a famous person. They are typically euphoric, but can be easily angered if challenged. This presentation is now relatively rare.

Simple dementing (~20–60 per cent of presentations) presents with clinical features of memory impairment, slowed thinking, apathy, lethargy and loss of insight. They tend to have a mild euphoria, and sometimes have persecutory delusions. The depressive form (~25 per cent) presents as a depressive episode but the affect may be shallow. Taboparetic is a combination of tabes dorsalis and the dementing types. The other presentations are rare and tend to mimic psychiatric disorders such as mania or schizophrenia.

Diagnosis depends upon a high index of suspicion combined with positive syphilis serology and examination of the cerebrospinal fluid. Current recommendations suggest that serology should be performed when neurosyphilis is suspected or clinically indicated. Testing patients for a sexually transmitted disease without informed consent raises ethical issues, especially when partners and children require follow-up. Treatment is intramuscular penicillin and the prognosis is generally good with symptom resolution in about half of patients.

Assessment and management of dementia

Assessment

The most important part of the assessment is the history. A good history will often give the diagnosis before any cognitive testing or other investigations. The patient might not tell you that anything is wrong and have no insight into their problems, or in the early stages they may be aware of some deficits, but may minimize the effects they are having. It is therefore imperative to get an informant history. As well as being able to provide useful information on the patient's symptoms, they can confirm or complete biographical details or provide necessary information, such as past medical history.

If the informant is present during the interview, they should be asked not to answer for the patient if possible, so that any differences in accounts can be ascertained (although this needs to be done tactfully and the reasons explained – this is particularly important during cognitive testing!). All the domains of a psychiatric history need to be covered as all are relevant to the differential diagnosis:

- Past medical history
  - current disorders that may affect functioning or cognition, or be risk factors for the dementia, previous disorders that are risk factors
- Past psychiatric history
  - risk factors of and for depression, other psychiatric illness that may be part of the differential diagnosis
- Personal history
  - looks at autobiographical memory and language abilities. The more severe dementia, the less coherent this becomes, with gaps, errors, mixing up of details and confabulations
- Drug history, including smoking and alcohol misuse
  - drugs that affect cognition, smoking as a safety issue (leaves burning stubs) and risk factor, alcohol as agent affecting cognition, risk for vitamin deficiency, delirium, possible primary cause
- Social history
  - vital for psychsocial aspects of care and risk factors for safety, self-care, care needs
- Premorbid personality
  - how were they before they developed the dementia? What has changed?

Mental state examination

This may show deterioration in self-care (unshaven, unwashed, food stains on clothes, disorganized clothing, unsuitable footwear, etc.), poor concentration, mood changes and any psychotic phenomena. Insight can be assessed.

Cognitive assessment

A good cognitive assessment is important to look for deficits in cognitive function that are not apparent from the history, to assess the level of impairment and to provide a baseline to monitor progress. The cognitive domains to assess are orientation in time, place and person, attention and concentration, memory (both anterograde and retrograde), language and praxis. A person's ability to complete the test should be optimized – hearing aids should work, glasses should be clean.

Screening tests

There are a number of screening tests for cognitive impairment. It is important to remember that these are not diagnostic and only show evidence of cognitive impairment. You should then look for the reason for that impairment, which may be dementia, but may be due to other causes, such as delirium, schizophrenia, etc. The results should be contextualized for the patient – someone who is illiterate may perform artificially poorly, those of high intelligence may not show deficits on screening tests until later in the illness.

Cognitive testing

Abbreviated Mental Test Score

The abbreviated mental test score (AMTS) is a 10-item, well-validated test that has been recommended by the the Royal College of Physicians and British Geriatric Society for routine cognitive assessment. A score of less than 10 suggests that further testing is warranted. The six-item cognitive impairment test (6-CIT) is also available for use in primary care.

Mini-Mental State Examination

This is a commonly used test, particularly in secondary care. The maximum score is 30, and a score less than 24 is said to indicate dementia; however, the score is susceptible to the effects of age, educational level, language skills and good vision and hearing, not to mention the method of delivery by the tester. It also has relatively little testing of memory and is not sensitive to early dementia, so patients may have a clear dementia but score more than 25 and further

---

Items in the Abbreviated Mental Test Score (Hodkinson, 1972)

- What is your age?
- What is the time to the nearest hour?
- Give the patient an address, and ask him or her to repeat it at the end of the test, e.g. 42 West Street
- What is the year?
- What is the name of the hospital or number of the residence where the patient is situated?
- Can the patient recognize two persons (the doctor, nurse, home help, etc.)?
- What is your date of birth? (day and month sufficient)
- In what year did World War 1 begin? (Other dates can be used but should be events reasonably distant in time.)
- Name the present UK prime minister or US president. (Alternatively, the question "When did you come to [this country]?" has been suggested.)
- Count backwards from twenty down to one.

---

memory testing should be undertaken. Studies have shown correlations between MMSE and AMTS scores and density of pathological lesions in the brains of patients with dementia.

Clock drawing

Although there are formal scoring schemes for this test, it is a quick and easy screening assessment. The patient is asked to draw a conventional clock face with the hands in separate quadrants, e.g. with the time at 3.55 or 7.10, etc. Patients with dementia will draw abnormal pictures; the more severe the dementia, the more distorted or incorrect the images becomes.

Other investigations

Bloods

A full battery of blood tests should be performed looking for treatable causes of dementia and for any other pathology that might be worsening the condition. Risk factors for vascular dementia can be monitored. This should include full blood count (looking for anaemias), urea and electrolytes (renal impairment), blood sugar (diabetes), B12 and folate, thyroid function tests, and possibly syphilis serology

Table 12.3   Computed tomography (CT) or magnetic resonance imaging (MRI) scan findings of common dementias

Dementia type	CT or MRI findings
Alzheimer's disease	Reduced brain volume and generalized atrophy (or involutional change), often more prominent in the medial temporal lobe Widened sulci, smaller gyri Enlarged ventricles
Vascular	Periventricular ischaemia Ischaemic changes in other areas, especially deep white matter Multiple infarcts
Mixed	Periventricular ischaemia Ischaemic changes in other areas, especially deep white matter
Lewy body	Generalized atrophy (though 40 per cent have preserved medial temporal lobe structures)
Frontotemporal	Atrophy of the frontal and temporal lobes

(if suspected, as this is no longer recommended routinely). In patients with vascular risk factors, it may also be worth testing blood lipids and cholesterol.

Imaging: computed tomography/magnetic resonance imaging

CT is valuable in establishing the cause of dementia, as there are characteristic changes in particular dementias. These may be more obvious on MRI scanning but these are not universally available. Characteristic findings on CT are given in Table 12.3. A CT scan may also show rare causes, such as normal pressure hydrocephalus or space occupying lesions. Functional scans such as single photon emission computerized tomography (SPECT) may also be useful in measuring cerebral blood flow but not in patients with Down syndrome as they may show SPECT abnormalities throughout life resembling those of Alzheimer's. Other investigations such as EEGs can be useful in CJD and frontotemporal dementia but are not routinely used.

Management

Managing patients with dementia can be challenging especially for hospital staff who may feel insufficiently trained or prepared for this type of work. It is important to consider how to provide a humane service that ensures that patients with dementia are helped to have as good a quality of life as possible.

Management may also entail working closely with family members (see further below). Whilst it is important to be mindful of the care that people with Alzheimer's might need, especially if they have behaviours such as wandering which put them at risk, it is important not to infantilize them, talk over them or not include them in the decisions about their care. Communication should be short and clear and there may be a need to gently steer it towards the main focus. It requires patience especially as more and more functioning and memory is lost. Distraction can be a useful technique to get back on track.

Patients with dementia often reminisce as they lose orientation in time and place. If they recall particularly distressing events, they may become acutely distressed as for them the event is happening at that time. Gentle reassurance can offer considerable support.

As a junior doctor, you are likely to be called to manage some of the behavioural problems associated with dementia in patients who have been admitted primarily for medical problems. It is therefore important to be aware of the risks of using medications to manage aggression as this may exacerbate rather than help the situation. Using the principles for managing acute distress is often helpful – keep calm, minimize the number of staff involved, reduce stimuli and provide reassurance. It can be helpful to use an ABC approach; that is consider the Antecedents (what is potentially causing the behaviour), the Behaviour itself (what does it mean? Who is distressed by it?) and

Consequences (is it bringing any rewards? e.g. contact with others). This ensures that if necessary these issues can be addressed before turning to medication.

Another point worth stressing is that people suffering with dementia should not be denied other medical care on the basis of their diagnosis. Whilst it may take more time, it is still important to investigate treatable problems for which even minor interventions can make significant impact on quality of life such as infections and pain management. Now we turn to more specific management interventions.

Biological

Any treatable cause of dementia and any comorbid conditions or risk factors need appropriate treatment or management. Any sensory disability should be minimized, so the correct glasses should be obtained and kept clean. Hearing should be optimized, by keeping wax to a minimum and using an appropriate hearing aid (with batteries that work!). Correct footwear and any mobility aids should be used to prevent falls and keep patients active.

Treatments for the dementia depend on the type. For Alzheimer's, acetylcholinesterase inhibitors were introduced in the late 1990s. These are designed to increase cholinergic transmission by reducing the breakdown of the acetylcholine at the synapse, allowing more to be available for the postsynaptic receptors. Three are currently available: donepezil, galantamine (which also interacts with nicotinic receptors) and rivastigmine. They should be initiated in secondary care and are subject to National Institute for Health and Clinical Excellence guidelines. They are not curative but they do slow the pathological processes and delay institutional care. Response is variable with about a third doing well, a third getting some benefit and another third not responding well. Treatment should be monitored and stopped if there is no benefit.

Adverse effects with these drugs include nausea, vomiting, diarrhoea, headache, anorexia, insomnia, syncope and increased confusion. Less commonly muscle cramps or urinary incontinence may occur. Caution is needed with these drugs in patients with renal or hepatic disease, sick sinus syndrome, conduction abnormalities, susceptibilities to peptic ulceration and asthma or chronic obstructive pulmonary disease.

In vascular dementia, drug treatment is usually aspirin, although its efficacy in preventing progression is not clear. Other agents such as clopidogrel or warfarin may be used. It is also important to introduce a tight control of risk factors for heart disease using the general health promotion ('healthy heart') advice. Given that most dementias are of a mixed type, this is actually important for all people with dementia, to minimize risk of future deterioration from CVD.

In Lewy body dementia, acetylcholinesterase inhibitors can be used, but antipsychotics should only be used to treat the psychotic symptoms with caution. Antipsychotics will frequently worsen Parkinsonian features, may cause unsteadiness and are associated with a marked increase in mortality in patients with Lewy body dementia. Frontotemporal dementia should be treated symptomatically.

Behavioural problems should be managed with non-pharmacological interventions if possible such as effective nursing care, establishing what may lead to distress and avoiding exacerbation of behavioural problems. Patience and gentle reassurance may be required. Many may become acutely distressed and confused and the principles for managing acute confusional state as discussed below and in Chapter 18 will need to be implemented.

If medication is required for behavioural disturbance, acetylcholinesterase inhibitors can be tried. Routine use of antipsychotics is not recommended in dementia. For patients with dementia and psychosis there may be a limited role for the use of antipsychotics in low dose with a suggested time limit of 3 months of use. Current evidence suggests no differences between the various antipsychotics but second generation drugs are preferable. Patients with dementia are at greater risk of adverse effects. Evidence of increased risk of cerebrovascular events in elderly patients on antipsychotics has driven guidelines advising restriction in their use. It was initially thought that these risks were greater with second generation drugs but recent data suggest it is a risk for all antipsychotics. Trazadone or carbemazepine may be helpful. Medication for sleep disturbance should be kept to a minimum as the risk of falls increases and daytime drowsiness may occur, exaggerating the underlying problem.

Psychological

Psychological therapies include reality orientation, reminiscence therapy, validation therapy and the use of memory aids, such as labels on items to remind the patient what they are. Various artistic therapies such as music and art therapy may also be beneficial. Patients should be encouraged to keep as active and stimulated as possible, as the adage 'use it or lose it' does seem to have some truth in it.

Social

Social treatment and support are the mainstay of dementia care. Quality of life should be prioritized, so that attention should be paid to adjusting or enhancing the patient's environment to ensure that they can manage. Most patients want to remain at home and, as retaining familiarity can help, this should be the goal for as long as it is safe and practical. In the early stages this is usually managed through support from family, but as the dementia progresses increased input via social services and home care teams, memory services or other services is required.

Safety needs to be reviewed. Gas appliances may need disconnection and instead microwave ovens used for cooking. Meals may need to be provided by meals-on-wheels services or prepared by home care. Heating (particularly use of fires) and access to shopping facilities need to be considered. Respite care (for example attendance at day centres, sitting services and full 24-hour residential care) may provide some support for carers. The carer role is discussed further below.

One important safety issue is driving. Patients diagnosed with dementia should be advised to inform the DVLA and may need to stop driving. Doctors may have to inform the DVLA directly if potentially dangerous driving continues against advice.

The ability to take medication correctly should be monitored. Concordance aids such as dosette boxes or electronic reminders can be used. Treatment regimes should be simplified, with reduced tablet numbers and frequency of administration. Medication may need to be supervised.

Financial and legal issues warrant early consideration because of capacity issues. Patients should be advised regarding benefits and Lasting Power of Attorney, for financial and health and welfare matters. Will arrangements should be made early. Day-to-day finances may be left with the patient initially but they may need to be taken over by carers as the disease progresses. Patients become vulnerable to exploitation and should be monitored for elder abuse both financially and socially – not every carer

has the patient's best interests at heart. Elder abuse is well known and it is now an offence under the Mental Capacity Act to wilfully neglect or mistreat a patient.

Accommodation issues need to be considered as the patient's own house may be too big and a move to a flat or sheltered accommodation may be required. The latter may be disorientating for patients but there may be few other options if the patient can no longer be managed at home because of deterioration or carer stress.

For patients presenting with challenging behaviours, admission to hospital may be necessary, and use of the Mental Health Act may be required. Some patients may require Guardianship to ensure that it either allows access to carers or to ensure they live in the most suitable accommodation. Other patients may need authorizations under the Deprivation of Liberty Safeguards (DOLS) in order to be managed in their best interests (part of the Mental Capacity Act legislation). If patients do not have the capacity to make decisions about their care, it should be provided in their best interests, which are identified through consultation with concerned parties, including carers.

Carers have high rates of stress and psychiatric morbidity so good support is required. Not only do carers have to cope with supporting the management of the tasks of daily living, they also have to cope with the loss of a loved one in the way that they knew them. Carers need support through education about the dementia along with advice on communication and management of difficult behaviours. Interactions with voluntary sector groups should be encouraged such as the Alzheimer's Society (www.alzheimers.org.uk), which can offer advice and carer support. As the population is now more elderly than before, the number of carers helping to look after people with Alzheimer's is increasing. This means that there needs to be a range of resources to help support carers varying from individual or group psychoeducation, peer support groups, telephone and internet support. There is obviously a need to involve family members in the care decisions but this should not replace the need to involve the person themselves.

Delirium

Delirium (often described as an acute confusional state) was recognized by Hippocrates, and its name comes from the Latin 'to be out of your furrow' (*de* away from and *lira* furrow in a field). Although it is easy to recognize in its florid form, it is often still missed and underdiagnosed (especially in elderly patients), with room to improve management. It presents as an acute confusional state, often associated with an underlying acute physical disorder. Typically, the patients present as agitated or overtly confused, but often missed are those who are withdrawn and do not display overt behavioural disturbances. A high index of suspicion is required in patients at risk, as early treatment has a positive effect on outcomes.

It is the most common acute disorder in general hospitals, and is a common cause of mortality (up to 20–25 per cent) and morbidity. It is common in older people and can occur at any age, including children. Its presence indicates more severe illness in younger patients, and it is well recognized on intensive care units.

Delirium is defined in ICD-10 as: 'An etiologically non-specific organic cerebral syndrome characterized by concurrent disturbances of consciousness and attention, perception, thinking, memory, psychomotor behaviour, emotion, and the sleep-wake schedule.' Core features include a rapid onset, global disturbance of cognitive functions and evidence of the physical cause. The incidence of and prevalence of delirium is variable depending upon the cohort studied and the criteria used. However, in community settings, delirium rates range from less than 0.5 per cent in working-age adults, increasing to over 14 per cent in those over 85 years old. In hospital the rates are much higher, with prevalence rates between 10 and 40 per cent on admission and 25–60 per cent developing it during their stay. Overall, the average is about 20–25 per cent in older adults, but unfortunately between 32 per cent and 66 per cent of all cases go unrecognized. Rates are higher in certain groups such as stroke (>30 per cent), hip fracture (40–60 per cent), vascular surgery (20–40 per cent) and terminal illness (>50 per cent). Delirium increases the risk of developing dementia about threefold and increases the length of stay in hospital. It increases morbidity and mortality, both short and long term. Mortality rates vary between 10 per cent and 20 per cent, double that of similar patients. The mortality effects continue even after discharge, with 2-year survival after an episode of about 40 per cent (see Fig. 12.1). Hence, the early diagnosis and treatment of delirium is a priority.

Risk factors

The underlying pathophysiological cause for the development of delirium is not fully understood and is multifactorial, but several premorbid factors increase the risk of patients developing delirium, especially age, dementia (both presence and severity), alcohol dependence and physical health problems. These are outlined in Table 12.4.

The exact aetiology of delirium is usually due to a combination of premorbid risk factors combined with precipitating causes. Drugs of any class affecting the nervous system, including psychotropics, are particular aetiological agents that should be considered, especially if there is polypharmacy (Table 12.4). When patients have mild cognitive impairment/reduced cognitive reserve their vulnerability to delirium may be increased especially if they suffer from any acute insults such as surgery, dehydration and so on. Even a move to unfamiliar surroundings may precipitate delirium.

Clinical presentation

Presentation is variable but is clearly illustrated in the definition, with disturbances across a wide range of cognitive and behavioural domains, combined with impaired consciousness and confusion, the latter succinctly defined as 'an inability to think with one's customary clarity and coherence' by Lishman. Onset is usually rapid, over hours to days, but may occasionally be a few months. Most of the features fluctuate and vary in their degree or intensity. Symptoms often tend to deteriorate towards evening and the sleep–wake cycle is reversed, with nocturnal insomnia and drowsiness during the day.

Disorders of memory are exemplified by disorientations in time and place, with difficulty following time. Patients have impaired anterograde memory, indicated by a reduced digit span and deficits in short-term recall (they will not recall a test address). Retrograde memory will be affected with poor long-term recall of biographical details or learned information. They may confabulate to fill the memory gaps.

Psychomotor changes are evident, with withdrawal or little activity in mild states or in hypo-alert states. Detection of delirium in these states is often missed. In more severe states, hyperactivity and agitation occurs, with illusions and hallucinations

Table 12.4   Delirium risk factors

Premorbid risk factors	Causative aetiological factors
Age	Infection (particularly urinary tract)
Dementia	Severe acute physical illness
Alcohol dependency	Hyponatraemia
Visual impairment	Hypoxia
Depression	Dehydration
Severe physical illness	Constipation or retention
Physical frailty	Pain
Stroke	Sepsis
Brain damage	Surgery (particularly cardiac and orthopaedic)
Metabolic abnormalities	Intensive care admission
(particularly renal impairment)	Multiple changes of environment
Polypharmacy	Physical restraint
Immobility	Drugs (particularly those with cholinergic side-effects)
	Opioid analgesia
	Withdrawal from drugs (particularly alcohol and benzodiazepines
	Cardiological, e.g. infarction, failure
	Respiratory, e.g. pulmonary embolus
	Endocrine dysfunction
	Acute brain injury, including stroke and trauma
	Neurological disorders

(commonly visual in nature) and other perceptual disturbances. Lilliputian hallucinations are characteristic. There may also be purposeless motor activity and emotional lability. In older patients hyperactive delirium is not necessarily more severe than the hypoactive form.

Diagnosis

The crux of the management of delirium is the detection and treatment of the underlying cause. It cannot be overemphasized that treating the underlying cause is the main treatment for delirium. It is important to emphasize that in elderly patients there may be several contributory causes, all of which will need attending to. In high risk groups, such as elderly surgical patients, being on alert for such states may help earlier diagnosis and reduced morbidity as well as putting preventive measures in place when possible.

To establish the correct diagnosis, a thorough history is needed. This may be difficult or not possible to obtain from the patient, so other informants must be used, e.g. relatives, or other sources such as the GP, old notes or care staff both before and since admission.

Much delirium has its onset during admission, so admitting ward staff are also key informants. The importance of communication within and between professional groups is important to gain a through history.

Important aspects of this history should include reasons for admission and any changes since admission, including medication and a comprehensive alcohol history. Any history should also ask about previous episodes of delirium and factors that might have been relevant.

A thorough examination should be performed if the patient's mental state allows. In agitated patients this may be difficult, but even observation may give important clues to the underlying disorder or exacerbating factor, e.g. hypoxia may be evident as cyanosis. It is important to check for problems such as dehydration, constipation or retention that can be remedied simply. Baseline physical observations and cognitive assessment should be recorded. This allows monitoring of progression of the course of the delirium.

Investigations for underlying cause are given in Box 12.2.

Sub-syndromal and fluctuating pictures are very

- dementia
- substance misuse
- withdrawal states, e.g. alcohol (delirium tremens), benzodiazepines
- schizophrenia or other psychotic disorders
- depression and other affective disorders
- conversion disorders
- temporal lobe epilepsy
- non-convulsive epilepsy.

Management of the delirious patient

Prevention is better than cure! It is important to look for and avoid potential risk factors as much as possible. Awareness of the risks and minimizing any potential areas of risk are important, e.g. in non-acute settings this may include volume replacement before surgery, ensuring electrolyte imbalances are reversed and correcting anaemia. Patients should have adequate hydration and nutrition, and should be given supplementary vitamins, particularly those with a history of alcohol misuse. It is advisable in elective settings to advise patients and carers about the possibility of delirium occurring, given its relative frequency. Consideration needs to be given to any medications the patient is taking. Patients should be mobilized and actively rehabilitated as soon as possible to prevent functional decline.

If delirium does occur, medical treatment and management of the underlying medical or surgical cause is a priority, and readers are referred to relevant medical and surgical texts for further details.

common, so if there is any doubt, one should proceed on the presumption that a degree of delirium is probably present. Delirium, like fever, is an important non-specific sign that there is something physically wrong with the patient, and it should be investigated accordingly and with a degree of urgency. Although, for most cases, the clinical diagnosis will be clear, the electroencephalogram (EEG) can be useful in determining the diagnosis and its continuing presence but is not usually used. It is also possible to use the Confusion Assessment Method (Box 12.3), which has been validated as a screening test for delirium, but is not a substitute for a history and examination.

The differential diagnosis includes the following causes but it is important to stress that in many cases many of these conditions co-exist:

Given the nature of delirium, treatment will require access to a full range of diagnostic, monitoring and treatment facilities, and a full range of physical treatments may be needed, including intravenous fluids and antibiotics, oxygen and electronic monitoring. Attention should be paid to areas such as adequate hydration and nutrition, ensuring homeostasis, including managing any hypoxia and electrolyte imbalance. Secondary complications such as dehydration, constipation or pressure sores should be prevented.

Symptoms tend to resolve as the underlying disorder is treated, but symptoms can persist and can take up to 6 months to fully resolve. If symptoms continue, then the possibility of an underlying dementia needs to be considered.

Non-biological management of delirium

As well as the physical aspects of care, it is very important to appropriately treat accompanying symptoms and behaviours. It is often these that cause the problems for staff and which may interfere with the treatments for the underlying disorder. Attention should be paid to communication and environmental aspects, although it may not be possible to have the ideal environment for the patient.

Delirium can be frightening for the patient. It is therefore important to communicate clearly and regularly with patients, orientating them and explaining what is happening. All care activities and particularly procedures should be clearly explained. Some patients are able to recall their experiences of delirium, and this may be quite disturbing, often like that of recalling dreams or nightmares.

Patients should be approached calmly and you should avoid startling or frightening them. You should try to minimize the possibility of any misinterpretations.

Exercise

The delirious experience:

Imagine that you are confused and frightened, thinking the staff are trying to harm you, and someone comes towards you with a needle and syringe.

How might you feel?

How might you behave?

How would you approach such a patient as a doctor?

To aid this, you should optimize the patient's sensory input, by ensuring that any glasses and hearing aids belonging to the patient work properly and are used correctly. They also need to be accessible and within reach of the patient. It is not unheard of for hearing aids not to have batteries, or for glasses to be in bedside lockers! If possible, patients should be managed in side rooms, with consistent input from the same members of staff. Noise should be kept to a minimum, and lighting levels need to be considered – well lit but not too bright or too dull as this may lead to misperceptions or illusions. Any clocks should be visible to the patient and kept to the correct time. In order to promote orientation, moves on or between wards and departments should be kept to a necessary minimum, which is often difficult in modern care settings.

Delirium can be frightening for the carers too, so they also need clear explanations of what may be happening. However, they can help manage the patient and should be encouraged to stay as much as possible with the patient, helping reassure and orientate the patient. They should be asked to bring in familiar objects, to promote reorientation and to help reassure patients.

Pharmacological management

The main causes of referral of delirious patients to psychiatrists are agitated or aggressive behaviour. These should be managed primarily with non-pharmacological means as outlined above but if pharmacological means are needed, care should be taken in deciding both the drug and the dose. Withdrawal of any drug that may be causing the delirium should be considered before adding psychotropic therapies. Drugs will not stop patients wandering and patients should not be restrained (unless as a temporary measure to prevent injury).

NICE suggests use of either haloperidol or olanzapine, preferably for no longer than 1 week. Haloperidol is recommended due to its relative lack of anticholinergic side-effects, but it can cause drowsiness or Parkinsonian side-effects, which may lead to falls. Haloperidol may be given intramuscularly if necessary but care needs to be taken with cumulative doses. Though olanzapine may increase risks of cerebrovascular events, this risk is felt to be low with short-term use. Drugs with anticholinergic effects should be avoided if possible. Alternatively, lorazepam can be used, especially if short-term sedation is needed (though traditionally advice has been to avoid benzodiazepines because of a potential to disinhibit, but this is rare). Regular small doses should be prescribed, particularly in older people, to help prevent oversedation (which may worsen the confusion). PRN treatment should only be used to treat acute flare-ups not responding to other methods; when used alone patients may develop alternating periods of sedation and agitation. Care should be taken not to exceed British National Formulary limits as this may lead to potentially serious unwanted side-effects, particularly oversedation.

Disturbed patients may respond to simple measures outlined above but if these do not improve the patient, help should be sought from liaison psychiatry teams. The patient may require additional pharmacological treatment, or even transfer to a psychiatric unit. Consideration also needs to be given to the impact of a disturbed patient's behaviour on the other patients in hospital settings. Capacity issues need to be addressed, for delirium is likely to render a patient incapacitous, particularly regarding treatment and restraint. Any treatment should be in the patient's best interests.

Delirium tremens

The link between alcohol and delirium has been recognized for centuries: 'A rigor and delirium from excessive drinking are bad' (Hippocrates 460–380 BC). It is considered separately by ICD-10, although it is essentially a delirium secondary to the absence of alcohol in dependent patients. It affects about 5 per cent of patients admitted to hospital who are dependent on alcohol.

Symptoms usually come on approximately 48–72 hours after stopping alcohol, although prodromal signs such as sweating, craving for alcohol and nausea may appear earlier. Patients typically have visual hallucinations, often frightening in nature, as well as tremors and autonomic disturbances.

Table 12.5   Differences between delirium and dementia

Characteristic	Delirium	Dementia
Onset	Acute (hours to days)	Chronic (months to years)
Progress	Fluctuant	Gradual deterioration
Variability	Changes over hours to minutes	Variable over days (good and bad)
Duration	Days to weeks	Years
Response to treatment	Usually good	Deteriorates despite treatment
Consciousness	Clouded or impaired	Clear
Psychotic features	Early	Late
Hallucinations	Common	Uncommon
Delusions	Common	Uncommon
Orientation	Marked early disorientation	Gradual loss, time and place early on
Memory	Impaired but variable	Early short term memory loss, long term lost later
Concentration	Fluctuant, marked inattention	Gradual deterioration
Psychomotor activity	Variable (increased, reduced or fluctuant)	Normal until later stages
Sleep–wake cycle	Characteristically disturbed	Variable
Language	Incoherent, inappropriate, psychomotor slowing	Good, some word-finding problems, expressive dysphasia

A thorough alcohol use history is therefore important in patients admitted to hospital, for although the frequency in dependent users is low, the rates of admission for alcohol-dependent people are relatively common. Treatment is different as there are two main complications from alcohol withdrawal that are important to prevent. These are grand mal seizures and Wernicke's encephalopathy. A reducing regime of chlordiazepoxide is prescribed for the prevention of seizures and other withdrawal symptoms associated with agitation and anxiety.

In order to prevent Wernicke's encephalopathy, high doses of thiamine and other vitamins are given (usually vitamins C and B). The encephalopathy usually presents with the classic triad of symptoms of ophthalmoplegia, ataxia and delirium. Failure to treat may lead to the development of Korsakoff's psychosis, which occurs in about 50–80 per cent of those with Wernicke's encephalopathy. Patients who develop Korsakoff's syndrome show apathy, loss of insight, the inability to learn new information and confabulation.

Earlier in the chapter, we asked the question 'What do you understand as the differences between dementia and delirium?' Even without investigations, we can determine whether someone has one or the other from key features in the history. These are illustrated in Table 12.5.

Summary

In this chapter we have seen that organic conditions are common, more so in older people. Physical disorders may present as psychiatric disorders, rather than physical ones, and should be excluded. Organic disorders have significant effects on mortality, morbidity and quality of life. The most common disorders are delirium and dementia. In delirium, early diagnosis and treatment of the underlying cause improve outcomes. In dementia, early diagnosis is key: much can be done now for Alzheimer's disease and other dementias. In managing dementia, a holistic approach should be taken, with emphasis on psychosocial carer support and quality of life and care issues.

Further reading

Burns A, Gallagley, Byrne J (2004) Delirium. *Journal of Neurology, Neurosurgery and Psychiatry* 75: 362–367.

Burns A, Iliffe S (2009) Dementia. *British Medical Journal* 338: 405–409.

Hodges J (2007) *Cognitive Assessment for Clinicians*, 2nd edition. Oxford: Oxford University Press.

Hodkinson HM (1972) Evaluation of a mental test score for assessment of mental impairment in the elderly. *Age & Ageing* 1: 233–8.

Jacoby R, Oppenheimer C, Dening T, Thomas A (eds) (2008) *Psychiatry in the Elderly*. Oxford: Oxford University Press.

Lishman WA (1998) *Organic Psychiatry: The Psychological Consequences of Cerebral Disorder*, 3rd edition. London: Blackwell.

Moore DP (2008) *Textbook of Clinical Neuropsychiatry*, 2nd Edition. London: Hodder Arnold.

Wattis JP, Curran S (2006) *Practical Psychiatry of Old Age*, 4th edition. Oxford: Radcliffe Publishing.

Websites for Alzheimer's can be very useful resources to support families.

CASE STUDY

Mrs V was an 84-year-old woman who lived with her husband in rented accommodation. She was noted by her husband to have become increasingly forgetful over the past 12 months but he became particularly concerned when she was brought home by the police after going shopping. She has a history of hypertension, diabetes and hypercholesterolaemia. On her way to the GP surgery, she trips, falls and fractures her left neck of femur.

How would you assess this lady?

What are you going to do to prevent her developing delirium in hospital?

As the pre-fall history is suggestive of dementia, she needs to have a full history and particularly an informant history from her husband. Although the gradual decline is suggestive of Alzheimer's disease, she has particular risk factors for vascular dementia. A CT scan would be helpful.

She requires surgery and preoperatively she should be hydrated, her blood pressure optimized and she should be given adequate nutrition, vitamins and analgesia prior to being nil by mouth. Postoperatively she is at high risk for delirium, and she should be monitored for this. Hydration, nutrition and analgesia should be maintained, and early mobilization should be encouraged. Electrolyte imbalance, anaemia and any infections should be assertively managed.

CHAPTER 13

PSYCHIATRIC ASPECTS OF INTELLECTUAL DISABILITY

Howard Ring

KEY CHAPTER FEATURES

- Importance of psychiatry and low IQ
- Manifestation of intellectual disability
- Intellectual disability and social context
- Outline of risk factors for the development of an intellectual disability
- Clinical descriptions and exemplars of intellectual disability
- Assessing and managing the health needs
- Delivering health care

Introduction

Approximately 2 per cent of the population of the United Kingdom have an intellectual disability (ID) and the individuals to whom this term refers manifest an enormous range of different abilities, diagnoses and comorbidities. However, they also share an array of challenges across intellectual, communicative, motor and social domains and have frequently been marginalized members of society, often poorly served by services that the rest of the community depend upon. Not surprisingly, people with ID demand from those working in mental health services a particular set of skills and knowledge and the aim of this chapter is to introduce these.

Why is this relevant to you?

Individuals with ID may present to any health service and often have multiple health needs. The evidence is that the care they receive can be less than optimal. It is important for all doctors to be aware of specific issues related to ID so that these can be managed appropriately. There may be limitations to how much people with ID can contribute to their own management plans. However, that does not mean they should not be involved in any aspects of their own care.

Terminology and definitions

Many terms have been used to describe those with lifelong impaired development characterized by clearly limited intellectual abilities to understand, participate in or to adequately safeguard their own basic needs in everyday life. Such terms have included imbecility, idiocy and mental retardation. The current choice of terminology aims to minimize the stigma associated with terms that have become prejudical while at the same time adequately reflecting the pervasive yet varied nature of such states. Although the description 'learning disability' is still widely used in the UK, the term 'intellectual disability' is becoming increasingly applied and reduces the risk of confusion, described below, with the very different diagnosis of a 'learning *difficulty*'. In this text 'intellectual disability' (ID) will be used.

> ### Exercise
>
> Consider what readily transferable clinical skills are critical in the practice of psychiatry with those with an intellectual disability.
>
> Could you explain the importance of taking anti-epileptic medication correctly to somebody whose verbal abilities may be at the level of a 3-year-old and to their carer whose main preoccupation up to now has been trying to support this patient to eat and drink adequately.
>
> How would you approach the issue of deciding what to do if you discovered a breast lump in a woman with a severe intellectual disability?

What is intellectual disability?

It means more than just low IQ. To have an ID is to have limited abilities across a wide range of everyday functions including cognitive, language and motor processes and social activities. ID is considered as a developmental disorder, in which the individual is either never able to acquire the educational and functional skills expected for their age or early in life suffers an insult that arrests their development such that they cannot go on to develop the expected level of functioning. Hence those with an ID include individuals with a developmental disorder that has been present since intrauterine development or birth and also those who were born with apparently normal brain functioning and intellect but who sustained a major insult to brain function in the first few years of life that subsequently led to pervasive limitations in cognitive development. Specific causes of ID include conditions in which there has been an abnormality in brain development, whether genetically determined (for instance Down syndrome) or arising from environmentally related pathological processes during pregnancy or birth (for instance in association with intrauterine infection or significant birth trauma) as well as major pathology sustained during infancy, arising for instance from brain damage caused by bacterial meningitis or a brain tumour and its

management. However, as is well known, intelligence is normally distributed in the population, with the implication that there will be some towards the lower end of the distribution who have a low IQ in the absence of any identifiable aetiological pathology.

Levels of intellectual disability

Although it is very important not to focus exclusively on IQ, this does provide a summary measure that, with various caveats, can give an indication of an individual's likely level of functioning. The IQ measure is calculated by dividing a person's mental age by their chronological age according to the formula (mental age/chronological age) $\times$ 100. In this context mental age is considered as performance on a range of standardized problem-solving tests that investigate a range of verbal and motor performance tasks. It is difficult, though, to develop tests that do not incorporate some educational or cultural bias. However, regardless of which tests are used, a person with ID will always function at a mental age considerably below their chronological age. Across the whole population intelligence as defined by IQ is normally distributed with a mean of 100. In practice, ID is considered to be present in those with an IQ of 70 and below. The ranges of disability are shown in Table 13.1.

As can be seen from Table 13.1, the size of each group diminishes as IQ falls. Hence the diagnosis of ID includes individuals with widely varying abilities, extending from those who can live more or less independently in the community and who may never formally be identified as having an ID to others with multiple complex disabilities severe enough to mean that they cannot communicate, self-care or indeed generate intentional activity of any kind.

Those with mild ID may be delayed in the rate at which they acquire abilities but will ultimately develop sufficient language function to be able to use speech for

Table 13.1 Ranges of disability

IQ range	Description	Proportion of ID population
50–70	Mild ID	75%
35–50	Moderate ID	20%
20–35	Severe ID	4%
<20	Profound ID	1%

everyday purposes. Many in the upper part of this band will lead largely independent lives, although budgeting, maintaining work and coping with complex social demands are likely to require support. With appropriate education some reading and writing skills may be developed. With moderate levels of ID, individuals will need at least some supervision throughout life and language skills are likely to be clearly limited. At lower levels of IQ, full support will be required for most or all aspects of daily living.

Intellectual disability and learning difficulties

It is important to note that ID (or learning *disability*) is *not* the same as learning *difficulty*. There are a wide range of specific learning difficulties (for instance dyscalculia, dyslexia) and they can occur in individuals with IQs in the normal range.

Epidemiology of intellectual disability

It is not easy to obtain accurate estimates of the prevalence of ID. A variety of agencies are involved in supporting those covered by this descriptive term. Some, even with moderate or severe ID, are looked after largely by their families, and a difficult to determine proportion of those with mild LD are unknown to services and live independently or supported by family, friends and their local social circles. However, various estimates of prevalence have been obtained, with results varying depending on how data were obtained and whether the studies were social care, health care or population based. In Western Europe, prevalence within the overall population of around 0.7 per cent has been estimated using national registers. Higher figures of around 1.6 per cent have been obtained in population studies, while health care-based research has reported approximately 0.4 per cent of patients to have an ID.

In 2001, the UK Government White Paper *Valuing People* stated that in England there were approximately 210 000 people with a severe and profound ID, of whom 65 000 were children and young people, 120 000 of working age and 25 000 older people. Additionally it was estimated that a further 1.2 million people had a mild or moderate learning disability. Research and examination of health trends also suggest that the number of those within society who have an ID will increase significantly in future years. The size of this increase has been estimated at 14 per cent by 2021. As the care for those with ID improves, much of this increase will be in the number of adults aged over 60 years and this will have implications for planning of future health and social care services. Further reasons for a likely increase in the prevalence of ID include the improved survival rates of very premature neonates and infants sustaining brain damage through trauma or disease and better management of significant comorbidities in those with ID, most commonly epilepsy and infections, leading to a general increase in life expectancy. At the same time, better education and increased genetic screening may somewhat reduce the magnitude of this expected increase in prevalence.

Historical context

To understand the issues raised and the approaches followed in providing care for those with ID it is helpful to be aware of the historical and cultural contexts within which this part of the population lives. From the later seventeenth century the move into the 'Age of Enlightenment', with critical aspects of humanity considered in terms of rationality, education and self-aware thought, emphasized the differentness of those with an ID and served to separate and diminish them with respect to the general population. This differentness was incorporated in a variety of social structures and laws. For instance, in the UK the Poor Laws of 1837 referred to idiots, imbeciles and those of weak intellect. In the earlier Victorian era, those with ID were not viewed as any threat to society. However, from the mid-nineteenth century concern emerged about a 'lack of moral sense' within that part of the population. Interestingly, in some circles the wider interpretation of Darwin's *Origin of the Species* in the later nineteenth century also increased concern about the 'debilitating' effect on society of those with intellectual disabilities, a concern that was also expressed in the eugenics movements of the earlier parts of the twentieth century. However, after the first half of the twentieth century demonstrated so clearly the inhumane and terrible consequences of philosophies espousing eugenics and an overly functional conception of society, more humane perspectives became widespread, although for those with intellectual disabilities this was often still translated into long-term institutionalization.

By the late twentieth century social and philosophical considerations suggested that society should empathize with those having an ID and that this would have a role in supporting the cultivation of humanity. In other words, the view developed that by looking after those who could not care for themselves, the general population were improving their own humane attitudes. Although such an approach may have benefited people with an ID to some extent, it did not acknowledge that people with ID could have rights of their own. Instead, it left them dependent on the wider population continuing to hold to the belief that looking after those with ID was a civilized thing to do.

Most recently, we have moved towards a human rights agenda. This has been a key step in developing social and health agendas to improve the lives of people with an ID in the UK and led to the development and publication of the Government White Paper *Valuing People*. This was based on the fundamental principle that people with learning disabilities have the same human rights as everyone else:

all people with a learning disability are people first with the right to lead their lives like any others, with the same opportunities and responsibilities, and to be treated with the same dignity and respect. They and their families and carers are entitled to the same aspirations and life chances as other citizens.

Risk factors

A very wide range of causes as well as no apparent cause at all can result in somebody growing up with an ID. Potential categories of causes with relevant examples of specific conditions are listed in Table 13.2.

Presentation and diagnosis

The presentation of an ID will, as indicated above, depend on the nature of the cause and severity of the condition. Those diagnoses associated with major structural anomalies may be diagnosed during intrauterine development or at birth. Others may be diagnosed by early abnormalities in development, for instance difficulties with feeding, abnormal muscle tone or failure to achieve early developmental milestones. Although in those with developmental ID of moderate or greater severity parents, health visitors or the family doctor will generally identify the likelihood of there being a problem in development in the neonatal period or early infancy, individuals with mild ID may never be identified or receive the extra help that they need. Problems may only come to light in later childhood or adulthood in the context of problems with learning, working or developing an independent life.

Table 13.2   Causes of intellectual disability

Cause	Example
Genetic causes	
Single gene disorder: X linked	Fragile X syndrome
Single gene: autosomal dominant	Tuberous sclerosis
Chromosomal disorder	Down syndrome
Imprinted gene disorder	Prader–Willi syndrome
Unknown but strongly hereditable	Autism spectrum conditions
Intrauterine causes:	
Toxins	Fetal alcohol syndrome
Infections	Rubella
Perinatal causes	
Hypoxia	Cerebral palsy
Brain damage in infancy	Meningitis, brain tumour
Environmental causes in infancy	Extreme deprivation

The nature of ID is such that, as well as often being associated with physical anomalies and delayed motor milestones, a large proportion of syndromes of ID are associated with abnormalities of various aspects of behaviour, and in some cases the precise pattern of behaviours may be relatively indicative of a particular genetic condition. A potentially useful concept in conceptualizing the presentation, diagnosis and management needs of genetically determined ID syndromes is the 'behavioural phenotype'. A behavioural phenotype is described as a behaviour consistently associated with and specific to a chromosomal or genetic aetiology where that phenotype is the result of the underlying genetic lesion. Examples of conditions in which a behavioural phenotype can be recognized include fragile X syndrome and Prader–Willi syndrome. Although this concept is valuable in making clear the existence of a relationship between an underlying genetic anomaly and observed behavioural symptoms, its limitations include the finding that the same behaviour is rarely found in every individual with the same syndrome and the very incomplete understanding that currently exists linking specific genetic consequences to particular behaviours or behavioural disturbances.

There are many different syndromes of ID and each of these will not only have a constellation of signs, symptoms and comorbidities that distinguishes it from other ID syndromes but also variations among individuals receiving a particular diagnosis. This variability between individuals within a specific diagnosis may arise for a range of reasons, including IQ level, presentation of comorbidity, unsuspected genetic variations and the modifying effects of early and later environment. The last point is worth emphasizing. It is well known that, particularly in childhood, adverse social pressures (for instance emotional or physical deprivation or abuse) can have a major impact on the pattern of later development including mental and physical well-being and intellectual functioning. This effect may be even more profoundly the case in people whose ultimate level of intellectual or emotional functioning is already impaired.

Clinical features of the more common intellectual disability syndromes

Key features of several well recognized syndromes of ID are described below.

Down syndrome

Down syndrome is the most common specific cause of ID, occurring in 1 in 700 live births. It develops as a result of trisomy of chromosome 21, and in 95 per cent of cases this is because of primary non-disjunction in maternal meiosis, the risk of which increases with maternal age (potentially occurring in 1 in 40 births to mothers aged over 45 years compared with 1 in 1400 births to mothers aged less than 25 years). Causative genetic lesions include balanced and unbalanced translocations and mosaicism. Balanced translocations are associated with a higher risk or recurrence. Mosaicism may be associated with milder forms of the condition that are not always diagnosed.

Down syndrome is associated with borderline intelligence or mild ID in 15 per cent of those with this condition, with the rest having moderate or severe impairments in intellect. As well as the intellectual impairment, Down syndrome is associated with a range of well-described anomalies of physical development, including congenital heart defects in 40 per cent, hypothyroidism and a characteristic facial appearance.

Psychiatric comorbidities are relatively common in those with Down syndrome, with ADHD and conduct disorder occurring at increased rates in children with the condition, while 25 per cent of adults with Down syndrome will have a psychiatric diagnosis, most commonly of depression. Down syndrome is the most common cause of early-onset dementia. Almost all the brains of those with Down syndrome over the age of 40 that have been examined have been found to have neuropathological changes of Alzheimer's disease and 40 per cent of those over 50 have acquired clinical manifestations of it. The amyloid precursor protein (APP) gene is located on chromosome 21, hence an additional copy is present in Down syndrome, leading to overproduction of β-amyloid and this is believed to be the mechanism underpinning the high rate of Alzheimer's disease. People with Down syndrome tend to have lower blood pressure than the general population, low levels of atheroma, and vascular dementias are uncommon.

Autistic spectrum disorder

Autistic spectrum disorder (ASD) is a pervasive developmental disorder, starting in early childhood and persisting throughout life. It is being increasingly recognized and current prevalence estimates across the whole population suggest a combined frequency for all ASDs (including atypical autism and Asperger's syndrome) of around 1 per cent. ASD is more common in those with an ID than in those with normal IQ.

Those with autism experience core features of absent, delayed or abnormal use of verbal and non-verbal language, difficulties in developing reciprocal social relationships, a narrow and restricted range of interests and absence of symbolic play. (The clinical features of autism are further discussed in Chapter 14 on disorders of childhood.) However, in those with severe ID the impairment of language and communication skills often associated with such severe intellectual deficits may make a specific diagnosis of autism more difficult. Language and social communication problems are central to many of the difficulties faced by people with autism, isolating them from those around them and leading to their exclusion from communal life. This is true not only for those whose IQ lies within the normal range but also for those who have an ID. In addition, in people with ID and autism there are increased rates of challenging behaviour, a collection of symptoms that may include aggressive actions directed at self or others, more fully described below. Clinical experience indicates that it is often difficulties in understanding and meeting the needs and concerns of people with autism and ID that lead to episodes of challenging behaviour.

ASDs are also associated with increased rates of psychiatric conditions and epilepsy. Studies suggest that in those with high functioning autism and Asperger's syndrome, there are slightly higher rates of schizophrenia than exist in the general population. In those with more severe autism and low IQ, epilepsy rates are particularly raised.

Prader–Willi syndrome

Prader–Willi syndrome (PWS) is a genetically determined neurodevelopmental disorder that results from the absence of expression of one or more as yet unidentified 'maternally imprinted/paternally expressed' genes located on chromosome 15. (Normally the PWS critical region of chromosome 15 is expressed from the paternally inherited allele, whereas the maternally inherited allele is silent. In PWS this region is not expressed at all, most commonly because there is a deletion in the PWS critical region in the paternally inherited allele.) PWS has a population prevalence of approximately 1:50 000. Infants with PWS are extremely hypotonic and fail to thrive, requiring assisted feeding. As early as 2 years of age, however, the presentation changes to the phenotype that characterizes the remainder of child- and adulthood. This comprises mild developmental delay, a tendency to skin-pick and, most significantly, obesity, which arises as a consequence of an extreme difficulty in controlling eating behaviour. Those with PWS find it very difficult to stop eating until they have consumed very high calorie loads. Later, short stature and a failure of normal secondary sexual development become apparent, as do behavioural and psychiatric problems. Most people with PWS have mild learning disabilities with an average full scale IQ score of 60, with good spoken language and adequate functional abilities. PWS is associated with diabetes mellitus, and sleep and respiratory disorders and has a yearly mortality rate of 3 per cent, largely associated with obesity-related morbidity.

Fragile X syndrome

Fragile X (FRAXA) syndrome is the most common cause of single gene ID, occurring in around 1 in 5000 males of European descent. Although an X-linked condition, it is also responsible for mild-to-moderate ID in 1 in 7000–10 000 females in the United Kingdom. In affected boys, physical signs include mild facial dysmorphia with long face and large ears and macro-orchidism by around the onset of puberty. However, these signs are not sufficiently constant or specific to be pathognomonic. Intellectual and behavioural signs include delayed language acquisition, impaired numerical and visuospatial skills and behavioural problems, including autism-like behaviours of social anxiety and aversion to eye contact in around 30 per cent (largely in those with lower IQ). Hyperactivity and self-injury when excited or frustrated (for instance hand-biting, scratching) are also recognized.

Comorbidities in those with ID

One of the most important aspects of supporting the health of individuals with ID is to recognize and treat the physical and psychiatric comorbidities that exist at higher rates in this group than in the general population and that historically have been underdiagnosed and inadequately managed. A variety of reasons underlie this relative neglect. These include difficulties experienced by those with limited communication skills in making their symptoms known, modification of symptoms and their expression by the presence of an ID and often the syndrome causing it and residence in a setting in which carers are either not alert to the possibility of comorbidities or inappropriately accepting of those they do notice as 'just part' of the individual's presentation. Unfortunately, there have also been and there continue to be reports of prejudices and uninformed attitudes in health care staff that have led to management decisions that would not have been made if the individual had not had an ID.

Physical comorbidities

The more common physical health problems in those with ID include poor oral hygiene with dental disease, gastrointestinal problems, including gastro-oesophageal reflux and constipation, and epilepsy. It should be readily appreciated that in those with limited communication skills the pain and discomfort associated with toothache and bowel symptoms may lead to a variety of manifestations of distress including behavioural symptoms ranging from self-injury (for instance hitting your own face repeatedly), to hitting out at those that try to get close, to apparent loss of previous skills). Surveys of those with ID have also revealed high rates of motor and sensory deficits. Whereas motor problems may be obvious in for instance an individual with cerebral palsy, possible partial sightedness and hearing disorders may not be diagnosed without specialist assessment and should be part of the management of children with ID, for if they remain undiagnosed they can significantly impair an individual from reaching their full potential.

Epilepsy is common in those with ID, its frequency increasing progressively with more severe intellectual impairment. Lifetime prevalence of epilepsy in those with mild to moderate ID (IQ >50) is 15 per cent whereas in those with severe ID (IQ <50) prevalence is 30 per cent. A recent population-based study of adults with ID reported a prevalence of epilepsy of 26 per cent. Hence more than 200 000 people in England have ID and epilepsy. As well as being relatively more common, epilepsy in those with ID has a worse

prognosis than epilepsy in the general population. Individuals are more likely to have multiple seizure types, to have lower rates of seizure freedom on antiepileptic medication and to have higher rates of sudden death in epilepsy (SUDEP). This means that even compared with those with ID but no epilepsy, who in any case have an increased standardized mortality rate (compared to the general population) of 1.6, those with ID and epilepsy have an even higher rate of 5.0. The frequency of epilepsy varies among different ID syndromes. In those with tuberous sclerosis (an autosomal dominant disorder involving one of two genes (TSC1 or TSC2) and leading to the development of multiple hamartomas in brain and other organs), severe seizures in infancy may be the presenting complaint.

Psychiatric comorbidities

Overall, psychiatric symptoms and psychiatric diagnoses exist more frequently in those with an ID than in the rest of the population. This is the case for both children and adults. Relatively common conditions include affective disorders and autism. Affective disorders and schizophrenia are both considered to occur at least twice as often in those with ID as in the rest of the population and ADHD also occurs more frequently in adults with ID than in adults with an IQ in the normal range. Several behaviours that are core features of autism, for instance obsessional need for sameness with intolerance of variation or unpredictability, also occur in various syndromes of ID, often in association with severe impairment of IQ.

As indicated in the above discussion of behavioural phenotypes, particular syndromes of ID may be associated with increased rates of a specific neuropsychiatric state. Down syndrome is associated with high rates of Alzheimer's disease and there is an increased prevalence of psychotic symptoms in people with Prader–Willi syndrome.

How do people with an ID manifest psychiatric symptoms?

It is more difficult to make psychiatric diagnoses in people with severe ID, who generally lack the language abilities to verbally describe their psychological experiences, than it is in people with mild or moderate impairments. Possible biological symptoms of depression such as sleep disturbance and change in appetite should be discussed with carers. Behavioural changes such as decreased social interaction, loss of interest in activities previously engaged in, apparent agitation or distress, tearfulness and a decrease in previous levels of functional abilities may all suggest significant lowering of mood. The reliable eliciting of these signs and symptoms involves patient, careful and clear questioning of family members and carers. To describe hallucinations or delusions requires significant language abilities and thought disorder may be difficult to identify in an individual whose behaviour and communications may already be difficult to follow. In these circumstances, information gathered from a family member or paid carer who knows the individual well may be invaluable. In addition, for those at the most severe end of the ID spectrum, it remains unclear whether behavioural disturbances that appear to indicate psychological distress reflect psychological states that are congruent with the depressive and psychotic states described in those with higher IQs. The diagnosis of psychotic states may be particularly problematic in this context and this may relate to the observation that there are increased rates of depression and psychosis in those with moderate compared with those with severe or profound LD.

Self-injury as a symptom is well recognized in the general population. It is also a common problem among those with more severe ID. In this group, however, it probably has a different meaning from that ascribed to it when it is carried out by those without an ID. In people with ID it often takes the form of biting, scratching or head-banging. It may at times be understood as a self-stimulatory behaviour and can occur for a significant proportion of the time and may be hard to stop. However, when it develops in an individual for whom it is not habitual, it is important to consider the possibility of physical health problems, environmental changes and mood disturbance.

Challenging behaviour

In addition to these psychiatric diagnoses there is in those with ID an additional diagnosis based on the occurrence of episodes of potentially damaging behaviour. This diagnosis is named 'challenging behaviour' and, even more than is the case for the better known psychiatric disorders referred to above, it is acknowledged that this is simply a term to describe particular classes of behaviour. The term does not convey any information relating to a possible basis to the presentation. In those with ID, behaviour can be described as challenging when it is of such an intensity, frequency or duration as to threaten the quality of life and/or the physical safety of the individual or others and is likely to lead to responses that are restrictive, aversive or result in exclusion. The prevalence of serious or aggressive challenging behaviour (CB) in those with ID has been estimated at around 10 per cent. Those with ID are the largest single group in society with lifelong disabilities and are among the most complex and heterogeneous group, requiring inter-agency, multidisciplinary and, often, expensive support. Despite the various comorbidities described above, it is the presence of challenging behaviour that is often a major factor in determining quality of life, cost of care and carer health. Within the heterogeneous population of those with an ID, although described as a diagnosis, challenging behaviour is very often a presentation resulting from any of a variety of physical or emotional causes or environmental triggers. These may include pain, for instance earache or toothache, changes in care staff or care routines or side effects from some prescribed medications. Although several studies and reports have investigated environmental and behavioural strategies to try to limit the development and intensity of these behaviours, the causes of what for individual patients are often repeated and relatively stereotyped outbursts has been the subject of only limited research and still remains poorly understood. This limited knowledge base has in turn severely restricted the development of successful management strategies.

Management

How to interact with people with an intellectual disability

As discussed above, in most branches of medicine a doctor will from time to time interact with individuals who have an ID. Although the level of interaction will clearly vary depending on the level of ability, there are some general principles that can be described.

Communicating with the patient using speech

- ID encompasses a wide range of intellectual abilities.
- Those with mild to moderate ID will understand some language.
- Those with very little speech will often be aware of many social conventions and may well be able to make use of signs or other communication aids.
- Before greeting a patient with ID whom you have not previously met, ascertain their level of ability with respect to communication.
- Speak clearly and not too quickly.
- Use short, clear and unambiguous sentences.
- Time should be allowed for the content of each sentence to be absorbed, particularly if the content is unfamiliar.
- Actual understanding of the communication should be regularly checked.
- It is also important, in terms of everyday politeness as well as in the interests of developing a useful therapeutic relationship, to engage in an appropriate social fashion.
- At least until the level of a person's awareness of their environment is established, it should be assumed that they expect to be greeted and where appropriate addressed directly and not simply referred to in conversation between you and an accompanying carer.

History taking from carers but keeping the individual involved

Initially it is generally better to assume that the patient can understand you. However, it is also important not to overestimate an individual's capacity to understand and to avoid doing this it may be necessary at an early stage, with the permission of the patient where appropriate and with clear explanations of what you wish to do to all concerned, to make enquiries of those accompanying the patient. As a clinician it is likely that you will need to acquire detailed information. Mismatches between receptive and expressive language abilities are common in those with ID and should be considered if conversations do not follow the expected course or if the individual's answers do not seem appropriate to the question asked. It will often be helpful to use communication aids such as pictures, gestures and signs. Other specialties within multiprofessional teams may also have specialist skills that can support communication and assessment, including speech and language therapy, occupational therapy, specialist ID nursing and psychology. If any written records or prescriptions are brought by the patient or a carer, then these should be reviewed. In addition, however, as with psychiatric histories in general, gathering a collateral account is frequently an important part of the clinical process. If the patient has the capacity to decide whether or not you can approach an informant, then you should be guided by their response.

Principles of management

Conditions leading to developmental intellectual disabilities are, by the time they are diagnosed (with the exception of rare conditions such as phenylketonuria, which is screened for), generally not directly treatable or reversible and management of the ID itself is aimed at ameliorating those aspects of the presentation for which treatment strategies may be available. In addition, however, and as noted above, the presence of an ID brings with it an increased risk for a range of physical, behavioural and psychiatric comorbidities. These comorbidities should be the focus of active management efforts. Sometimes the treatment approach will be similar to that used for the population without ID, but in other circumstances management strategies will need to be altered. However, in all circumstances it is important that the person with ID, if at all possible, understands what they can of the treatment and why they are receiving it. In the case of pharmacological or other physical treatments, it is critically important to be aware that the individual may be unable to report the presence of a side-effect. Carers and clinicians should discuss the nature of possible effects, consider how these may be manifest in a particular individual and be on the look out for these as well as for any other changes. On some occasions, it may also not be immediately obvious whether a treatment has led to changes warranting either continuation or cessation. It is generally very helpful for clinicians, informed by the patient where possible and by the carers, to develop a written record in which the effects of the intervention can be reported day by day by the patient or their carers. This is often invaluable in determining how successful treatment changes are.

These principles of management are equally applicable to treatment of comorbid physical, psychiatric and behavioural symptoms. Bearing this in mind, the treatments available for management of psychopathology in the general population will in many cases be applicable to those with an ID. People with IQs in the mild to moderately disabled range can often make good use of cognitive behavioural approaches as long as these are pitched at levels appropriate for them. For those with more severe impairments of function, behavioural management programmes can frequently lead to clinical improvements, although these will need to be developed by clinicians skilled in working in this area. Clinical indications for the use of psychotropic medications generally resemble those in the wider population. It is essential to resist therapeutic nihilism: even if the ID syndrome, physical circumstances and life opportunities faced by an individual are not likely to be amenable to change or treatment, any additional symptoms of affective or psychotic disorder must be actively treated and may well respond just as such symptoms do in the rest of the population. Careful explanation, appropriate psychoeducation and ongoing support will be very important, but then they always should be, regardless of who the patient is.

Decision-making and mental capacity in people with ID

Physical examination and investigation of individuals with ID raises several very important and potentially complex issues. On all occasions as full an explanation as possible of what you wish to do is critical, although for some patients this will still be very limited. Where possible use visual aids or mime what is intended before carrying it out. Issues of capacity to consent to examination, investigation and treatment are of enormous importance and can get quite complicated. In the UK these issues have now come under the auspices of the Mental Capacity Act (2005), which all doctors need to be aware of.

Simply having a diagnosis of an ID does not necessarily mean that an individual is unable to make decisions for themselves, although as the severity of the ID increases this becomes much more likely. The principles discussed in Chapter 5 are important to bear in mind.

With respect to an individual with ID the following points should be considered.

- An individual should be presumed to have capacity unless shown not to.
- Capacity should be assessed in relation to the particular issue in question.
- When assessing somebody with ID simply considering their IQ or 'mental age' is not sufficient. An assessment relating to the particular decision to be made should be carried out.

Information describing the relevant issues may be presented by any means appropriate, including spoken language, images, gestures and signs. Similarly, the individual's decision may also be communicated by any of these means. When assessing capacity in an individual with ID, the following approach is appropriate:

1 Obtain relevant background information: personal and medical history and accounts from informants.

2 Consider any current psychiatric/medical diagnoses.

3 Consider intellectual level, the presence of ID does not necessarily preclude capacity, and examine intellectual functioning with respect to the specific decision to be made.

4 Enhance capacity if possible, for instance by providing information at the appropriate level of complexity and in the most accessible form for that individual. Assistance of a skilled speech and language therapist or psychologist may be appropriate.

5 Keep full clinical notes of the assessment.

If an individual lacks capacity for a specific decision then whoever must make the decision in their place must follow the principle of 'best interests'. In the context of the inability to make a decision about medical treatment, the treatment finally decided upon must be for life, health or well-being and it must represent a necessity. Where there is a choice of treatments possible, the least restrictive or invasive alternative should be chosen. However, it is *very important* that the need to follow the 'best interests' approach does not end up disadvantaging the individual by excluding them from a treatment that might otherwise have been indicated had they not had an ID. Over the years there have been well described accounts of people with ID being excluded from potentially life-saving treatments not because it was not in their best interests but purely because they have had an ID. Such an approach would be discriminatory.

How and where should health care be delivered?

In the UK, until the latter part of the last century, most health care for those with moderate and more severe ID was delivered in institutional settings, often large long-stay hospitals or 'communities'. These original institutions have now almost all been closed down and the vast majority of their residents have moved into a variety of 'community settings', including hostels, group homes and supported living projects. Others with ID continue to live with their families, and in all these settings they may, when required, be supported by clinicians working in multidisciplinary community ID teams.

In addition, arising out of a series of White Papers, from *Valuing People* (2000) to *Valuing People Now* (2008), a more assertive model of general health care delivery has been developed. This includes the registering of all those known to have an ID with their local GP surgeries and the development of individual and regularly reviewed health action plans.

Mental health care is generally delivered by community-based multidisciplinary teams comprising professionals with a range of skills, including psychiatry, psychology, specialist ID nursing, behaviour therapy, speech and language therapy, occupational therapy and expressive therapies, including drama and music. The social care provided for people with ID, including everything from accommodation to daytime activities to 24-hour staff support if required, is the responsibility, in the UK, of local council social service departments. The well-being of people with ID is often critically dependent on these aspects of care and therefore it is commonly the case that the health teams work very closely with social service agencies.

Summary

In this chapter the nature and range of intellectual disabilities, the more common conditions associated with ID and their most frequent comorbidities have been reviewed. Because of the history of marginalization and discrimination that have characterized the lives of many with an ID over the years, a brief social history of the relationship between people with an ID and society at large has been provided. People with an ID present in all branches of medicine and therefore this chapter has also provided some guidance in how to approach an individual and how to go about gaining a history. The point is also made that most of the skills that will support a successful interaction with a person having an ID are readily transferable to the rest of medical practice.

Further reading

Department of Health (2001) *Valuing People: A New Strategy for Learning Disability for the 21st Century.* London: DoH.

Emerson E, Hatton C, Thompson T, Parmenter TR (2004) *The International Handbook of Applied Research in Intellectual Disabilities.* Chichester: John Wiley and Sons.

Fisch GS (ed.) (2003) *Genetics and Genomics of Neurobehavioural Disorders.* Totowa, NJ: Humana Press.

CASE STUDY

Each new set of information is followed by one or more questions. Think about possible answers to each set of questions before proceeding to the next set of information.

A 19-year-old man with mild learning disabilities, autism and epilepsy is becoming increasingly agitated. At his day placement, he is unwilling to cooperate with anybody and he stays in a corner and shouts at people to go away.

a. What other information would you obtain in order to construct a differential diagnosis?

b. Based on the information above, what conditions/situations may have contributed to this presentation?

continued ≫

CASE STUDY continued

2. There have been no changes to his environment, no changes in timetable, and no changes in the mental states of the other people he is surrounded by. However, he is observed to repeatedly shout 'leave me alone, go away'.

a.   What might be causing this?

3. When you go up to him he is willing to talk to you and he tells you that he is shouting at the angels to go away and leave him alone.

a.   What do you think may be causing this state?

b.   What aetiological factors do you think there may be?

4. He tells you that the angels have been calling him since his older brother died in a motor bike accident some months ago.

a.   What treatment options would you consider?

b.   What role do you think psychological interventions may have in these circumstances?

c.   You decide to prescribe an antipsychotic medication. How will you explain your planned course of action to the patient?

d.   How might you check that he understands what you are saying?

5. Once he has been treated and appears no longer to be psychotic, he tells you that in order to help him remember his brother, he would like to take all his money out of the bank and use it to buy a motorcycle. He tells you that he knows that he should not drive it as it can be dangerous and because he has epilepsy but he would just like to keep it in his front garden and look at it and clean it and occasionally sit on it.

a.   What factors would you consider when deciding how to respond to his request?

b.   How will you respond to this request?

c.   How would you determine whether he should be able to make such a decision?

CHAPTER 14

DISORDERS OF CHILDHOOD AND ADOLESCENCE

Nisha Dogra

KEY CHAPTER FEATURES

- Behavioural problems in the under fives, children and adolescents
- Attention deficit hyperactivity disorder
- Autistic spectrum disorder
- Emotional disorders specific to childhood (such as attachment disorders, separation anxiety and school refusal)
- Self-harm as a presentation
- Family problems
- Major mental illness and the differences in children and adolescents

Introduction

In this chapter we cover the disorders that are usually identified in childhood and adolescence or are specific to that developmental period. It is probably most helpful to categorize the disorders as behavioural, neurodevelopmental and emotional, although there is often overlap. It is also helpful to divide childhood into under fives, childhood and adolescence (over 12 years of age). This enables the disorders to be seen in the context of expected developmental stages. It may be obvious but in assessing for child disorders, child development (physical, social, emotional, cognitive, moral) and family relationships are crucial components of the process. The aetiology chapter will have alerted you to the environmental factors that influence the development of mental health problems. For children the key environmental factors that may be significant are the family and school. For each disorder a definition is provided before describing the prevalence and risk factors. The presentation features, any issues pertaining to assessment and management are then discussed. A clinical case scenario is presented to provide a clinical picture.

We begin with behavioural disorders in the under fives and then consider oppositional defiant disorder before discussing conduct disorders. We then review two major neurodevelopmental disorders, attention deficit hyperactivity disorder (ADHD) and autistic spectrum disorder (ASD). In emotional disorders we consider anxiety disorders specific to childhood. Phobias present in childhood as they do in adults, and treatment options that are more widely used in child mental health are discussed. Self-harm is considered separately as it is a behaviour that presents relatively frequently but is more often related to distress than mental health problems *per se*. We also discuss family problems, as these can cause quite significant distress to children. Major mental illness is only discussed in relation to issues specific to this age group as the diagnostic criteria for schizophrenia and bipolar disorder are the same as for adults. Depression may present in young people as it does in adults, but there are variations which are discussed briefly. Eating disorders are also not uncommon in this age group; however, these are covered in the chapter on eating disorders. Finally we mention substance misuse, as it often presents in conjunction with other problems.

Dependence can and does occur in young people but often not to the same extent as in adults and often there are other underlying issues such as family problems.

Why is this relevant to you?

You may be wondering why you need this information as a medical student who is not even thinking about working with children, let alone children with mental health problems. Whatever area of clinical medicine you enter, you will come across children or parents, and understanding about child mental health may help you deliver better care even if it is not for the child's mental health problem itself. In your foundation training years you are very likely to come across deliberate self-harm in young people and again having some awareness of the issues the young person may be experiencing can help improve the care you provide. Up to 25 per cent of young people may suffer from mental health problems with about 10 per cent suffering from severe mental illness. However, only a fraction of these (approximately 10 per cent) have access to services and in many countries child mental health is not even considered.

When is a problem a problem?

There are several aspects to the young person's presentation that are helpful in establishing whether there is a problem or not as the symptoms are likely to be on the spectrum of everyday experience, and these are outlined in turn.

Age

A behaviour that was appropriate at one age can become a problem if it continues (for example, temper tantrums may be okay at 3 years but are not okay if they continue when the child is 10 years old).

Frequency

Something happening once may not be a problem, but happening more regularly it can be – such as panic attacks.

Severity

Feeling a little anxious may not be a problem, but extreme anxiety may be very disabling.

Individual characteristics or temperament

A particular event may be managed appropriately by one child, but another child, because of his/her temperament or personality, can develop problems.

Impact on others

Behaviour may not be seen as a problem if adults around the child are managing it. The same behaviour can be seen as a problem if it cannot be managed or if it begins to have a negative impact on others (for example, a child's aggressive behaviour may be presented as a problem if it is a risk to other family members). Child psychiatry also has another issue to contend with and that is when parents are convinced the child has a psychiatric diagnosis to explain behaviours that they are struggling to manage. There are concerns that children may be being over-labelled with disorders such as ADHD as adults displace their own responsibilities. Clinicians should only make a diagnosis if there is the evidence to support this and not because of pressure from parents or other adults (for example teachers).

Family/social circumstances

Behaviour may not be seen as a problem if the family are managing, but a change in family circumstances (such as parental depression, unemployment, financial difficulties) can mean the family's ability to manage is compromised. In addition, the presence of another disorder can compound already existing behaviours that previously were not seen as a problem (for example, a withdrawn child may not be a problem; however, a withdrawn child who refuses to go school may be a problem). Sadness is another example: being sad following bereavement is to be expected but sadness out of the blue may be a problem that needs addressing.

It does not necessarily follow that a referral to specialist services is indicated as there are increasingly resources being placed in the community to try and help the prevention of problem development through early recognition and support.

Behavioural problems in the under fives

These are mentioned here as they occur commonly and most are not severe so that they can usually be managed with relative ease in primary care contexts and sometimes community paediatric services. It is important to note that the prevalence of actual behaviour problems is probably similar across different cultures but what differs is how these are perceived. Asian families in the UK have in the past been less likely to present with sleep problems but may have greater concerns about non-compliance. Much of the work in assessing and treating children with such problems is really through educating their parents/carers. Severity can usually be decided on by considering the factors discussed above in 'When is a problem a problem?' Only severe cases and cases that fail to respond to treatment (if treatment is effectively implemented) warrant more specialist interventions (which may or may not be specialist child psychiatric services).

Sleep problems

Settling to sleep

The child either does not settle when put to bed or is constantly up during the night. The behaviour is usually perpetuated by parents inadvertently reinforcing it by responding to the child when they leave the bedroom.

Nightmares

These can occur at any age and may be associated with specific life events such as an accident or abuse. They may occur in association with flashbacks and anxiety. A child who has had a nightmare is usually able to give a vivid account of their experience. Management usually involves identifying potential causes for the nightmare and addressing those issues (e.g. if the child is being bullied and the nightmares reflect this, tackling the bullying will help the nightmares). Reassurance can be helpful. Recall and discussion of a nightmare may lead to anxiety and reassurance needs to be provided in a way that does not reinforce the anxiety.

Night terrors and sleep walking

These are most common between the ages of 6 and 9 years. Night terrors present with a history of the child sitting bolt upright while still asleep and appearing terrified. They may awake with no recall of what has just happened, but if awake are often disorientated and they can be difficult to engage. Children may sleep walk in the presence and absence of night terrors. Both occur in the same stage of sleep. Most children outgrow both problems. Management largely consists of reassuring the parents and helping them ensure the child is safe if they sleep walk. They also need to know not to try and wake the child during a night terror as this is likely to distress the child and also disorientate them.

Feeding problems

About 10 per cent of preschool children can show difficulties or problems with their feeding at some stage.

Weaning

There may be problems weaning the child and for various reasons breastfeeding may go on for longer than needed (the length of time breastfeeding continues will be dependent on several factors such as cultural, familial and economic).

Faddiness

The child is faddy and will eat a very limited repertoire. If given other foods they may be vomited back up, raising parental concerns. Parents worry about the child not growing but these concerns are often unfounded. If faddiness is humoured, it is likely to continue. The most severe faddiness may lead to non-organic failure to thrive (that is when there is no identified medical explanation for why a child is failing to grow). This may need to be monitored. It is important to recognize that faddy eaters are not usually concerned with weight gain or such issues. Often they initially did not like the textures or tastes. Often the parental responses shape further faddiness. Difficulties with feeding are common in children with autistic spectrum disorder, discussed later in this chapter. They are often also present in children with physical illness.

Behavioural problems

The child is presented as being uncooperative, with unwillingness to comply with adult requests and they have 'temper tantrums' when they do not get their own way. The behaviour is often described as wilful, defiant and may also be aggressive. This is most marked between 2 and 4 years, when the child is gaining a concept of self but does not yet have the skills for independence.

Risk factors for behavioural problems:

- parents who lack confidence
- parents who received indifferent parenting so struggle with setting clear boundaries
- conflicting expectations by different adults involved in the child's care
- family conflict, especially witnessing violence and aggression
- child temperament
- comorbidity with ADHD or ASD
- child abuse
- organic problems (such as anaemia, lead poisoning).

Management

Parents who have not received adequate parenting themselves (for example having grown up in care) may need basic education about limits and boundaries. Parents who were brought up by very strict parents may feel that they do not want to be as strict with their own children but then struggle as the child is in charge of the family. Understanding the different experiences of both parents can also be a useful exercise, as it can reveal much about the dynamics of what the child has to understand and negotiate their way through.

Simple behavioural therapy is usually the most effective frontline treatment. However, parents often require considerable support, especially if the problems have been longstanding, as they can lack confidence. Underlying issues such as parental conflict may also need to be resolved. For most behavioural problems in young children, the approach is straightforward. However, the application may not be, for carers may struggle to hold their own. There is a need to be clear with the child in terms of what is expected from them, and the expectations have to be specific. It is unhelpful to say the child has to be 'good' as the behaviour that constitutes what is good will vary from adult to adult, and even from day to day. The adult responses to the child have to be consistent. It is unhelpful to young children if the same behaviour elicits different responses at different times as they

then have no clarity about what is expected of them. The child also has to learn that there are consequences for unacceptable behaviours. The rewards and punishments (if used) must be meaningful to the child and realistically attainable for their developmental stage. It is unhelpful to expect young children to wait for weeks for rewards when they have little conceptual understanding of the future beyond a few days. It is also important for the adults involved in the child's care to be consistent, for the same reasons that they need consistency from the same individual. This can be especially difficult if children have to cope with growing up in two or more households.

When implementing the behavioural strategies, it is important that the adults remain in control and do not show emotion and engage in justifying what they are doing to the child. An under five should not be treated as an equal. If a child is told not to do something and their response is to cry, the adult should not seek to comfort the child at that point as it leads to a lack of clarity about what is happening. If children learn that their crying distracts the parents, they will use this strategy again. Some parents worry that this will scar the child – it rarely does but what it does do is help the child learn appropriate behaviour. The scarring is prevented by being emotionally responsive to the child at other times rather than while they are exhibiting undesirable or unacceptable behaviour. Parents may also need to ensure that their expectations are age and/or developmentally appropriate (for example, a 1-year-old child is unlikely to have the skills to eat their dinner without some degree of mess).

For sleep issues, it is useful to have good and clear sleep hygiene, which should resolve most sleep issues. Sleep hygiene is essentially the factors that interfere with falling and remaining asleep. For young children, a consistent routine is often required and limiting excitement before bedtime can be helpful.

A review is warranted if these simple techniques do not work; it may be that other disorders need to be excluded. It is worth noting that behavioural problems that are not addressed when children are young do not simply resolve themselves, and most will develop into oppositional defiant disorder and then into conduct disorder. The older the child is the harder it becomes to makes effective interventions. In long-established presentations, family therapy may be warranted to help the family change the way they think about the situation and the role the child has come to be known by. It is not unusual for families to ascribe certain roles such as 'the naughty one', the mischievous one' to children that can be difficult to change.

Oppositional defiance disorder

This is the continuance of many of the features described above such as temper tantrums, defiance, aggression and so on. It will extend beyond the family into school life to such a degree that it may impact significantly on learning and peer relationships. It can be diagnosed from toddler years up to age 10.

Conduct disorder

Oppositional defiance disorder beyond 10 years of age is usually defined as conduct disorder. It is included in both ICD and DSM classifications but there is considerable debate about whether this is appropriate. Conduct disorder is grouped into socialized and unsocialized types, with some overlap. Socialized conduct disorder is usually viewed as less serious and tends to be phasic in nature. Unsocialized conduct disorder is more serious and potentially leads to criminality and a later diagnosis of antisocial personality disorder.

Attention deficit hyperactivity disorder

ADHD is a heterogeneous behavioural syndrome characterized by the core symptoms of hyperactivity, impulsivity and inattention (Box 14.1). If the ICD-10 criteria are used, the prevalence is approximately 1–2 per cent of children and young people. Using the broader DSM–IV criteria, ADHD prevalence rises to

---

Box 14.1: Key features of ADHD

Triad of hyperactivity, poor concentration and inattention impulsivity

Not situation or context specific so assessment needs to reflect this

Onset before age 6

Mild cases do not require medication

Moderate and severe cases require methylphenidate, plus psychoeducation and supportive therapies

---

possibly 3–9 per cent of school age children, and 2 per cent of adults. Prevalence also varies across different samples (community versus clinical, and in different countries). However, as a condition it is not culturally specific but it is likely that different families may tolerate different levels of symptoms.

Risk factors

Children with birth injury are more prone to ADHD as are children with learning disability and ASD. Fetal alcohol syndrome babies are also at risk. There is some genetic risk but this is unclear. ADHD is more common in boys than in girls.

Clinical factors

The key is a triad of impulsivity, hyperactivity and poor concentration. These features are pervasive in all contexts and are not situation specific. Onset is by 3 years of age, although may not be identified at that stage. Children are however often presented because of secondary problems related to these symptoms, such as lack of academic attainment, aggressive and other behavioural problems, poor peer relationships.

Assessment

Different localities will have different arrangements for who initially assesses children with possible ADHD. The assessment needs to be of a reasonable length of time. Distractibility for a few minutes does not indicate ADHD! Even if the child appears to have ADHD in the clinic context, a diagnosis should not be made unless there is evidence that this also occurs in other contexts (such as school and home). School observations are a useful adjunctive assessment context. There are many questionnaires that can be used to indicate various symptoms, but the diagnosis should be made on clinical assessment and not questionnaire completion.

Management

Once the diagnosis is made and an explanation given to the child and carers, mild ADHD can be managed with behavioural strategies and psychoeducation of the child, carers and teachers. Moderately severe and severe cases usually require medication. The first-line medication is methylphenidate, and atomoxitine is another option.

Medication if it is used is only part of the treatment. Psychoeducation and behavioural strategies are also still required. Parent and child support groups are also recommended, but availability varies. This enables parents to learn appropriate management strategies and for the child to learn appropriate social skills and management of their impulsivity.

Children on methylphenidate need regular monitoring because it can affect growth. As it is also a stimulant, it can cause psychosis, so any treatment should only be initiated by a specialist.

Autistic spectrum disorder

ASD is a lifelong condition that affects how a person communicates with, and relates to, other people. It also affects how they make sense of the world around them. ASD is a term that is used to describe a group of disorders, including autism and Asperger's syndrome (which was assumed to be a milder form without all aspects of the impairments being present). The word 'spectrum' is used because the characteristics of the condition vary from one person to another. Those with autism may also have a learning disability. There was a view that those with Asperger's syndrome tend to have average, or above average, intelligence, and thereby would be less seriously affected. However, as they still have social interaction difficulties but can understand that they do not fit in, the problems they face can in fact be greater. It is probably most helpful just to use the term ASD rather than try and guess where someone will be along the spectrum. The prevalence of ASD is around 1 per cent. There have been concerns that the prevalence has been increasing but this is probably most likely to be due to improved identification and less rigid application of the diagnostic criteria. It is significantly more common in boys (around four times as common) and indeed some experts have commented that the mild end of the spectrum is fairly typical male behaviour!

Risk factors

- The aetiology is unclear but there is a genetic risk and it does appear to run in families.
- Children with learning disability are at increased risk of ASD.

- The condition is present before 3 years of age but those with less marked features might not be identified until adolescence.
- There is no credible evidence to link ASD with the measles–mumps–rubella triple vaccine.

Clinical features

This disorder also has a triad of key clinical features that are shown in Box 14.2.

Box 14.2: Clinical features of ASD

Impairment of social interaction

Impairment of communication

Restricted, repetitive and stereotyped patterns of behaviour, interests and activities

There is also a school of thought that has impairment of imagination as part of the triad of impairment

No cure

Management involves providing appropriate supportive therapies and helping the child's perspective to be understood

In the under fives ASD may present through delayed development, especially language development. There may also be odd behaviours such as intolerance of specific textures, distress at apparently minor changes, an indifference to pain, a lack of engagement with primary carers, a baby or toddler who is difficult to settle.

There may also be adult concerns about the child's social relationships – for example poor eye contact, thought to be deaf as do not respond to social interactions, often do not want to play with others and appear not to understand social cues and rules. They are unable to pick up the subtleties of non-verbal language or understand the fine nuances of language. They often do not understand jokes, sarcasm or a play on words.

In school age children, presentation is likely to be through behavioural problems, which are an indication of the child struggling with expectations within a new environment and increasing expectations that the child should be learning to work with peers. The relationships they have are usually on their terms and they struggle to understand other people's perspectives. They may have some very obscure interests and talk to people about them without realizing that the other person does not share their interest.

In adolescence anxiety, features of OCD and behavioural reasons are often the features that lead to presentation at services. In all these situations, the young person rarely sees that they have a problem and usually feel the issue is for others to address.

Some individuals with less marked features or features that those around the individual have adapted to may not present until adulthood.

Treatment

Despite many claims, there is absolutely no evidence that ASD can be cured. Management is a case of helping the family to understand the young person and helping the young person learn to operate in a world they do not really understand. Many of the interventions are educational and based in educational settings, or behavioural strategies to manage difficult behaviours. One of the key clinical features is that children with ASD struggle with change so can present with anxiety or what appears to be obsessive compulsive disorder. A thorough history and assessment will identify the underlying problems. Cognitive behavioural therapy by the very nature of how it works is less useful in children with ASD, but they can be helped to manage their feelings in socially appropriate ways.

Emotional disorders of childhood

These may include anxiety, worry, fear, sadness and depression, and anger. Anger is not in itself a mental health disorder but an inability to manage anger and other emotions in appropriate ways can be a problem as it may impact on the young person's development.

Only those anxiety disorders specific to childhood are covered here as the features of the other disorders (such as generalized anxiety, phobias and obsessive compulsive disorder are similar to those in adults). Interventions will usually involve parents as co-therapists but similar techniques and strategies are employed. They are not generally treated with medication.

The disorders that will be covered here are attachment disorders, separation anxiety and school refusal. Before we discuss these, it will be helpful to consider the concept of attachment.

Attachment refers to a specific type of biologically based relationship, which provides a secure base from which children can explore the world. Work by Mary Ainsworth and colleagues in the early 1970s and then others has enabled attachment to be classified as either secure or insecure, with three types (ambivalent, avoidant or disorganized) of insecure relationships identified.

When children have secure relationships with their primary caregivers, they feel secure and safe in the understanding that they will have their needs (physical and emotional) met. They form a sense of confidence about themselves and the world around them and are able to explore the world beyond their immediate surroundings in the knowledge they have a secure base to which they can retreat for safety. They separate easily from their caregivers, although they may be upset, as they trust that the caregiver will return.

Children who for various reasons (such as primary caregivers with a history of postnatal depression, unwanted pregnancy and/or other adverse perinatal events, other parental illness, abuse and neglect, temperament clash between child and primary caregiver) do not develop secure attachment are described as having ambivalent, avoidant or disorganized attachment. These bring different types of behaviours and may have different consequences, but common to all will be that the child's psychological development is limited and their ability to develop appropriate relationships with others will also be affected.

Ambivalent attachment tends to lead to very anxious and clingy individuals who fear trying anything new and lack confidence. Even when the parent seeks to offer comfort, they are likely to remain distressed and may be aggressive towards the caregiver. They are wary of strangers and as adults often struggle to trust others but at the same time are very needy.

Children with avoidant attachment styles tend to avoid parents and caregivers and appear to be unaffected when they are left by them. These children might not reject attention from a parent, but neither do they seek comfort or contact. Children with an avoidant attachment show no preference between a parent and a complete stranger. They are often very friendly and seem to be socially skilled. This is often seen in children who have experienced multiple caregivers and in some ways may be a way of protecting themselves. As adults, those with an avoidant attachment tend to have difficulty with intimacy and close relationships. They struggle to share feelings, thoughts and emotions with partners and others and may appear very self-reliant.

Children with disorganized attachment show a combination of ambivalent and avoidant features that reflect lack of consistency in the care given.

Attachment disorders

Attachment disorders appear under disorders of childhood and give the false impression that the disorder lies within the child. A diagnosis is a reflection of the child developing and presenting particular symptoms that reflect a failure for the child to have developed appropriate attachment. However, the reasons for this lie in the adults caring for the child. It is important that attachment disorder is not diagnosed without clarity of context, as attachment is a two-way process.

Presentation

Broadly two types of attachment disorder have been identified: those where children are indiscriminate about who they form 'attachment' to – they are inappropriately friendly with everyone and show little wariness; and another group whose attachment is more defined in relation to the child's behaviour towards the caregiver. Children with insecure attachment, especially disorganized attachment, are at significant risk of later emotional and behavioural problems.

Children will show developmentally inappropriate social relationships and may also present as having an anxious relationship with caregivers and/or disinhibited behaviour (behavioural problems, inattention, poor concentration, aggression) or asocial behaviour (lack of empathy or ability to see another perspective) in which ADHD or ASD may be mistakenly diagnosed. Learning disability may also need to be excluded, because children who demonstrate friendliness to strangers may be doing so as they do not understand the contexts for different social relationships.

Management

To date there is no known effective treatment for attachment disorders, although several psychotherapeutic techniques are used on the basis of very little evidence. Therapies such as holding therapy have gained popularity despite the lack of evidence. Family therapy may be appropriate in some contexts but would be inappropriate if there is ongoing abuse (emotional or otherwise). Social cognitive treatment approaches may be more beneficial given that there is greater evidence of efficacy for changing specific behaviours (such as peer rejection).

Separation anxiety

This is anxiety when the child is separated from their primary caregiver. Separation anxiety is part of normal development but is considered a disorder when it persists beyond about 15–18 months. Prevalence is approximately 4 per cent, but definitive rates are difficult to establish as many do not present to services. It most commonly presents in preschool or early school years and is characterized by features of anxiety associated with actual or anticipated separation from a particular adult, usually the mother.

Insecure attachment relationships, coupled with high levels of parental anxiety, are associated with increased risk of anxiety disorders generally in children and particularly separation anxiety. Temperament may be of relevance, as may previous experience.

Presentation

At separation or the thought of separation the child becomes distressed and exhibits signs of anxiety such as hyperventilation, feeling sick, panic and alarm. The anxiety may result in difficulty settling at night, and reluctance to go to school or to be alone – this can be to the extreme of refusing to be alone in a room even when others are in the house. Parents may report that the child follows them everywhere and may even physically cling to the parent. The parent may also experience anxiety at the prospect of separation. Children may be the ones who decide on the rules in the family as the parents struggle to cope with the child's distress.

Assessment should explore the presenting features and likely precipitants especially parental anxiety, which may exacerbate the problem. The dynamics of the parent–child relationship need exploration, particularly the transmission of anxiety between them and to identify parental behaviours and anxieties that perpetuate the problem.

Management

Some work with the family is usually indicated, with individual work with the child dependent on age and cognitive development. Specific interventions are mostly behavioural and usually involve graded exposure to separation starting in the situations defined by the family as least distressing. Unintentional rewards for clingy behaviour should be identified and avoided. Separation should be rewarded with positive comment and praise. If the features re-emerge (as they may do at times of transition and stress), cognitive behavioural therapy may be warranted. Family work should address parental expectations, anxiety or behaviours which in themselves may exacerbate the anxiety. There is insufficient evidence to support the use of medication.

School refusal

School refusal presents throughout childhood especially at times of transition, for example when starting or changing school. School refusal usually peaks during early adolescence, when it may represent a combination of adolescent stress and the revival of an earlier overdependent parent–child relationship. The increased need for independence and autonomy posed by the demands of secondary school may precipitate an avoidance of school. It may sometimes follow difficult experiences at school, such as bullying or being told off by a teacher.

The problem can manifest after a time of change at school or a period of illness. The unwillingness to go to school is often expressed openly and the young person may say there is a particular student or lesson that they dislike or find anxiety provoking. Younger children especially may complain of headaches and abdominal pain to avoid school. There can be reluctance to accept that the anxiety rather than school is the problem.

Delay in the recognition of the underlying psychological basis for the problem greatly exacerbates the difficulties and by the time young people are referred to specialist services (in those where mental health is an issue) the patterns are long established and may be difficult to change.

Management

School refusal is most appropriately managed by the education welfare service unless anxiety is a key feature. There should be a clear and consistent approach to returning young people to school. The school should involve the parents, and if appropriate the child, in devising programmes or plans. Parents need to support the programme to introduce the child or young person back to school. A phased return into the school environment especially when absence has been prolonged can be a useful way to start the return. The longer it is left, the more the young person will feel that getting back is insurmountable. Parents need to be firm about what is expected of the young person and resist the temptation to accede to the young person's distress. Cognitive behavioural techniques to help with the anxiety may be indicated. Tuition at home is usually an unhelpful strategy, as it can perpetuate the problem and impedes appropriate social and educational development.

The problems may manifest themselves after school holidays and parents need to ensure that their management remains clear and firm.

The prognosis is not good for a significant minority of adolescents. Up to one-third of school refusers fail to maintain regular school attendance and may have a predisposition to anxiety or agoraphobic symptoms. If there are concerns about parental commitment, this may be appropriately discussed with social services or addressed legally.

Self-harm

It is important to emphasize that self-harm is a symptom or behaviour and not a diagnosis. This is common in adolescence but does occur in younger children. Exact prevalence rates are hard to state as so much of it does not present to services. There is now some good evidence that most young people who self-harm are not mentally ill but that self-harm is usually related to life problems and there is generally low suicidal intent. There is a tendency for non-mental health professionals to hear the term 'self-harm' and make an immediate assumption that this then falls under the remit of mental health services. All doctors should be able to undertake a basic psychiatric history and risk assessment to identify those that need specialist help and those that might be managed through psychoeducation and help with the problem that has led to the self-harm. Repetition of self-harm is common and appears to be most likely where there is significant psychosocial disadvantage or mental health issues. Asking young people about self-harm does not increase the likelihood of them self-harming. In fact the effect can be quite the contrary as in asking about it, the young person may be relieved of guilt for having such feelings and of feeling understood. Also, assurance that feelings of self-harm are not uncommon can also be helpful.

Risk factors

Factors associated with self-harm include:

- previous self-harm
- substance use
- presence of a mental health problem such as depression
- being in a vulnerable high-risk group
- physical, emotional or sexual abuse
- being lesbian, gay or bisexual
- loss of relationship
- poor or inadequate coping skills
- family history of self-harm and suicidal behaviour
- availability of means (availability of firearms increases likelihood of completed suicide)
- family discord
- parental mental illness and/or parental substance use
- intercultural stressors, especially for South Asian females
- school and peer problems
- unemployment
- poverty/homelessness.

Clinical features

- Self-harming behaviour or indication that they are considering self-harm.
- Self-harm can be cutting, overdose, strangulation.
- Recent common adverse events, such as relationship break-up, falling out with parents or peers.
- Chronic psychosocial problems such as family problems, bullying, peer relationships.
- Substance misuse.
- A small number may have mental illness.

Young people who self-harm typically exhibit:

- feelings of insufficiency and low self-esteem
- lack of supportive relationships and low family cohesion
- cognitive distortions and attribution styles
- responses to problems using maladaptive cognitive strategies relating to expectancies, commitments and explanations for events.

Management

Self-harm requires assessment and it may be that increasingly more of the less serious self-harm assessments are undertaken by non-specialist health care staff. There is a need to undertake a risk assessment. For most young people and their families, the assessment is an opportunity for the young person's perspective to be heard. It is really important not to be dismissive of the young person's actions or feelings. Most young people self-harm because they lack appropriate coping skills and humiliating them does not help them develop the relevant skills. Few young people who have self-harmed are likely to need specialist CAMHS but can be directed towards counselling support or family support depending on the underlying issues.

Family problems

The reason for mentioning this here is that young people often present with potential 'mental health symptoms' such as self-harming, low mood, general unhappiness, irritability, behavioural problems (such as petty criminality, substance misuse). An assessment shows that the underlying problems are family issues or a difference between parental expectations for the young person and the young person's own wishes. Cultural issues in the broadest sense can be quite significant in these types of problems.

Issues that may give rise to problems are:

- pressures to conform to practise their family's religion or other practices that do not sit comfortably with the young person;
- pressures to conform to expected gender roles (boys wanting to pursue careers generally considered to be in the female domain such as nursing, child care and vice versa);

- pressures to conform to the social norms, e.g. the expectation that a young person will go on to further education despite this not being what the young person wants;
- pressures to conform to family expectations that differ from what the young person wants (e.g. an expectation that the young person work in the family business);
- sexual orientation;
- impending forced marriages;
- difficulty in reconciling the culture in the private and public domains of their lives (feeling they have to be a different person in the two contexts but not being able to do that comfortably).

Exercise

Consider your own teenage years. Were there areas of conflict between you and your parents? How were these differences resolved?

Differences between parents and young people can be a part of the process of growing up as adolescents establish their own values. These only tend to come to the attention of services when the young person responds with maladaptive coping strategies (self-harm or conduct disorder) or if they present with emotional problems (such as anxiety or depression).

Mental disorders

Depression

Depression is the persistence of low mood that lasts over several weeks. The issues of definition of depression and the accuracy of screening methodologies may be even more salient than they are among adults, but estimates of prevalence are in the range of 1–2 per cent for prepubertal children and 3–8 per cent for older adolescents. From the age of 14 years onwards, the adult preponderance of females with depression emerges. There is reasonably consistent evidence that the prevalence of depression in young people, certainly among adolescents, has increased in recent years. Changing social contexts of expectations of young people and family structures may be plausible explanations.

Risk factors

As with most disorders of childhood there is no single aetiological factor. Family history is a risk factor, although sometimes it can be difficult to differentiate whether the risk is family history or that family members experience the same adverse circumstances. With the exception of physical illnesses, risk factors for depression in young people are not too dissimilar from those among adults, although the aetiology is generally held to be more psychosocial than biological. That being said, although parent–child relationships will clearly play an aetiological role, one review estimated that parenting accounted for only 8 per cent of the variance in the liability for childhood depression.

Clinical presentation

Presentation varies with the young person's developmental stage. Symptomatically, adolescents and adults do not differ greatly, although adolescents report fewer of the features of somatic syndrome. Irritability and anger are more commonly observed than in depressed adults. Associated with the low mood, there may be biological features such as sleep problems, poor concentration and motivation, appetite disturbance (in young people increased appetite may be present or the usual loss of appetite), anhedonia and negativity. Issues of self-esteem and poor confidence are also common in adolescence. In some young people the depression can be severe enough to present with psychotic features – delusions of worthlessness are not uncommon. Thoughts of self-harm are very common in adolescents and suicidal ideation common in those with low mood. Asking young people about their self-harm can be very helpful as it may help the young person from feeling isolated and alone. Comorbidity is not uncommon and young people may use alcohol to treat their low mood without realizing that the alcohol actually worsens the situation. Depression and anxiety copresenting is not unusual, and it can be difficult to identify the primary problem. Young people with depression may have self-esteem issues and it can be difficult to tell if these lead to relationship difficulties which cause depression or result from the low mood.

Depression can occur in younger children but exploration often shows them to be unhappy with the world around them rather than being depressed. Younger children may present with changes in behaviour, becoming more irritable and moody. As with adults, they may also present with physical symptoms such as headaches and stomach aches.

In both groups, there may be deterioration in their academic work and social relationships. There may be family arguments because the family does not recognize the young person's problems.

Management

For depressed young people, psychotherapy and/ or counselling are the usual treatments of choice. Family involvement (often with a strong educational component and involving parents as 'co-therapists') is frequently deployed. From the age of about 10 years and over, cognitive behavioural therapy is the more usual first-line treatment and there is evidence of its efficacy in adolescents both in the short and in the longer term. There is no good evidence that antidepressants are effective in childhood depression.

For severe to moderate depression in adolescents the first-line treatment is medication. Only fluoxetine is licensed for the treatment of depression in young people under the age of 16 years. Alongside the medication there is a need to offer counselling or supportive psychotherapy to help resolve some of the issues that precipitate or perpetuate the illness. Dependent on the relevant factors, family therapy may also be required. Initially cognitive behavioural therapy may be difficult as the young person is not in a state where this can be utilized, but as their mood improves cognitive behavioural therapy is a very useful adjunctive treatment. There is a slight but statistically significant increase in self-harm (but not suicide) among young people who are prescribed SSRIs, and this gave rise to warnings about their use. Prescriptions of SSRIs fell, but sadly suicide rates rose thereafter among young people in Holland and the USA, suggesting that untreated depression is the major risk factor for suicide.

Psychosis

Like self-harm, psychosis is a symptom and not a diagnosis in itself. The most likely causes of psychosis in young people are substance misuse, depression, organic medical problems, bipolar disorder and schizophrenia. A thorough history and assessment is required. Medication is used to manage the psychosis and then appropriate treatment is given for the diagnosis. Psychosis may present with risk to the young person and/or others dependent on the nature of their perceptual symptoms.

Bipolar disorder

Bipolar affective disorder is relatively uncommon in children and adolescents. A young person may be treated for an episode of depression but then later turns out to have bipolar disorder when a manic episode occurs. The diagnosis of bipolar disorder in children is a contentious issue and it is more commonly diagnosed in the USA. A more conservative diagnostic approach is generally adopted in Europe. Conservative diagnosis would require a typical episodic picture of adult manic symptoms, whereas liberal criteria would consider irritability and mood fluctuations/lability to be symptomatic of possible bipolar disorder. Differentiating such symptoms from adjustment difficulties in various phases of development is clearly problematic, and there is the additional complication of possible comorbidity.

Schizophrenia

The prodomal phase of schizophrenia may begin in adolescence. The family may describe something not being quite right and the young person often insists all is well. Assessments are helpful to establish the history but it can be difficult to provide a definitive answer. The presentation and clinical features are as for adults and not discussed any further.

The management is as for adults in that medication is used to help manage the psychosis. Psycho-education of the young person and their family is crucial. For understandable reasons, clinicians can be reluctant to make the diagnosis at the time of the first presentation given the long-term implications. However, it is important to identify this early to be able to provide the necessary support.

Substance misuse

Young people are unlikely to present with dependence on substances, although this is changing. In most young people substance misuse is related to adverse personal and social circumstances. Alcohol is often used to manage the symptoms of anxiety and/or depression. Substance misuse may lead to affective presentations that necessitate referral to specialist services. A joint approach between specialist services for substance misuse and child mental health services is usually appropriate as the former can address any substance misuse issues and the latter any individual or family issues.

Anorexia nervosa and bulimia nervosa

These are not covered here as they are addressed in Chapter 11. Presentations are increasingly occurring in younger children. Family therapy has proven efficacy in children under the age of 14 years and is the treatment of choice. It is often supported by individual work with the young person.

Summary

In this chapter the most common mental health disorders of children and young people have been covered. Although a detailed knowledge of them is not needed for most doctors, awareness of the conditions is relevant, as early identification and referral to appropriate agencies can ensure that the potential negative impacts are reduced.

Further reading

Dogra N, Parkin A, Gale F, Frake C (2009) *A Multidisciplinary Handbook of Child and Adolescent Mental Health for Front-line Professionals*, 2nd edition. London: Jessica Kingsley.

CASE STUDY 1

Oliver is 3 years old and his mother presents to you as her GP at the end of her tether. She and her husband have been having marital problems and she feels Oliver maximizes the tense situation. Oliver defies his mother in all aspects refusing to cooperate with any bedtime routine and being uncooperative at meal times. Playschool staff also have some problems but not as often and of the severity as experienced by his parents.

What is the likely diagnosis?

What would be the most appropriate management?

The most likely diagnosis is oppositional defiance disorder.

There is a need to implement straightforward behavioural therapy. The parents need to agree on the rules and enforce them consistently. They need to ensure that they do not reinforce unacceptable behaviour by giving into Oliver's demands and undermining their own roles.

CASE STUDY 2

John, aged 16 years, was referred to CAMHS as he had told the GP he was unhappy and wanted to die. John was offered the opportunity to meet with the child psychiatrist alone but was unable to make a decision so was seen with his mother. John thought he had been referred to CAMHS because 'I get depression' and 'I find school very uncomfortable'. When the concept of depression was explored with him, he felt he did not want to live but also did not want to die. He had not tried any self-harm but often wondered what drowning might be like. He thought life was useful but did wonder about the point of it given we all ultimately die. His unhappiness stemmed from difficulties with peers. He had never had good peer relationships and his mother recalled that he had never really had a friend. John felt he did want friends but none of his peers at school met his high expectations or standards. He does not enjoy school because of the problems with peers but manages some of the academic work.

There were no problems with John's pregnancy. He was an irritable baby compared with his siblings. His mother recalled that he had always been a picky eater and had a very small, rigid and limited repertoire. He was always very sensitive to smells, textures and noises. As a toddler in playschool he preferred to play alone than with peers. He liked to play with the same toys and would often spend hours lining up the toys in a particular order and become distressed if the order was disrupted. His mother could not recall if he was an affectionate baby but she felt he was less responsive than his sisters.

continued ≫

CASE STUDY 2 *continued*

John was cooperative with the assessment. When he
struggled with a question he was even more inclined to avoid
eye contact, which was poor throughout the interview. He
struggled to express himself clearly and often used words such
as 'depression', which he could not describe further. It was
as though he had heard the words but did not really have an
understanding of the concept. His speech was monotonous
with no variation in tone or pitch. He did not appear depressed
and was not suicidal as exploration revealed that he saw life as
pointless on a philosophical level rather than because of how
he felt.

What is the most likely diagnosis?

What would be the most appropriate management?

What would be the place of counselling using a psychotherapeutic
approach?

ASD is the most likely diagnosis and John fulfils the triad of
impairment.

An explanation of the disorder was given to John and his mother.
This included explaining the impact of the clinical features on
everyday life. The diagnosis with permission was communicated
to the Educational Psychologist who was able to initiate school
interventions to help John better manage school. His mother
was also advised of a support group for parents to help manage
some of John's difficulties and also develop strategies to
manage aspects of his difficult behaviour. His mother learned
that it was important to be aware that John did not understand
concepts such as compromise and understanding other people's
perspectives.

John's mother queried the possibility of individual work with John
using a psychotherapeutic approach. Given John's very rigid and
inflexible thinking it was agreed that this would not be helpful. A
more behavioural approach was taken to help John learn socially
acceptable behaviour.

CHAPTER 15

DISORDERS OF PERSONALITY

Nisha Dogra and Stephen Cooper

KEY CHAPTER FEATURES

- Definition and prevalence of personality disorders
- Characteristics of the subtypes and their presentation to services
- Impact of having a personality disorder
- Management of personality disorders

Introduction

Issues relating to different traits and types of personality, how these may be factors in increasing risk of mental illness and how they may modify its presentation were discussed earlier in Chapter 2. There is no clear dividing line between the point where particular features suggest someone has a particular personality trait and the point where similar features suggest a diagnosis of personality disorder. Indeed, some would argue that the concept of a disorder of personality is inappropriate for something that may perhaps be seen as relating to traits on a continuum from mild to severe. There is also considerable debate about how far 'treatment' is effective and indeed whether it is appropriate to attempt to change what is a person's essential personality. Indeed, in Soviet Russia in the mid-twentieth century, those with dissident ideas, who disagreed with the communist state, were sometimes described by the authorities as suffering from some form of mental disturbance, which could range from personality disturbance to mental illness, and were subsequently placed in mental institutions. The argument has become political in more ways than one. Successive UK government Home Secretaries have sought to make responsibility for people with 'dangerous and psychopathic personality disorders' the domain of mental health services. They wish us, as mental health professionals, to assess risk, provide treatment and protect the public from such

individuals. In the mind of the general public, it is often the disturbed, impulsive, aggressive psychopath who seems to be *mentally ill* rather than those we as doctors may regard as much more ill.

Thus, we cannot avoid having to face the issues involved. Perhaps the most useful way to try to define the point where a personality trait becomes a disorder is as below:

It is where maladaptive patterns of behaviour, modes of thinking and relating to oneself, the environment and other people result in impairment of social functioning for the individual or others affected by their behaviour.

In general, the features defining an individual's personality disorder are present during adolescence and are persistent throughout their life. ICD-10 defines 10 main personality disorders (Box 15.1) as well as a category of Enduring Personality Changes, where features do not easily fit one of the 10 specified categories.

Why is this relevant for you?

As students you will only encounter a few people with clearly established personality disorder, but some of those encounters may be the most challenging that you experience. Knowing something about the types of disorders can help you understand how different types of people may access help and present to services and how to ensure that the care you provide is professional despite the challenges. It may also help you in understanding their perspectives and being more objective if you are aware of the potential problems. It is also important because there can be a tendency to label people by their major trait and overlook other possibilities on the basis that they are just anxious or such like.

Assessment and diagnosis of personality disorder

Diagnosis of any particular personality disorder needs to be made carefully. First, it is often difficult as individuals sometimes have features present in more than one type of disorder. It also depends in part on gaining a good account of an individual's general demeanour and behaviour from an informant (family member, friend) as one cannot rely solely on the person's own account. (We do not always see ourselves as others see us.) Finally, given the variability in how any of us behaves over time, it is important to be able to establish that the features being used to make the diagnosis are consistently present. The evidence for having a personality disorder is that the person consistently displays evidence of behaviours, cognitions and emotions that cause problems for him or her and others around them. These difficulties are evident in a number of different situations and appear to have persisted throughout life and begun in childhood.

A diagnosis of personality disorder may co-exist with diagnosis of another mental disorder. Sometimes other disorders are secondary to the personality disorder, arising because the personality disorder results in conflicts between the individual and the world around them, leading to depression or anxiety. Sometimes the disorders are coincidental. As with personality traits, it is best to view a diagnosis of personality disorder along a separate axis to the diagnosis of another mental disorder and to list one as the main diagnosis and the other as a secondary diagnosis, rather than as another differential diagnosis.

Types of personality disorders

As outlined in Chapter 2 and shown in Box 15.1 there are several personality disorders. It is perhaps simplest to classify people into one of three broader categories:

Box 15.1: ICD classification of personality disorders

F60 Specific personality disorders

Paranoid – includes previous categories such as sensitive and querulant personality

Schizoid – not the same as schizotypal disorder (related to schizophrenia)

Dissocial – more used term is antisocial, psychopathic or sociopath

Emotionally unstable – either impulsive or borderline type

Histrionic (was hysterical)

Anankastic (was obsessive)

Anxious (also called avoidant)

Dependent (was asthenic, inadequate or passive)

Other specific personality disorders, including narcissistic personality disorder

F61 Mixed or other personality disorders

- odd/eccentric types (paranoid, schizoid)
- emotional, erratic types (dissocial, emotionally unstable, histrionic)
- anxious/fearful types (anankastic, anxious, dependent).

We will not describe all of the different personality disorders in detail but talk about them generally. However, two particular types merit some detail given their impact on the community and health services.

How common are personality disorders and what causes them?

Prevalence is thought to be around 10 per cent. It is difficult to be precise as many may not present to services and some may present through presentations other than their personality. Although many people may not have personality disorders, many individuals do have traits but not to the extent of being a disorder as discussed earlier. Having a trait and significant other aetiological factors may increase the risks of developing mental health problems even for those without a personality disorder.

The aetiology of personality disorders is unclear but it is likely that as with other types of mental disorders the aetiology is multifactorial. Having a predisposition to develop an antisocial disorder is more likely to materialize in the context of being raised in an aggressive, violent and abusive background. Being 'mollycoddled' and having anxiety traits may make avoidant personality disorder more likely.

Before we discuss the potential impact of having a personality disorder, we will discuss the broad characteristics of the key groups. Dissocial personality disorder is more frequently found in men whereas emotionally unstable personality disorder is higher in women. As well as biological differences, this may also reflect societal expectations and gender roles.

Odd/eccentric types (cluster A)

People with paranoid personality are by their nature paranoid; they are suspicious and mistrustful of others often believing themselves to have been unfairly treated or maligned. They tend to be very negative in their views about the external world and when these negative ideas prove themselves to be true, they feel justified in their original views. They are unable to see how their own behaviour may lead to the pattern of events. There is little if any evidence to support their suspicions about others. They are more likely to be involved in legal actions as a recourse for their perceived injustices, as reasoning with them can prove to be difficult as they do not trust others. They tend to have difficulty developing close and warm relationships.

People with schizoid personality are loners who struggle to make appropriate social relationships. They tend to be emotionally detached and have little involvement with others and the external world in socially acceptable ways.

Schizotypal personality, which is classified under schizophrenia rather than personality disorder, is different in that not only are these people socially and emotionally detached (as are those with schizoid personality) they can often show oddities of thought, perception and communication. Some individuals who go on to develop schizophrenia are thought to have this type of personality, although most with this disorder do not develop schizophrenia.

It is important, as with schizophrenia, not to confuse this type of disorder as 'split personality'. These people do not have many different types of personality but are socially withdrawn and isolated.

Emotional, erratic types (cluster B)

The two major ones are discussed in some depth as they can present significant challenges to health care providers. Also both tend to stabilize and/or diminish with age.

Dissocial/antisocial personality disorder

This is the disorder that is most often in the news headlines because it is more likely to lead to violent or extreme behaviour. The most severe form of this is psychopathy, which makes up about 20 per cent of this group. The main features are listed in Box 15.2 and the diagnosis is made more often for men than women.

The history of many of these people may reveal a number of features that should make you consider the possibility of such a diagnosis. Typical are bullying behaviour at school, leaving school early, convictions for assault, poor employment record, substance misuse, cruelty to animals and fire-setting.

In recent years, there has been increased interest in looking for underlying biological factors in these individuals. For example, there is evidence that impulsivity in some circumstances may relate in part to disturbances of serotonin function. Some

---

Box 15.2 : Features of dissocial personality disorder

More common in males

Evidence of conduct disorder in childhood (required for DSM-IV diagnosis of Antisocial personality disorder but not for ICD-10 Dissocial personality disorder)

Callous unconcern for the feelings of others and no remorse for behaviour

Gross and persistent irresponsibility and disregard for social rules, norms and obligations

Unable to form stable or enduring relationships although has no difficulty in establishing them

Low tolerance to frustration and easily becomes angry or aggressive

Incapacity to experience guilt or profit from experience

Marked proneness to blame others for difficulties

Often behaves impulsively

May have a criminal record

functional MRI studies suggest possible areas of brain dysfunction. However, most theories relating to all forms of personality disorder focus on psychological and developmental factors and are beyond the scope of this book.

As would be expected from the clinical features, they are at increased risk of engaging in criminality and violence. They are also at increased risk of death from suicide, accidents and violence.

A diagnosis of dissocial personality disorder does not absolve an individual of responsibility for any criminal acts that they commit. The criminal justice system (police, prisons, courts and probation service) frequently manage such individuals (although they may not necessarily be labelled as having this disorder). It is important to maintain clear boundaries and rules when treating these patients. Any associated criminal offending is often best managed by the criminal justice system rather than mental health services.

Emotionally unstable personality disorder

Borderline personality disorder is a commonly used term for emotionally unstable personality disorder (EUPD). It is a condition characterized by impulsive actions, rapidly shifting moods, and chaotic relationships. There are two types (impulsive and borderline type) and in both there is:

- a marked tendency to act impulsively without considering the consequences of these actions, for example engaging in unprotected sex or substance abuse;
- an inability to plan ahead, coupled with a lack of self control and outbursts of intense anger, which can lead to violence and other extreme behaviour, especially if impulsive acts are challenged or prevented by people around them.

The impulsive type is characterized by emotional instability and an inability to control impulses, with episodes of threatening behaviour and violence occurring particularly in response to criticism by others. Women are more likely to receive a diagnosis of this disorder than men.

In addition, people with this type of personality disorder may experience severe doubts about their self image, aims and sexual preferences which cause upset and distress. The main features are a chronic feeling of emotional emptiness, emotional instability, a pattern of forming very intense, but usually unstable, relationships, outbursts of anger, acts of self-harm

and threats of suicide. When these individuals do experience emotions it is often in a very intense way but this rapidly turns to an inability to cope with these emotions, leading to some of the features above. They are liable to become involved in intense but unstable relationships that can cause them continual emotional crises, which they will endure to avoid being abandoned. Pseudo-hallucinations may be described by some in states of acute crisis. It is more common in females and a history of sexual abuse is often elicited. Completed suicide occurs in around 8–10 per cent of individuals with this disorder, and acts of self-mutilation (e.g. cutting or burning) and suicide threats and attempts are very common. Recurrent job losses, interrupted education and broken marriages are common.

Comorbidity with mood disorders, substance misuse, eating disorders (usually bulimia) and post-traumatic stress disorder is common. Very stressful or chaotic childhoods are commonly reported (e.g. physical and sexual abuse, neglect, hostile conflict, and early parental loss or separation). For this reason multi-axial classification systems can be helpful in designing interventions. This often means that the features leading to the presentation are longstanding so long-term therapeutic interventions may be helpful.

Some of these individuals present frequently to A&E departments, to their GPs and to crisis teams in the community. There are often strong pressures for their admission to hospital, but this is rarely helpful in the long term as it leads to increased dependence on others and further failure to develop coping mechanisms.

The terminology 'borderline' stems from the idea that borderline disorder lay somewhere between the older notions of neurotic disorders and a psychosis. This is not the case hence the move towards EUPD.

Anxious fearful types (cluster C)

Cluster C has different types of personality disorder within it with three types being most prominent. Individuals with avoidant personality disorder worry about doing anything new for fear of being rejected of failing. They are desperate for acceptance and approval yet at the same time can be crippled by fear of rejection or being disappointed. They actively seek relationships and want them so an added component is frustration with the fact they are unable to make successful relationships or be the person they might actually want to be.

Individuals with dependent personality type have difficulty in taking any responsibility for themselves and almost need to be given direction. They lack any ability to fend for themselves. A point worth bearing in mind is that in some cultural contexts (and even the broader UK context less than a generation ago), dependency by women on men is actively encouraged as 'cultural norms' deemed women unable to make decisions regarding their own future. A trait is not a personality type if it is within a cultural norm.

An individual with obsessive compulsive personality is preoccupied with order and control. They often seek perfection and thereby are great non-finishers as the end product is never judged to be good enough. However, as they take their responsibilities seriously they can become very stressed especially as they are generally indecisive and inflexible. People with obsessive compulsive disorder (OCD) differ from those with obsessive compulsive personality disorder in that those with OCD experience anxiety related to specific preoccupations, which are perceived as threatening. They then carry out rituals in an attempt to dispel that threat. Unlike individuals with OCD, those with obsessive compulsive personality generally do not have repeated, unwanted and/or ritualistic behaviour.

Impact of having a personality disorder

Clearly from the above descriptions it will be evident that some disorders have more obvious social impact than others. However, personality disorders do share some commonalities and these relate to how the individual with a disorder relates to others and the external world. Many people with a personality disorder do not recognize that they do indeed have a personality disorder, although this may not be the case when the disorder is used to absolve responsibility for one's own behaviour. Different disorders carry different degrees of risk but people with personality disorders are at a high risk of undertaking behaviours that do not conform to expected societal norms. They may be particularly vulnerable to developing specific psychiatric problems as they do not tend to have a range of coping skills and at times of stress may be even less adaptable than usual. They may resort to their key trait and become even less functional. Developing and maintaining relationships may be

particularly challenging and not just for those with DPD or EPUD. If an individual is an odd, eccentric person and is also suspicious of others, it becomes clear that relationships are likely to be strained, as they may well be in someone who constantly seeks reassurance. In particular, relationships with health care providers can be especially fraught. This may be true for all the personality types. Those in the odd/eccentric cluster may be frustrated by the needs of others to get them to access help when this is not something they feel they need. The more dramatic personality types can frustrate health care providers by their behaviours and recklessness. The anxious types can be demanding on health services and yet never satisfied with the responses they receive. It can also be an issue that individuals with personality disorders do not do as well as they might expect and then become frustrated. An example of this may be the obsessive type of person who becomes stuck in tasks but never actually finishes them because of circularity in their thinking. However, with these negative sequelae the individual is likely to become more entrenched and thereby exacerbate the problem.

Not only are individuals with personality disorder at risk of developing mental health problems, their personality can have a detrimental impact on their ability to parent and thereby be a factor in their children's mental health. A parent with an anxious personality type may because of their own fears restrict the child's exposure to the external world and thereby instil in the child a sense of fear rather than sense of mastery. For reasons that relate to their personality, parents with personality disorder may be inconsistent, detached, over-intrusive, over-permissive and/or inflexible. All of these may be important aetiological factors in whether children develop problems or not.

Individuals with a personality disorder may be more likely to use a more limited range of defence mechanisms than others. The defence mechanism of projection (attributing one's own feelings or thoughts to others) is typical of cluster A type personalities and type B when under pressure. Splitting is typical of EPUD and often used with clinical staff. Acting out (expressing an internal impulse through an external behaviour) is characteristic of type B personality types.

Management of personality disorders

Most people with personality disorders, especially dissocial personality and EUPD, are often challenging to manage and can evoke strong negative feelings in others (for example through repeated self-harm, through aggression). Recognizing these feelings (countertransference) is important and helps in establishing and maintaining a professional relationship to ensure that they still receive any care they require. Despite many efforts, treatment for personality disorders is often unsatisfactory.

The most appropriate approaches are generally forms of psychological therapies. A few 'Therapeutic Community' treatment programmes have been successful for a proportion of patients. The aim of these is to provide a supportive and trusting environment in which the patient can learn better ways to cope. However, these all require a considerable commitment from the patient – something which is often lacking in the above two types of more severe disorder. It is worth remembering that many individuals with personality disorder do not necessarily agree that they do have a disorder. Various psychotropic drugs have been used and some have been subject to reasonable quality clinical trials. In general, evidence for their effectiveness is poor. Those most examined have been SSRIs for impulsivity, antipsychotics and mood stabilizers. In general, these really only seem to be useful if appropriate target symptoms are present (e.g. depression, marked paranoid ideation) and even then are not very effective.

Summary

There are three major subtypes of personality disorders and two that can present with significant challenges to health services. Although personality disorders have a prevalence rate of about 10 per cent, the traits are more common and may still lead to problems. As future doctors, it is helpful to be aware of the potential presence of a disorder as it may help how you relate to the patient to provide them the care that they require.

Further reading

Coid J, Yang M, Tyrer P, *et al.* (2006) Prevalence and correlates of personality disorder in Great Britain. *British Journal of Psychiatry* 188: 423–431.

Fonagy P and Bateman A (2006) Progress in the treatment of borderline personality disorder. *British Journal of Psychiatry* 188: 1–3

McMain S and Pos AE (2007) Advances in psychotherapy of personality disorders: A research update. *Current Psychiatry Reports* 9: 46–52.

CASE STUDY

A 32-year-old man presents to casualty having got into a fight with a neighbour. He accused the neighbour of spying on him. He is known in the neighbourhood as being someone who keeps himself to himself but every now and again there are incidents when altercations occur.

What would you do as a doctor working in casualty?

What might your differential diagnosis be?

The first action needs to be to treat any injury that might have occurred in the fight. The man is likely to be argumentative and suspicious so it is important to be aware of this when treating him. Once the injury has been treated, it is important to take a history and see if you can establish what might be making him suspicious at this point. Before a diagnosis of personality disorder is considered, you need to ensure that a psychotic illness has been excluded.

CHAPTER 16

COMMONLY USED PSYCHOLOGICAL TREATMENTS

Ian Collings and Nisha Dogra

KEY CHAPTER FEATURES

- Common components of psychological treatments
- Features of counselling, behavioural therapy, cognitive behavioural therapy, family therapy, group therapy, interpersonal therapy and psychodynamic psychotherapy
- Clinical indications for these types of therapy

Introduction

Psychiatrists do not just prescribe pills! We have a further armoury to call on, that of the psychological therapies. These therapies usually involve an interaction between an individual or group of individuals and a therapist or therapists, although, increasingly, psychological treatments are being delivered with limited therapist input. Examples include guided self-help, where an individual is given written or computer materials to follow with only limited therapist contact, or pure self-help, where the individual does not interact with a therapist. Over the years many different types of psychological treatment have been developed, all of which share some important features as summarized by Jerome Frank (Box 16.1). In this chapter only the commoner forms of psychological treatment will be considered.

All of the therapies discussed in this chapter can be used in any age group dependent on development levels. At times, therapies will require adaptation for use with particular groups or not be suitable for them (e.g. very young children and individuals with severe learning disabilities).

Psychotherapies may be as much about helping someone to be able to manage the life they have as about changing aspects of it. There is also often an

Box 16.1: Common features of psychological therapies

Listening and talking

Release of emotion

Giving information

Providing a rationale

Restoration of morale

Suggestion

Guidance and advice

Therapeutic relationship

impression that 'talking therapies' do not carry any risk, after all no potentially dangerous medicines are used. However, therapy that is poorly carried out can be damaging. Therapy that is mistimed may lead to the patient suffering more if their coping mechanisms (albeit that they may be maladaptive) are stripped away but they are left with nothing to replace them.

Exercise

Do this with your colleagues if possible so you can discuss your responses.

What frightens you? Think about something that makes you feel scared or anxious. It might be a spider or a rat. How do you think you might get over that fear? Talk it through with your colleagues.

You probably know how to explain a physical treatment to a patient, such as a medication or surgical intervention. Think about how you might explain a psychological treatment to a patient. What words would you use? How would you explain its mode of action?

Exercise answer

Think of the psychology you learnt in your first or second year at medical school. Remember Pavlov and his dogs? Every time a bell was rung the dogs would salivate because originally the bell was rung at the same time as the dogs got food. The food was called the unconditioned stimulus and the salivation the unconditioned response. The bell was rung so many times at the same time as the food was given, that it became the conditioned stimulus. Removing the food and ringing the bell, Pavlov noticed that the bell still produced the salivation. However, continued ringing of the bell without the food resulted in the response dying out, this is called extinction.

Now think of that thing that scares you. Why does it scare you? Have you had a bad experience in the past? Maybe if you continue to face the object of the anxiety either all at once (flooding) or in steps (systematic desensitization) the anxiety associated with it will eventually die out. These are two important psychological treatments, the second of which is still in use today.

Psychodynamic therapies

Although there are various types of psychodynamic treatment, it is commonly agreed that many were developed out of the original work of Sigmund Freud and others. Freud developed a technique known as psychoanalysis, which often took place over many years, with an individual meeting their analyst five or more times a week. This form of psychotherapy is often referred to in the media and popular culture. Think of the patient lying on the couch, the caricatured therapist analysing their dreams or shouting out random words and asking the patient to respond with the first word that comes to mind. These techniques of dream analysis and free association were classic components of Freud's psychoanalysis. This form of therapy is still used today, although less commonly than in the past. Psychodynamic therapies can be a difficult concept for many students, as the processes taking place are often less transparent than in other therapies. It can also appear to be rather unstructured and random. It is also more dependent than some of the other therapies on the relationship between the patient and therapist. Some students struggle to identify how the therapist evaluates change. As with other interventions there should over time be a reduction in symptoms or their impact on the individual. It might be useful to try and think about the principles that have arisen out of psychotherapy that are applied in everyday clinical practice, such as taking a patient-centred approach and understanding the patient perspective better through exploring what meaning the issues have for them. It may also be useful for you to think at a more basic level about how unresolved conflict with a friend or partner leaves you feeling and how it impacts on you the next time the same situation arises.

Brief forms of psychodynamic psychotherapy are now more widely used and usually take the form of once weekly sessions (or fewer) with a psychotherapist. The therapist is aiming to help the individual explore and understand their unconscious motivation. Various defences are used to deal with intrapsychic conflict and the aim is to give the individual insight into their presentation as discussed in Chapter 3. Some of these defences are reiterated for convenience below (Box 16.2). An unskilled therapist can let transference and countertransference issues affect the therapy in a detrimental way; care should be taken to prevent this from happening.

Psychodynamic therapy tends to focus on unconscious processes as they are manifested in a person's present behaviour. The goals of psychodynamic therapy are to raise the patient's self-awareness and understanding of how events in the past may be influencing current behaviour. In this way the patient is able to explore past unresolved conflict (which is what leads to the current behaviour that is causing them problems or symptoms) such as dysfunctional relationships, unresolved feelings. In doing so the current problems can be better understood and enable more effective change. For example, a female who may have had a difficult relationship with her father may have a tendency to enter relationships with males that lead her to feeling

Box 16.2: Defence mechanisms

Repression: pushing away of unacceptable ideas or thoughts

Denial: denying external reality of unwanted information

Displacement: uncomfortable emotions or thoughts are moved from a bad object to a more acceptable one

Projection: unacceptable ideas and thoughts are transferred on to another person

Regression: moving to a lower level of complexity when under stress

Reaction formation: taking the opposite attitude to oppressed wish

Rationalization: explanation of things in a logical or ethical way

Sublimation: creative activities which are motivated and driven from sexual instincts and drives

Identification: attributes of others are taken on to oneself

bad about herself. Through therapy she may have insight that these relationships have come about because she has unresolved issues regarding her father. This is a fairly simplistic example, but indicates the way that psychotherapy tries to work. Through therapy the woman may recognize the defence mechanism she uses to try and deal with the internal conflicts that the relationship with her father has left.

The main forms of psychodynamic treatment now last from around 12 sessions through to 40 sessions, but for some patients the process is much longer.

Brief psychotherapy is felt to be most appropriately suited to highly motivated individuals of above average intelligence who are psychologically minded. There is some evidence that brief psychodynamic psychotherapies can be helpful, but the evidence base is far less developed than that of other brief psychotherapies, such as cognitive behavioural therapy (CBT) or family therapy.

Cognitive behavioural therapy

There are various forms of CBT. Aaron Beck is considered to be the originator of cognitive therapy. He developed a therapy for depression, arguing that individuals develop basic or core beliefs/schemas from early experiences, for example feelings that

they are not good enough, perhaps they experienced harsh paternal criticism, or considered people to be judgemental. This leads to conditional dysfunctional assumptions, for example 'If I get anything wrong I will be punished'. Many negative events lead to negative automatic thoughts, for example 'It's my fault; I'm a failure; Things will never go right for me', which then result in the development of depressive symptoms. It is argued that these negative thoughts maintain the depression and a vicious cycle is established. The main function of therapy is to break this cycle by getting individuals to recognize how their thoughts and feelings impact on each other. In cognitive therapy it is common to use dysfunctional thought records to challenge these views. Individuals are asked to rate their emotions, what they were thinking about at the time and the thoughts that were running through their mind, i.e. the negative automatic thoughts. They are asked to challenge these automatic thoughts with alternative, more positive views and then rate the outcome according to how far the individual now believes the original thoughts. By continually doing this, it has been shown that individuals are able to challenge their thoughts and feel brighter as a result.

This cognitive approach is often coupled with a behavioural approach. The key behavioural feature of depression is reduction in usual activity, often as a result of loss of interest, motivation and pleasure. Behavioural techniques encourage an individual to re-engage with activities, often referred to in therapeutic terms as 'behavioural reactivation'. This is often done by encouraging individuals to keep a weekly activity schedule and list exactly what they do, including rating how much pleasure they gain from it and how much of an achievement that was. This can also be used to help individuals plan what they are doing and to set goals that are achievable for individuals.

In addition to CBT for depression, CBT has been developed and used for a wide variety of other disorders, including most anxiety disorders, stress-related disorders and somatoform disorders. It has also been used in the treatment of schizophrenia in an attempt to help individuals deal with hallucinations and delusions, although the evidence for this is less convincing at present than for CBT for depression or anxiety disorders. Of particular research interest during recent times is the use of CBT to help patients manage symptoms of chronic physical disease.

Research suggests that CBT can help patients deal with chronic pain and life-altering diagnoses such as HIV infection and cancer.

Trauma-focused CBT is a specific treatment used for the management of post-traumatic stress disorder. This involves an individual focusing on the trauma. For example, individuals are often asked to develop a detailed present tense account of exactly what they have been through, make a recording of this and listen to it over and over again. It is believed that individuals are helped by the repeated exposure to what happened, which allows the mind to habituate to the experience.

Eye movement desensitization and reprocessing

This treatment involves an individual with post-traumatic stress disorder focusing on the worst picture of the trauma, coupling that with a thought, for example 'I am out of control', their feelings at the time, for example anxiety, and the part of the body where the anxiety is felt, for example in the pit of the stomach. While holding these four separate things together, bilateral stimulation, for example through asking the patient to follow the fingers of the therapist from side to side or alternating hand tapping, the individual is asked to allow their mind to go where it wants to, i.e. a form of free association. It is not known how eye movement desensitization and reprocessing works, but randomized controlled trials have shown that it is an effective treatment for post-traumatic stress disorder (NICE guidelines: www.NICE.org.uk). Some individuals argue that it works by a similar mechanism to trauma-focused CBT, whereas other individuals believe that there is a different as yet unknown mechanism.

Other forms of behavioural therapy

Relaxation training

This is a useful form of therapy for people with stress or anxiety disorders. Here patients are asked to use techniques such as progressive muscle relaxation, where the individual moves through different muscle groups tensing and relaxing them, or guided imagery, when at times of stress or anxiety the individual learns to take themselves off into a situation they find relaxing, such as walking in a meadow or alongside a stream on a warm summer's day.

Systematic desensitization

In the treatment of phobic anxiety disorders, systematic desensitization is often used. In this an individual is gradually exposed to more stress-inducing situations on a hierarchy they have developed in conjunction with the therapist regarding their phobia. The list below shows a graded hierarchy for an individual with a fear of spiders:

1 Discussion of a small spider.
2 Picture of a small spider.
3 Picture of a bigger spider.
4 Film of a small spider.
5 Film of several spiders.
6 Real life exposure to a small spider in a jar.
7 Exposure to spider out of jar.
8 Exposure to bigger spider in jar.
9 Exposure to bigger spider outside jar.
10 Visit to zoo to see spiders through window.
11 Entry into spider exhibit within zoo.
12 Progress to contact with spiders.

The aim of a graded desensitization programme is to gradually move through the steps, asking individuals to rate their level of anxiety at each step, often using diaries similar to those described above for depression. As the levels of anxiety reduce, i.e. the individual habituates, they are asked to move up to the next level of the hierarchy. This has been shown to be a very effective treatment of phobic disorders if individuals are able to fully engage with it.

Exposure with response prevention

In this type of therapy, which is particularly used for obsessive compulsive disorder, the patient is asked to think of a hierarchy of situations that may fuel a particular ritual and expose themselves in a controlled way without engaging in the ritualistic behaviour. It is anticipated that if the patient can hold off engaging in the ritual for upwards of an hour the anxiety and drive to do it will eventually habituate and die out.

Interpersonal therapy

Interpersonal therapy was developed to treat individuals with depression but is now also used for the treatment of other conditions, such as anorexia nervosa. There are numerous positive studies showing the effectiveness of this form of therapy in depression. This therapy is based on interpersonal theory from the work of Adolf Meyer, Harry Stack Sullivan and later John Bowlby and other individuals. The theory argues that life events occurring after the formative years influence psychopathology. The focus is on an interpersonal problem, for example a complicated bereavement, relationship difficulty or an interpersonal deficit, using techniques from different psychotherapies. It has some overlap with psychodynamic therapy and CBT, and deals with four interpersonal problem areas: grief, role dispute, role transitions and interpersonal deficits.

Problems in a patient's life are split into one of these four areas and strategies are developed to help the patient to cope with difficulties or to think about them in a different way. As with CBT, homework is often used to enable the patient to experiment and try out these strategies in their day-to-day lives.

Group therapies

Group therapies often use components of other therapies, for example psychodynamic groups and cognitive behavioural groups. It has been argued that there are many advantages to working in groups, making it a superior form of treatment to individual therapy, although most research studies do not convincingly show group therapy to be better than individual therapy. Groups may be closed and run for a specified period of time with the same members, or open with members coming and going depending on their needs. Irvin Yalom described a list of seven factors associated with the effectiveness of group therapy but several of these are more widely discussed.

1. Universality

Universality describes the shared experiences among clients. It helps the clients overcome their sense of isolation, validates their experiences and raises self-esteem. For many, it may be the first time they feel understood and like other people.

2. Altruism

As members are able to help each other, they identify their own strengths but also learn from each other, thus improving their own self-esteem, and develop better coping styles and interpersonal skills. By being able to help others their own sense of worth is likely to increase and for many it might be the first time they have felt useful or as if they have something to offer.

3. Instillation of hope

The group members are able to learn from each other and gain hope through the experience of others. As each member in a therapy group is inevitably at a different point on their therapy (this would only be the case for open groups), watching others cope with and overcome similar problems usually instils hope and inspiration. New members or those in despair may be particularly encouraged by others' positive experiences.

4. Cohesiveness

Cohesiveness is often referred to as the most therapeutic factor from which all of the other factors flow. Humans have an instinctive need to belong in groups, and some personal development can only occur in interpersonal relationships. Cohesiveness brings belonging, acceptance and validation to the counselling process.

5. Corrective recapitulation of the primary family experience

Members of a group will often unconsciously identify other members of the group as similar to their own immediate family. In this way through the therapy process, they can deal with these unresolved issues and address unhelpful patterns in their relationships. For example, a dominant member of the group may remind them of their authoritarian father and their need to rebel. Through this identification they may be able to address their feelings in a more appropriate way than for example with substance misuse.

6. Self-understanding/interpersonal learning

Members of group counselling may achieve a higher level of self-awareness through interactions and observations of others. They may also achieve greater levels of insight about the origins of their own problems and their maladaptive coping strategies.

7. Catharsis

Catharsis is defined as the experience of relief from emotional distress by expressing emotion. This is often a very positive part of the group therapy process and relating their experiences and not being judged by them can be a way of helping people move forward.

Group therapies may be particularly useful for problems people have with relationships. Because of the group situation an important caution in group therapy would be any form of anxiety particularly associated with a group setting such as social phobia.

Counselling

Counselling is a widely used term that has been defined as 'the means by which one person helps another to clarify his or her life situation and decide further lines of action'. In fact, various forms of counselling are used.

The humanistic or client-centred approach was developed by Carl Rogers, who emphasized the importance of recognizing that individuals already have the ability to work through their problems and that a counsellor's role is to facilitate this process by providing conditions of warmth, empathy and unconditional positive regard.

Other forms are more therapist led. For example, problem-solving counselling purely focuses on identifying and formulating problems, setting clear and achievable goals, generating alternatives for coping and then allowing an individual to problem solve as necessary. Problem-solving counselling is very much recommended for many types of less severe mental illness such as mild forms of depression and anxiety.

Other forms of counselling use techniques developed separately as therapies, for example cognitive behavioural counselling and interpersonal counselling, which would be virtually indistinguishable from CBT and interpersonal therapy. Psychodynamic counselling is another form of counselling that uses psychodynamic theory, and one of the most widely recognized forms of counselling is grief or bereavement counselling, which is widely used to help individuals with the loss of a loved one to help them work through the different stages of grief (denial, anger, bargaining, depression and acceptance).

Family therapy

Most children and adolescents live within families. Families are an environmental factor that can influence the presentation and maintenance of mental health problems, so it is perhaps unsurprising that there is a treatment modality which is specifically aimed at working with families. A child mental health assessment should include a brief assessment of family functioning, which will identify any need for more detailed exploration.

Family therapy is one of the most effective therapies available, with good evidence for its use. It is the first-line treatment for several disorders of childhood, including eating disorders. However, it also has a place in anxiety, bereavement disorders, conduct problems, substance misuse, chronic illness and psychosomatic disorders. The success of family therapy in the classic sense is less proven in substance misuse and conduct problems, but in conjunction with other therapies it can be useful.

Family therapy was developed on the basis that there was a 'right' way for families to function and family therapy helped the family negotiate this right way. Over time, the approach has changed and there is a greater focus on collaboration and seeing family therapy intervention as a way of helping families find their own solutions. However, in practice family therapy remains about helping families find better ways of being or functioning.

Principles of family therapy

There are clear principles at work for most of the models.

- Children need parents (or carers) who love and care for them, are emotionally responsive to their needs but also set clear and appropriate boundaries (this is culturally and socially dependent).
- Most people take a fairly pragmatic approach to defining a family and let the family decide for itself who is part of their family.

- Parents take on adult roles and responsibilities and set limits and boundaries. Where the adults fail to do this, intergenerational boundaries are considered too fluid. Where there is no understanding of a need to be flexible, the boundaries are considered too rigid.

- The family is an interdependent unit with flexibility to adapt to changing life stages and circumstances.

- There is a healthy balance between individuals in the family caring about each other but also having relationships outside of the family (depending on age).

- Families in which members are overly dependent on each other without a sense of individual autonomy are described as 'enmeshed'. It is mindful to be aware of cultural expectations, but even families that subscribe to a collective sense of self have individuation within a context.

- It is important not to attach blame but help families understand that they function the way they do for a host of reasons, and family work helps unpack some of these reasons and allow for improved family functioning.

Summary

This chapter described the common components of psychological treatments and outlined the features of behavioural therapies, cognitive behavioural therapy, counselling, family therapy, group therapy, interpersonal therapy and psychodynamic psychotherapy. The clinical indications for these types of therapy have been explained.

Further reading

Jacoby R, Oppenheimer C (2002) *Psychiatry in the Elderly*. Oxford: Oxford University Press.

Tyrer P, Silk KR (2008) *Cambridge Textbook of Effective Treatments in Psychiatry*. Cambridge: Cambridge University Press.

Weisz JR, Kazdin AE (2010) *Evidence-based Psychotherapies for Children and Adolescents*, 2nd edition. New York: Guilford Press.

CASE STUDY 1

David is a 35-year-old doctor who has suffered with two episodes of depression in his life. The second one started 2 months ago. He has low mood, decreased energy, sleep problems and appetite loss. This has impacted on his work and he is currently taking sick leave. He was commenced on an antidepressant by his GP. There has only been a partial response and his GP has suggested a course of CBT.

Explain the term CBT to David.

Advise him how it will work to improve his depression and any side-effects of the treatment. CBT or cognitive behavioural therapy is a structured form of talking therapy that has been proven to be very effective in treating a number of mental health problems including depression. It works on the premise that when you are suffering from mental illness your thinking pattern is different. Cognition is another word for thought. The different thinking pattern is characterized by a number of cognitive distortions. For example, if you are depressed you may minimize all the positive things in your life and maximize (blow them out of proportion) the negative things.

As a consequence of this different pattern of thinking there is an emotional response (feeling low in depression or anxious with a phobia) and this in turn leads to a behaviour associated with the disorder. In the case of depression the negative thought pattern will lead to feeling down which may lead to not going out or seeing friends which perpetuates the difficulties.

CBT looks at altering the thought patterns that are seen in the mental illness in a hope to change the emotional response and subsequent behaviours. By challenging the negative thoughts and offering behavioural exercises like activity planning this can improve your depression.

CBT rarely has side-effects. It does demand a lot of work on the part of the patient though (it isn't as easy as swallowing a pill every day)! There are usually homework assignments and the individual has to continue with the techniques they have learnt long after the formal therapy has finished.

CASE STUDY 2

Marianne is a 26-year-old barrister. All her life she has had an irrational fear of pigeons. This started as a child when she was taken to Trafalgar Square by her parents to feed the pigeons and two of them landed on her head and pecked her. Now she gets panicky even if she sees pigeons on the television. The phobia has never been a problem as she lives in the country and went to university in Cambridge, where there weren't too many pigeons; she could always detour around them. However, in the past month she has been offered a job with a prestigious law firm in the city of London. She is terrified about encountering a flock of pigeons and wonders whether she can take the job or not. She doesn't want this irrational fear to prevent her career progression. She has heard that there may be some help available for her in the form of a talking therapy.

What kind of therapy might be useful for Marianne?

Devise a structure to her treatment. Marianne may well respond positively to a systematic desensitization approach which is often used to successfully treat phobic anxiety disorders. Below is a hierarchy that may be used to address her pigeon phobia.

Systemic Gradual Desensitization Approach

1. Discussion of pigeons
2. Picture of a pigeon
3. Picture of a flock of pigeons
4. Film of a pigeon
5. Film of a flock of pigeons
6. Real life exposure to a pigeon at a distance
7. Exposure to a flock of pigeons
9. Exposure to a flock of pigeons flying
10. Close exposure to a flock of pigeons
11. Pigeons eating seed out of her hand
12. Pigeons landing on her head

You probably know how to explain a physical treatment to a patient such as a medication or surgical intervention. Think about how you might explain a psychological treatment to a patient.

continued ≫

CASE STUDY 2 *continued*

What words would you use? How would you explain its mode of action?

We all explain medications to patients routinely every day, why not use the same template as we use when talking about medication? Talk about modes of action, side-effects, how long you have to take the treatment for. It's not as difficult talking about psychological treatments as you may think. Remember don't use jargon or big medical words. Give the patient an opportunity to ask questions and if you don't know the answer to the questions just say so and tell the patient you will find out.

Here are some words and phrases that you may be able to use:

Talking therapy

Thoughts

Feelings

Behaviours

Relaxation

The mode of action of psychological treatments may include words like:

Listening and talking

Release of emotion

Giving information

Providing a rationale

Restoration of morale

Suggestion

Guidance and advice

Supportive and therapeutic relationship

CASE STUDY 3

Alexa is an 11-year-old girl referred by her GP for features of obsessive compulsive disorder. The history from the mother reveals that over the last 4 months Alexa has developed counting rituals and also has to complete some activities a specific number of times. The rituals do not appear to be present at school but it is unclear if she is just better at hiding them there. Alexa appears to be constantly angry and not interested in anything. Alexa herself believes something bad will happen if she does not complete the rituals. The background is that Alexa has suffered from chronic airways disease for several years. She has at times become cyanosed and needed emergency oxygen. She is currently using a continuous positive airway pressure machine to prevent her from becoming cyanosed when asleep because of sleep apnoea. Alexa heard the paediatrician say that she requires further operations and this has caused some anxiety. She does not appear to understand her medical condition except that is worrying for the adults. Alexa presents as a very anxious girl. She also expressed some distress around family arguments related to her tantrums.

What is likely to be the primary diagnosis?

The primary diagnosis is likely to be anxiety and the OCD features are a way of managing her anxieties rather than OCD *per se*. Having rituals helps emotional containment.

What interventions might be helpful in this case and why?

The intervention involved individual work with Alexa to help her think about what her worries were and how they might be addressed. The work with her parents involved helping them to help each other as a couple contain their anxieties about Alexa's medical problems. In doing this, they were able to be firmer and clearer with Alexa when she had a tantrum. During the tantrum they focused on ensuring they remained firm and consistent. However, they were also able to identify times when they could be responsive to Alexa and discuss her worries in an appropriate way.

CHAPTER 17

PSYCHOPHARMACOLOGY

Stephen Cooper

Introduction

The general aim of this chapter is to give you an understanding of the mode of action and adverse effects of those drugs commonly used in the management of psychiatric illnesses. The drugs used under this heading are often termed 'psychotropic' drugs. Alcohol and a wide variety of drugs of abuse, such as cannabis and cocaine, also have potent effects on brain neurotransmitter systems and these may also be termed 'psychotropic' agents. However, this chapter will focus on therapeutic drugs.

The drugs to be discussed achieve their effects through alteration of function in neuronal systems in the brain. The main general mechanisms by which they achieve this are:

- alteration of neurotransmitter availability or release
- antagonism or agonism at neurotransmitter receptors
- by effects on second messenger systems in neurones or directly at ion channels.

Various aspects of the pharmacokinetics, mechanisms of action, adverse effects and drug interactions are discussed for each group of drugs. It is important to understand these basic issues in order to better understand how to use these drugs in practice and be able to inform patients, who now expect to be involved in discussion of their drug treatment. Ensuring good adherence (compliance) with treatment is very important to achieve a good clinical response and this depends on good communication with the patient about their treatment.

Anxiolytics and hypnotics

It is only when anxiety or sleep disturbance become more persistent, severe or disabling in terms of daily functioning that pharmacological treatment is required. The most universally effective treatment for anxiety symptoms is a benzodiazepine (BDZ), but these drugs must not be used indiscriminately.

Mechanism of action

Gamma amino-butyric acid (GABA) is the principal inhibitory neurotransmitter in the central nervous system and acts via $GABA_A$ receptors to increase the opening of chloride ion channels. An influx of Cl^- ions results in hyperpolarization of the post-synaptic neurone, making an action potential more difficult to achieve. $GABA_A$ receptors are linked to benzodiazepine receptors in the GABA–BDZ receptor complex, which is made up from five macromolecular subunits. These subunits are arranged around the chloride ion channel (Fig. 17.1). Opening of the ion channel requires binding of two GABA molecules to the two GABA receptors. When a BDZ binds to its receptor site on the complex, the ion channel opens for a longer period. Thus, BDZs enhance the inhibitory effects of GABA.

Standard benzodiazepines act as agonists at this BDZ receptor. Points to note are: (a) BDZs act only to enhance the effect of GABA and will do nothing in the absence of GABA or if the GABA receptor is blocked; (b) the binding sites for GABA and BDZs are separate; (c) the presence of a BDZ enhances the binding of GABA to its receptor.

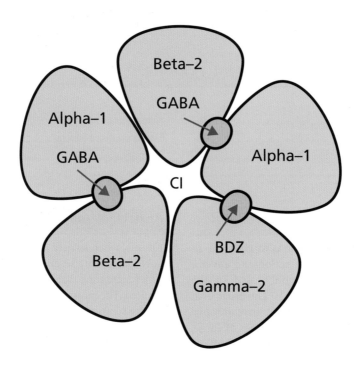

Fig. 17.1   A diagrammatic representation as though looking down onto that part of the receptor complex that is on the outside of the neuronal membrane. It shows the arrangement of the five subunits (in this case two alpha-1, two beta-2 and one gamma-2) around a chloride ion (Cl⁻) channel. The two GABA binding sites are at the interface between the alpha-1 and beta-2 subunits and the benzodiazepine (BDZ) binding site is at the interface between the alpha-1 and gamma-2 subunits. Opening of the Cl⁻ channel depends on the binding of two molecules of GABA. Binding of a BDZ molecule will increase the amount of time GABA maintains the opening of the ion channel.

Although the typical BDZ drugs, such as diazepam, act as full agonists at the receptor, having sedative, anxiolytic and anticonvulsant effects, other compounds may have different effects. Full inverse agonists have the opposite effect, being proconvulsant and anxiogenic. (Such compounds are largely of experimental interest only.) Neutral competitive antagonists block the effects of both agonists and inverse agonists and have no intrinsic activity of their own. Flumazenil acts as such a drug in most situations and is thus used to reverse the effects of overdosage of BDZs. Partial agonists and partial inverse agonists occupy the receptor but have only some of the effects of the 'full' agonists/inverse agonists.

There is evidence for a number of endogenous GABA–BDZ receptor ligands in the central nervous system. However, these are only present in small amounts and do not have any clear physiological significance.

Older drugs

Before BDZs became available, barbiturates, first synthesized around 1900, were the most widely used drugs for anxiety and sleep disturbance. (Barbiturates were also widely used as anaesthetic induction agents until the late 1990s.) They were very potent and, as well as having marked anxiolytic and hypnotic effects, also caused significant impairment of psychomotor function. This potency, the rapid development of tolerance to their effects and marked induction of their own metabolism led to escalation in dose by many patients as the effects would appear to wear off.

Dependence occurred in a high proportion of patients. Barbiturates can also cause marked respiratory depression and are thus extremely dangerous in overdose. At normal doses they act at a receptor site on the GABA–BDZ receptor complex to enhance the effects of GABA (like BDZs). However, in overdose they open the chloride ion channel independent of GABA, causing marked and prolonged neuronal depolarization and thus marked central nervous system depression. This does not occur in overdose with BDZs (whose effects are always dependent on GABA) making them relatively much safer.

Benzodiazepines

The greater safety of BDZs in overdose and the fact that, when used properly, they are less prone to dependence resulted in them rapidly supplanting the barbiturates when they were introduced in the early 1960s. Despite concerns about tolerance and dependence with BDZs, they remain one of the most effective and safe treatments for symptoms of anxiety. Death or serious morbidity from overdose of BDZs alone is rare and is only likely to occur if they are combined with other central nervous system (CNS) depressants. BDZs became used a little too ubiquitously during the 1960s and 1970s, leading to some patients becoming dependent. This led to a considerable reduction in their prescription from the early 1980s once this issue was recognized. A consequence of this was a rise in using other drugs for overdose (e.g. paracetamol) that carried greater risks in overdose.

Pharmacokinetics

Diazepam is the most widely used BDZ and its kinetics are summarized in Table 17.1. Absorption is good with oral use but is erratic and slow with intramuscular administration. Lorazepam, which has greater water solubility, is the BDZ recommended for intramuscular use. The principal active metabolite, desmethyldiazepam, has a very long elimination half-life, and gradual accumulation of active metabolites is one of the main reasons for many of these drugs having 'hangover' effects throughout the following day when given as hypnotics. The elimination half-life of diazepam is age dependent, resulting in greater hangover effects in older people. Some BDZs undergo Phase I metabolism, which results in production of active metabolites, and some only Phase II metabolism, resulting in inactivation. This and other pharmacokinetic properties of some of the commonly used BDZs are summarized in Table 17.2.

Physiological and adverse effects

The relative potencies of different BDZs as agonists at the GABA–BDZ receptor complex correlate with their potencies as anxiolytics and hypnotics. The inhibitory effects in the brain then cause the anti-anxiety, sedative and anticonvulsant effects. At normal therapeutic doses, BDZs have little effect on cardiovascular, respiratory or autonomic function. Respiratory depression and reduction in systolic blood pressure may occur, but principally with intravenous administration or overdose. Leucopenia and eosinophilia are rare. In the 1980s there was a

Table 17.1 Pharmacokinetic properties of diazepam

Bioavailability	Almost complete with oral dosing
Peak concentration	30–90 minutes
Renal excretion	Negligible for unchanged drug
Elimination half-life	Young adults: 20 hours
	Elderly people: 30–100 hours
Metabolism	Active metabolite:
	Desmethyldiazepam: half-life 30–90 hours

Table 17.2   Comparison of the pharmacological properties of common anxiolytics and hypnotics

Drug	Absorption	Metabolic phases	Parent drug $t1/2$ (h)	Important major metabolites $t1/2$ (h)
Diazepam	Rapid	I+II	20–100	30–90
Chlordiazepoxide	Intermediate	I+II	5–30	30–90
Lorazepam	Intermediate	II only	10–20	None
Nitrazepam	Intermediate	I+II	24	30–90
Temazepam	Slow	II only	10	None
Zolpidem	Rapid	II only	2	None
Zaleplon	Rapid	II only	1	None
Zopiclone	Rapid	I+II	3–4	3–6

$t1/2$, elimination half-life.

suggestion of increased risk of breast cancer but a large case–control study refuted this.

The more common adverse effects are listed in Table 17.3. Sedation is common and occurs with all BDZs. Tolerance to this effect generally occurs. Psychomotor impairment can be demonstrated in real life as well as in laboratory testing. It is partly related to sedation and impairment of central information-processing ability. Research is equivocal on whether or not tolerance develops over time to these impairments. The effects of BDZs on memory were first noted in 1965, when they were being used as premedication before general anaesthesia, many patients demonstrating amnesia for events prior to their surgery. This appears to be an anterograde amnesia, with no impairment of previously stored information. Sedation also plays a part in this.

It seems likely that different subtypes of the GABA–BDZ receptor complex may mediate different actions of these drugs. The different subtypes have different anatomical distributions, but may overlap in different brain regions. However, at present the available BDZ drugs are not particularly specific for individual receptor subtypes and therefore influence a number of functions.

Tolerance and dependence

The phenomena of tolerance and dependence are perhaps best illustrated by the effects of BDZs on rapid eye movement (REM) sleep. In the first week of taking BDZ hypnotics, REM sleep is suppressed from around 25 per cent to around 10 per cent of total sleep time. Over the following 14 days, adaptation occurs (probably due to resetting of receptor sensitivity) and REM sleep returns to around 25 per cent of total sleep time. Thus, tolerance has developed to the suppression of REM sleep. However, if the BDZ is now suddenly stopped a rebound increase in REM sleep to around

Table 17.3   Adverse effects of benzodiazepines

Common	Occasional	Rare
Drowsiness	Ataxia	Amnesia
Dizziness	Headache	Restlessness
Psychomotor impairment	Reduced blood pressure	Skin rash
	Dry mouth	
	Blurred vision	
	Gastrointestinal upset	

40 per cent of total sleep time occurs. This results in increased awakenings through the night and thus a tendency for the patient to restart and continue the BDZ believing their original sleep problem remains. If the patient remains off the drug, the increase in REM sleep takes around 6 weeks to return to normal.

Although tolerance appears to develop to the effects of BDZs on REM sleep, it is not clear that it occurs for the hypnotic, or sleep-inducing, effects of these drugs. There is certainly evidence, using subjective measures, of effectiveness being maintained for up to 6 months. With regard to the other effects of BDZs, there is evidence from human and laboratory animal studies for the development of tolerance to the sedative, muscle relaxant and anticonvulsant properties. However, evidence is equivocal with regard to tolerance to the anxiolytic and psychomotor effects. It seems clear that only some patients with anxiety disorders will begin to escalate their doses over time. The mechanisms underlying the development of tolerance seem to be partly pharmacodynamic, related to alterations in receptor sensitivity, but also cognitive, related to behavioural adaptation to the effects.

In the late 1970s it became clear that a withdrawal syndrome occurred after sudden cessation of normal therapeutic doses used for 6 weeks or more and not just following prolonged use of very high doses. The appearance of withdrawal symptoms will often lead to the patient recommencing the drug. The symptoms of this are listed (Table 17.4), the most common being symptoms similar to those of the anxiety disorder for which the drug was probably first prescribed. Thus, withdrawal of a BDZ should be gradual, particularly if the person has been on it for some weeks. A dose reduction by 25 per cent every 1–2 weeks is recommended for long-term users. A beta-adrenoceptor antagonist, e.g. propranolol, may reduce the intensity of the symptoms of withdrawal but does not actually improve success in coming off and remaining off BDZs.

The existence of a BDZ withdrawal syndrome can be interpreted as indicating that the patient has developed a degree of tolerance to some of the effects of the drug and that they have become addicted. This problem was recognized in the 1980s, when BDZs were very widely, and almost indiscriminately, prescribed (31 million GP scripts per year across England and Wales in 1979). Thus, during the 1980s there was a campaign to decrease the use of these drugs and ensure more careful use. Guidelines for their prescription can be found in the relevant section of the British National Formulary.

Clinical use

BDZs are used where moderate to severe anxiety symptoms arise due to acute stress, and in such situations their use should be short term and preferably for no longer than 2 weeks. Their main use, however, tends to be in patients presenting with generalized anxiety disorder (GAD). This is often a fluctuating condition with exacerbations at times of stress and chronic, milder symptoms on a longer term basis. Ideally use of BDZs for GAD should be for short periods, maximally 4 weeks, with the dose tailored to the severity of symptoms. Inevitably, some of these patients use BDZs chronically. BDZs can also be useful as a short-term adjuvant to cognitive behaviour therapy for phobias but are of limited use for panic disorder and obsessive compulsive disorder, except when patients are very acutely anxious.

BDZs are commonly used to assist withdrawal from alcohol, where a long elimination half-life drug is best. Chlordiazepoxide is the most widely used. In acute psychotic states short-term use of a high-potency drug, such as lorazepam, can be helpful in managing acute anxiety, agitation or aggression.

Hypnotics

Hypnotics are drugs that help to induce sleep. BDZs are useful in the treatment of insomnia, particularly

Table 17.4   Benzodiazepine withdrawal symptoms

Anxiety type	Disturbance of perception
Anxiety	Hypersensitivity to stimuli
Tremor	Abnormal bodily sensations
Dysphoria	Abnormal sense of movement/body sway
Sleep disturbance	Depersonalization
Muscle pains	Visual disturbance
Headache	**Severe but rare**
Nausea, anorexia	Paranoid psychosis
Sweating	Depressive episode
Fatigue	Seizures

for initial insomnia, when patients have difficulty falling asleep. As in the treatment of anxiety, they should only be used for short periods, as prolonged use will result in difficulties in withdrawal. However, it is relatively rare for patients to escalate the dose of hypnotic they use, and since 1980 prescribing of hypnotics has been stable at around 12 million scripts per year across England and Wales. They will generally assist induction of sleep within 30–60 minutes. Some of the original BDZ hypnotics had active metabolites with long elimination half-lives that caused significant 'hangover' effects the next day. However, some have no active metabolites (e.g. temazepam) and thus have advantages.

During the last 10 years several new hypnotics have become available (zolpidem, zopiclone and zaleplon) that are not chemically benzodiazepines but which nevertheless act via the GABA–BDZ receptor complex. They generally have shorter elimination half-lives, reduced risk of tolerance and dependence, and reduced psychomotor and hangover effects and are thus now the most usually prescribed hypnotic agents.

Other drugs used for anxiety

Antidepressant drugs, both the older tricyclic antidepressants (TCAs) and the newer drugs, have been demonstrated to have anxiolytic effects in mixed anxiety–depressive patients, GAD and panic disorder. Those antidepressants acting principally via the 5-HT system also seem to be useful for the symptoms of obsessive compulsive disorder. Thus, selective serotonin reuptake inhibitor (SSRI) antidepressants and others are now quite commonly prescribed for anxiety, as the patient can be maintained long term without the problems of tolerance and dependence that sometimes occur with BDZs.

In the late 1960s, beta-adrenoceptor antagonists, particularly propranolol and atenolol, were shown to be effective for the physiological symptoms of anxiety, particularly in situational anxiety and GAD. It was generally thought that their effectiveness was due to a primary reduction in peripheral symptoms, such as tremor and tachycardia, and that reduction in the unpleasant experience of these symptoms then reduced 'negative' feedback to the individual making it easier for them to manage the psychological aspects.

Buspirone, an azaspirodecanedione, an agonist

at 5-HT$_{1A}$ receptors, also seems to have anxiolytic effects. Initially it probably has no net effect as it acts to stimulate postsynaptic 5-HT$_{1A}$ receptors but also to reduce 5-HT release through its effect on cell body 5-HT$_{1A}$ receptors. However, over a 2–3 week period the effect on the cell body receptors wears off and the net effect becomes an increase in 5-HT transmission. It is less potent than the BDZs and the effects take up to 3 weeks to become evident. There is high first-pass metabolism and a considerable proportion of the effect is due to a metabolite (1-PP). The principal adverse effects of buspirone are nausea, gastrointestinal upset and headache. Because of its low potency it is not widely used.

Flumazenil

Flumazenil is a competitive antagonist of BDZs at the GABA–BDZ receptor and is used to reverse the CNS depressant effects of benzodiazepines when taken in overdose. It can only be given intravenously and has a short elimination half-life of 1 hour. Thus, its action to counteract the potentially life-threatening effects of an overdose may well wear off before there is a large fall in the plasma level of the BDZ taken in overdose. It is thus important to maintain the patient under observation until it is likely the drug taken in overdose has been washed out.

Antidepressants

These drugs are used for the treatment of depressive illness but are best reserved for patients with moderate and severe depression (see Chapter 6). Since the development of the first antidepressant drug in 1957, there have been considerable advancements in our understanding of probable mechanisms of action of these drugs. This has resulted in development of drugs with greater safety in overdose and profiles of adverse effects that most patients find easier to tolerate. There are now over 20 drugs licensed for use as antidepressants in the UK.

After a first episode of depression, prophylaxis is required for at least 6 months, and ideally 12 months, to reduce the risks of relapse or recurrence. This should usually be with the dose of antidepressant to which the patient initially responded. Those with recurrent episodes require prophylaxis over many years.

Neurochemical theories

Current theories of the biological mechanisms underlying depressive illness are largely derived from observations of the neurochemical effects of effective antidepressant drugs and ECT. Dysregulation of the serotonergic and/or adrenergic systems is thought to be important. This may itself result from disturbance of signal transduction and gene expression within neurones and will certainly affect such processes. Other evidence demonstrates disturbance of the corticosteroid system and potential interactions between this and the monoamine systems. Where the initial disturbance lies is not yet clear, and indeed pathways may differ between patients.

Classification of antidepressants

These drugs are most commonly classified according to their principal pharmacological effect rather than by specific chemical structure (Table 17.5).

The exceptions to this are the TCAs, which share a common chemical structure and also common pharmacological effects. The other group of drugs used in the treatment of mood disorders is the mood stabilizers (lithium compounds and some anticonvulsants), which are discussed later.

The SSRIs are the most widely prescribed antidepressant drugs in the UK. Their development during the 1980s and 1990s represented one of a series of steps in the wider development of antidepressant drugs with more specific pharmacological effects. For 25 years prior to this the TCAs had been the mainstay of antidepressant treatment, but they had a wide spectrum of pharmacological effects and were associated with many adverse effects. They remain in use for more treatment-resistant patients, and to understand the place of the newer drugs it is useful to have knowledge of what preceded them. The monoamine oxidase inhibitors were another of the first generation of antidepressant drugs. They also suffer a number of drawbacks compared with newer drugs and are thus

Table 17.5 Classification of antidepressant drugs

Group	Principal pharmacological effects	Examples
Tricyclic antidepressants (TCAs)	Inhibition of reuptake of 5-HT and NA in synapse Anticholinergic effects	Amitriptyline Clomipramine Imipramine
Selective serotonin reuptake inhibitors (SSRIs)	Inhibition of reuptake of 5-HT in synapse	Citalopram Fluoxetine Paroxetine Sertraline
Noradrenalin reuptake inhibitors (NARIs)	Inhibition of reuptake of NA in synapse	Reboxetine
Serotonin and noradrenalin reuptake inhibitors (SNRIs)	Inhibition of reuptake of 5-HT and NA in synapse Lack other effects of TCAs that give rise to many of their adverse effects	Venlafaxine
Atypical	Have some amine uptake inhibition but also antagonize one or more of 5-HT$_2$, alpha$_1$-NA, alpha$_2$-NA receptors. These receptor effects increase amine availability in the synapse	Mianserin Mirtazapine Nefazodone Trazodone
Monoamine oxidase inhibitors (MAOIs)	Inhibition of MAO types A+B and thus reduce metabolism of 5-HT and NA (These older drugs are non-selective and the effects are irreversible)	Isocarboxazid Phenelzine Tranylcypromine
Reversible inhibitors of MAO-A (RIMAs)	Inhibition of MAO-A in a competitive and reversible manner	Moclobemide

also confined mainly to treatment-resistant patients. However, it useful to understand their pharmacology as newer, safer versions have been developed.

Tricyclic antidepressants

These were so named because of the three-ring structure that is central to all of these drugs. However, if they were being named now they would more appropriately be called non-selective monoamine uptake inhibitors. Their principal pharmacological effects are inhibition of serotonin (5-HT) and noradrenalin (NA) reuptake into the presynaptic terminal, thus enhancing the effects of these monamine neurotransmitters at the postsynaptic receptors. All TCAs inhibit reuptake of both 5-HT and NA but they vary in their potency of effect for each. For example, clomipramine is about 1000 times more potent in its inhibition of reuptake of 5-HT than NA, whereas desipramine is about 100 times more potent in its effects on NA reuptake than 5-HT. Most of these drugs will also inhibit dopamine (DA) reuptake to some degree and are potent antagonists of the muscarinic cholinergic receptor, the H_1 histamine receptor and alpha$_1$-adrenoceptors.

Although reuptake inhibition occurs immediately on commencing these drugs, onset of the therapeutic effect is classically delayed to between 10 and 21 days. Studies in laboratory animals and humans demonstrate a number of other pharmacological effects occurring with longer term (in the experimental context) use. There is downregulation of postsynaptic 5-HT$_{2A}$ receptors, presynaptic and cell body 5-HT$_{1A}$ receptors, presynaptic alpha$_2$-adrenoceptors and beta$_1$-adrenoceptors. This means that the increase in synaptic concentration of neurotransmitter results in an adaptive response by the neuron. Given the interactions in the CNS between the serotonin and noradrenalin systems, the end result of these effects is difficult to determine but is thought to be an overall enhancement of serotonin function and a stabilization of noradrenergic function, which is probably dysregulated in depressive illness.

Kinetics

These drugs are all lipid soluble, are well absorbed from the gut and are widely distributed in the body. Peak plasma concentrations are reached 2–6 hours after a single oral dose, and elimination half-life is between 8 and 36 hours, generally allowing once daily dosing. Most have active metabolites, also with relatively long half-lives. They are highly bound to plasma proteins (75–95 per cent) and undergo extensive hepatic metabolism.

There is no evidence for a clear relationship between plasma concentration and clinical response. An approximate 80–180 µg/l 'therapeutic window' has been suggested for migraine, with levels below this being unlikely to induce response and levels above being unlikely to induce additional improvement. However, routine use of plasma levels is not of value in monitoring treatment.

Adverse effects and toxicity

Sedation is common, especially early in treatment, and is largely related to antihistamine and anti-adrenergic effects. Weight gain may also be related to antihistamine effects. Some recent evidence suggests there can be impairment of psychomotor function but in the treatment of patients with depression this must be balanced against improvements in function likely to occur in conjunction with improvement in the illness.

The antimuscarinic properties result in what are usually the most troublesome adverse effects: dry mouth, blurred vision, constipation and (mainly in older males) urinary hesitancy and retention. Pupil size, and hence risk of glaucoma, is determined by a balance between anticholinergic (mydriatic) and sympthomimetic (miotic) effects.

Sympathomimetic effects (from NA reuptake inhibition) and antimuscarinic effects can cause a sinus tachycardia. Postural hypotension may occur as a result of sympatholytic alpha$_1$-adrenoceptor antagonism. These drugs can also have a direct effect on cardiac muscle, causing impairment of cardiac conduction, and this is the principal risk factor in overdose.

These drugs lower the seizure threshold and can occasionally result in convulsions. In patients with bipolar affective disorder (manic depressive illness) mania can be precipitated, possibly partly related to their DA reuptake inhibitory effects. They should be avoided if possible in cardiac disease and are contraindicated after recent myocardial infarction. There is no specific evidence of teratogenicity towards the fetus but, like most drugs, they should be avoided if possible during pregnancy. Care is required in elderly people as they are more sensitive to the adverse effects, have a lower rate of metabolism and excretion and are more likely to have concurrent physical disease (e.g. cardiac disease).

Drug interactions

Co-administration with monoamine oxidase inhibitors (MAOIs) will result in increased adverse effects, particularly antimuscarinic effects, and can lead to a dangerous toxic interaction, 'serotonin syndrome' (see below). Although in the past such a combination might have been used in hospital for very treatment-resistant patients it would be very rare to consider it now.

TCAs potentiate the pressor effects of directly acting symphomimetic amines, such as adrenalin or noradrenalin, to cause hypertension. Small amounts of these, such as are present in dental anaesthetics, can be dangerous. TCAs will inhibit the antihypertensive effects of the older antihypertensive drugs, such as adrenergic neurone blocking agents (e.g. guanethidine), α-methyl-DOPA and clonidine.

Taken with alcohol, they potentiate the sedative effects and impairment of psychomotor performance. Hepatic enzyme induction by anticonvulsants or nicotine may reduce plasma levels. Cimetidine may increase levels by enzyme inhibition. Some antipsychotic drugs may compete for similar metabolic pathways.

Selective serotonin reuptake inhibitors

These are now the most widely prescribed antidepressant drugs, essentially because of their safety in overdose and their relative lack of adverse effects compared with TCAs. These are all inhibitors of reuptake of 5-HT with no significant effect on reuptake of NA. They are well absorbed and elimination half-lives for most people are in the region of 15–40 hours. There are active metabolites but except for fluoxetine these do not contribute greatly to the therapeutic effect.

The response rate reported in clinical trials is around 55–70 per cent, with a delay in response as for the TCAs. However, with TCAs it is often necessary to increase the dose gradually to allow for tolerance to the adverse effects. With SSRIs there is rarely any need for this as they can be started at full therapeutic dose because of the lack of adverse effects. Dosing is usually once daily.

Adverse effects

Nausea and sometimes vomiting may occur because of activation of 5-HT_3 receptors. Diarrhoea and headache may also occur. Tolerance generally develops to all of these effects within 7–10 days. Sexual dysfunction is reported, principally delayed ejaculation and anorgasmia. Antimuscarininc effects are rare. SSRIs increase the risk of gastrointestinal bleeding, particularly in the elderly. This is probably because they can alter platelet function. Care is required in patients on warfarin, aspirin or non-steroidal anti-inflammatory drugs.

A syndrome of restlessness or agitation, which seems very similar to the akathisia sometimes induced by antipsychotic drugs, may occur early in treatment in up to 5–10 per cent of patients. This may be accompanied by increased suicidal ideation. It is an indication to stop the SSRI immediately and seek advice from a more senior doctor. Some studies have suggested that increased suicidal ideation *per se*, in isolation from the above restlessness, occurs in some patients, particularly adolescents. As a result, careful clinical monitoring is required early in treatment. For depressed patients under 18 years of age only fluoxetine is licensed, as current evidence suggests it carries less risk in adolescent patients. It should be noted that controversy surrounds this area with analysis of certain types of clinical trial suggesting there may be an effect on thoughts of suicide but other epidemiological studies not suggesting a link with suicidal behaviour. This uncertainty is not a reason not to use SSRIs but is a reason to ensure good monitoring and clinical care.

Sedation is uncommon and some patients find that these drugs prevent them getting to sleep, which is why the dose is best taken in the morning. Effects on psychomotor function can occur but are uncommon compared with TCAs.

Occasional patients have a small reduction in heart rate, but otherwise effects on the cardiovascular system are rare. Epileptic convulsions can occur but are rare and much less common than with TCAs. There is some evidence for potentiation of ECT-induced seizures. Reduction in plasma sodium can occur, particularly in elderly people, and needs to be borne in mind should potentially related symptoms be described.

Drug interactions

Co-administration with other drugs acting to enhance serotonin function can result in development of the 'serotonin syndrome'. This almost invariably occurs if co-prescribed with MAOI antidepressants. It can occur with TCAs, lithium and L-tryptophan, but combination with these drugs for treatment-resistant patients is acceptable as long as they are carefully monitored in the early stages of treatment. In 'serotonin syndrome', the patient is initially restless and may have nausea or diarrhoea. Hyperthermia, rigidity, tremor, myoclonus, autonomic instability and convulsions may develop with fluctuating levels of consciousness. Death may ensue.

Fluoxetine and paroxetine inhibit cytochrome P450-2D6 and thus may affect metabolism of opiates, many antipsychotic drugs and TCAs.

Monoamine oxidase inhibitors

The enzyme monamine oxidase exists in two forms: MAO-A (intestinal mucosa and intraneuronally in the brain) and MAO-B (platelets and mainly extraneuronally in the brain). Serotonin is preferentially metabolized by MAO-A, and noradrenalin, dopamine and tyramine by both forms. The original MAOI antidepressants (phenelzine, tranylcypromine and isocarboxazid) inhibit both MAO-A and MAO-B and are thought to work through increasing the availability of 5-HT and NA in the synapse – with longer term adaptive effects occurring as for the TCAs. These MAOIs are 'irreversible', that is they permanently inactivate MAO. Thus, recovery of activity after stopping the drug occurs slowly, over days, as new MAO molecules are synthesized.

Recently drugs selective for one or other form of MAO have been developed as well as drugs that are reversible inhibitors of each form. The aim of these strategies is to develop drugs less prone to the tyramine interaction ('cheese effect') and which can be withdrawn or changed to another drug more rapidly. The only one of these in regular use is moclobemide, a reversible inhibitor of MAO-A (RIMA).

These drugs are rapidly absorbed and achieve peak plasma level 2 hours after a single dose. Although elimination half-lives are generally short, the irreversibility of the effect on MAO makes this largely irrelevant. Slow acetylators (approximately 50 per cent of the Caucasian population) may develop toxic plasma concentrations.

Tyramine interaction (the 'cheese effect')

The clinical effect of a tyramine interaction ('cheese reaction') is a hypertensive crisis: flushing; severe throbbing headache; severe hypertension; tachycardia; pallor. This is a dangerous condition and there is a risk of cerebral haemorrhage. Treatment is by alpha$_1$-adrenoceptor antagonist (phentolamine or chlorpromazine), which is usually given by slow intravenous injection.

Tyramine acts as an indirect sympathomimetic to cause release of catecholamines from nerve terminals. Tyramine is found in a number of foods: mature cheeses, yeast extracts, some red wines, hung game, pickled herrings, broad bean pods. Normally MAO-A in the intestinal mucosa will metabolize tyramine absorbed from the gut. In patients on the older MAOIs, considerable amounts of tyramine will enter the circulation and will act to release the increased amounts of catecholamines stored in nerve terminals – increased because of the effects of the MAOI to prevent their metabolism. For patients on the RIMA drugs, high concentrations of tyramine can compete for MAO-A, thus mitigating some of the effects, and MAO-B is still available to metabolize noradrenalin. MAO-B however has relatively much less effect on 5-HT and thus 5-HT function is still enhanced.

Adverse effects and toxicity

These drugs are best avoided in patients with cerebrovascular, cardiovascular and hepatic disorders. Some sympathomimetic effects may occur, mainly mild tremor and occasionally cardiac arrhythmias. Apparent 'anticholinergic' effects may also occur but these are mainly the result of sympathetic potentiation in tissues with dual cholinergic/adrenergic innervation, e.g. pupil. Sympatholytic effects can also occur, principally postural hypotension, because of synthesis of relatively inactive 'false' transmitters (e.g. octopamine) in nerve terminals following inhibition of MAO and activation of alternative metabolic pathways.

Other adverse effects noted are restlessness, insomnia, peripheral oedema and sexual difficulties.

Drug interactions

Tyramine-containing foodstuffs must be avoided. Indirectly acting sympathomimetic amines, such as phenylpropanolamine or phenteramine, that are used as nasal decongestants or bronchodilators also pose a risk. These may be found in over-the-counter cough mixtures and will release the enhanced neuronal stores of pressor amines. Combination with SSRIs carries a high risk of 'serotonin syndrome'. Use with TCAs carries some risk of this and should be avoided except for occasional inpatient treatment of the most treatment-resistant patients.

MAOIs also potentiate the effects of opiates, particularly pethidine. This is in part a pharmacokinetic interaction and may result in a syndrome of excitement, hyperpyrexia, muscle rigidity, sweating, respiratory depression and hypotension. If opiates must be given to a patient on an MAOI the dose should be 10 per cent or less of the usual dose.

Other antidepressant drugs

Their principal pharmacological actions include inhibition of reuptake of NA, 5-HT or both and they generally have some additional direct effects on specific receptors, which in theory should assist their therapeutic action. For example, mirtazapine has alpha$_2$-adrenoceptor antagonist properties that should enhance NA activity and also have a secondary effect of enhancing 5-HT activity through adrenergic effects on the serotonergic raphe nuclei. Venlafaxine enhances NA and 5-HT reuptake but lacks the antimuscarinic effects of the older TCAs. The adverse effects of these drugs are potentially the same as for the TCAs but tend to be much less frequent and severe. Similar drug interactions may occur but are generally less likely.

L-tryptophan, the amino acid precursor of 5-HT, has been used as an antidepressant as its administration may enhance serotonin function. There is considerable doubt whether on its own it is an effective antidepressant but it has been used successfully to augment the effects of other antidepressants in treatment-resistant patients. Mild sedation is the main adverse effect. Some years ago there were concerns that this might be associated with an eosinophilia-myalgia syndrome, so it is wise to monitor eosinophil count initially after starting L-tryptophan.

Mood stabilizers

Patients who have experienced an episode of hypomania, or full mania, have an 80 per cent risk of a further episode of illness – which may be either of hypomania/mania or depression. Similarly, patients who have had a first episode of severe major depressive disorder with associated somatic symptoms and/ or psychosis have an 80 per cent risk of recurrence at 3 years. Following a second episode of either type

of illness the risk of further recurrence rises to well over 90 per cent. Thus, prophylaxis is very important for both bipolar and unipolar affective disorder and is more or less mandatory if a second episode occurs within 2 or 3 years of the first. Immediately following the first episode, prophylaxis is necessary for at least 6–12 months and further continuation will depend on clinical circumstances and patient attitude.

For patients with bipolar affective disorder (manic depressive illness) lithium, usually in the form of lithium carbonate, has been the main prophylactic agent for the last 50 years. However, during the last 15 years certain anticonvulsants (sodium valproate, carbamazepine) have also been found effective and are now regularly used, particularly for patients with 'rapid cycling' illness. For patients with recurrent depressive disorder, prophylaxis is equally effective with either continuation of the antidepressant which was effective for the first episode (at the effective dose) or with lithium carbonate. Where these are not effective, anticonvulsants may be helpful and some recent evidence favours lamotrigine.

Lithium

Lithium carbonate (e.g. as Priadel® or Liskonum®) and lithium citrate (e.g. as Camcolit®) are the most commonly used compounds. Lithium has effects on cation transport, on individual neurotransmitters (including 5-HT) and on intracellular second-messenger systems. It may also have neuroprotective effects. Which of these is key to its therapeutic efficacy is not entirely clear but, as for the antidepressant drugs, the net effects seem to be to enhance serotonin function and to stabilize the noradrenergic system.

Once lithium treatment is established it is very important that it is not suddenly stopped as this may result in rebound hypomania in patients with bipolar disorder and increased risk of suicide in patients with all types of mood disorder.

Kinetics

Lithium is rapidly absorbed. Peak serum concentrations are reached in 2–3 hours. It is excreted unchanged by the kidney at a rate proportional to the glomerular filtration rate (GFR). It is best given as a single daily dose around 22.00 hours and steady-state serum levels are reached after 5–7 days of dosing, with the elimination half-life being around 10–24 hours for most people. Most formulations of lithium are in the form of a slow-release preparation. There can be variations in kinetics between different proprietary brands and it is best for individual patients to remain on the same brand.

Monitoring lithium treatment

Lithium has a narrow therapeutic range. The gap between minimum effective serum concentration (0.4 mmol/1) and that at which toxicity may begin to appear (1.2 mmol/1) is low. Plasma concentrations can rise quite rapidly with even small changes in dose within this range. It is therefore important to monitor serum lithium regularly. When establishing a patient on lithium, or restarting treatment after a gap of more than a few days, monitoring must be done weekly until the final dose is established and steady-state serum lithium has been achieved. Blood samples for serum lithium should be taken 12 hours after the last dose. For patients on regular dosing, serum concentrations are fairly stable from around 12 hours after the last dose. Fluctuations of ±0.1 mmol/1 between tests are acceptable but greater than this should prompt some concern. A common cause, however, is often the patient varying the time of dosing or omitting a dose. Patients well established on lithium require a serum level approximately every 3–4 months, unless they show signs of lithium toxicity.

Renal function must be assessed before starting lithium for two reasons. First, long-term treatment with lithium may sometimes impair renal function. Second, lithium is excreted entirely via the kidney, and patients with any impairment of function require greater care in their management. Assessment is now usually by serum creatinine and estimated glomerular filtration rate (eGFR), which is calculated automatically and reported with standard laboratory electrolyte and renal function screens by most laboratories. If eGFR is not available then a 24-hour creatinine clearance should be carried out. Serum creatinine and eGFR then require to be monitored twice annually. Thyroid function (T_4 and thyroid stimulating hormone (TSH)) must also be assessed before treatment and every 6 months, as lithium can induce hypothyroidism in 10–15 per cent of patients.

The total daily dose of lithium required to achieve a therapeutic serum concentration is usually between 400 and 2000 mg. Initiation of therapy should usually be with 400 mg per day. Not all patients will achieve clinical response at the lower end of the therapeutic range and in acute mania a higher concentration may be required to speed response. However, serum concentrations above 1.2 mmol/1 must be avoided. It should also be remembered that toxicity can occur in a few patients at concentrations below 1.2 mmol/1 and that identification of lithium toxicity is always a clinical diagnosis – it is simply much more likely to occur above 1.2 mmol/1 and almost invariable above 1.6 mmol/1.

Adverse effects

These are best considered in three groups: *minor*, often occurring at the beginning of treatment with

Table 17.6   Adverse effects of lithium preparations

Minor effects to which tolerance generally develops	More persistent effects, some of which require to be monitored	Signs of toxicity which require urgent action
Fine tremor	Polyuria and polydipsia	Dysarthria
Mild GI upset	Hypothyroidism	Ataxia
Metallic taste in mouth	Lethargy	Coarse tremor
	Weight gain	Marked GI upset
	Persistent tremor	Impaired consciousness
	T wave flattening on ECG	Epileptic seizures
	Mild cognitive impairment	
	Change in hair texture	
	Mild leucocytosis	
	Exacerbation of psoriasis	

tolerance frequently developing; *persistent* and requiring monitoring during treatment; *toxicity*, requiring immediate cessation of lithium. These are summarized in Table 17.6.

Lithium toxicity is an extremely dangerous condition. Even suspicion of this requires immediate attention and, if confirmed, usually admission to an acute medical ward. The management of toxicity requires monitoring of electrolytes, regular CNS observations, use of anticonvulsants should seizures occur, increased fluid intake to promote excretion (unless renal function is impaired) and cardiac monitoring. Haemodialysis should be considered if conservative measures are ineffective or serum lithium is above 3.0 mmol/1.

Normal use of lithium may result in permanent renal impairment in a small proportion of patients. Polyuria occurs in 20–40 per cent and is due to inhibition of the action of antidiuretic hormone by lithium. It usually resolves on cessation of lithium as do any effects on glomerular function. Evidence suggests that once-daily dosing is preferable with regard to renal function, unless the daily dose is very high. There is evidence that a few patients may develop renal tubular damage. If eGFR is found to be falling below 60 ml/minute and continuing to fall over time, then a renal physician should be consulted and consideration given to stopping lithium.

Interference with thyroid function is due to inhibition of the action of TSH and is easily managed by prescription of thyroxine. Lithium is contraindicated during pregnancy (major vessel anomalies in the fetus) and during breastfeeding.

Drug interactions

Thiazide diuretics considerably reduce renal clearance of lithium and should be avoided. Loop diuretics, such as furosemide, seem to have less likelihood of such effects, but any drug affecting fluid and electrolyte balance should be used with care and with careful monitoring.

Non-steroidal anti-inflammatory drugs (NSAIDs) inhibit prostaglandins and can therefore reduce sodium and lithium excretion. This may result in lithium toxicity and patients need to be warned about use of NSAIDs, as these can now be obtained over the counter. Paracetamol is safe.

There are reports of interactions between lithium and carbamazepine, haloperidol, digoxin and verapamil, resulting in a variety of neurotoxic and cardiotoxic effects. These are not common interactions but clearly indicate a need for caution if such drug combinations are unavoidable. Prolonged apnoea has been reported when patients on lithium were given succinylcholine or pancuronium during anaesthesia.

Anticonvulsants

Carbamazepine and sodium valproate have been found effective both in the treatment of acute mania and in prophylaxis, particularly for patients with 'rapid cycling' illness (four or more episodes per year). Further clinical trials are required to fully establish their role in prophylaxis of more usual forms of recurrent affective disorder, but existing data suggest they are an effective alternative to lithium and are now widely prescribed. Evidence is also accumulating for lamotrigine. The mechanism of action is unknown. It is not appropriate here to go into the details of the pharmacology of anticonvulsants.

Anticonvulsants may interact with other psychotropics either through enzyme induction or displacement from plasma protein binding.

Antipsychotics

These drugs are used for the treatment of psychosis in whatever context: schizophrenia, mania, psychotic depression, drug-induced psychosis, other organic disorder induced psychoses (e.g. through dementia or toxic confusional state). In schizophrenia, it is only the positive symptoms that show consistent, significant response to antipsychotics. Antipsychotics are useful for agitation in the context of depressive illness. Historically, low-dose first-generation antipsychotics, such as chlorpromazine, were frequently prescribed in the management of anxiety disorders, but the evidence base for this is poor. There is some evidence to support the use of second-generation drugs, such as risperidone, as adjuncts to antidepressants in some patients with anxiety but this use should be reserved for care supervised by a psychiatrist. They have also often been used for the management of agitation occurring in a variety of situations in elderly people. This is not strongly evidence based and there is evidence that all antipsychotics in elderly people may increase the risk of vascular events such as stroke.

Mechanism of action

All effective antipsychotic drugs antagonize dopamine (DA) receptors (principally the D_2 subtype) and this led to considerable investigation into possible abnormalities of DA systems in schizophrenia. *In vivo* functional brain imaging does not support earlier claims, from studies of post-mortem brain tissue, of an increase in DA receptor density, but does support a subtle alteration in DA turnover in the brain. There may also be subtle disturbances in glutamate and serotonin systems.

Positron emission tomography studies of D_2 receptor occupancy in patients demonstrate that clinical response is normally achieved with 50–70 per cent occupancy with no additional benefit above 70 per cent. However, above 70 per cent occupancy extrapyramidal side-effects (EPSE) become much more prevalent. Clozapine and the second-generation drugs rarely achieve occupancy greater than 70 per cent, even at maximum doses, whereas this is relatively easy to achieve with the first-generation drugs at medium to high doses.

Classification of antipsychotics

The first antipsychotic drug was chlorpromazine, introduced in 1952. This and others are listed in Table 17.7. Chlorpromazine is moderately potent in antagonism of D_1 and D_2 types of DA receptors but also antagonizes a wide variety of other receptors – serotonergic, adrenergic, cholinergic, histaminergic

– resulting in a wide variety of adverse effects. Other first-generation (often called 'typical') antipsychotics also had a wide spectrum of effects beyond the desired antipsychotic effect. Among the most problematic adverse effects of these drugs were the EPSE related to DA receptor antagonism in the caudate–putamen region: drug-induced pseudo-Parkinsonism, acute dystonia, tardive dyskinesia and akathisia. Drug design to eliminate these problems is difficult because the antipsychotic effect is primarily due to DA receptor antagonism as well.

However, there are now a number of second-generation (often called 'atypical') antipsychotics that have much reduced propensity to induce EPSE. These drugs differ from the first-generation antipsychotics in two main ways: (a) most are less potent in their antagonism of dopamine receptors (see above) and (b) they have a high ratio of 5-HT$_2$ receptor antagonism to DA receptor antagonism (often referred to as a high 5-HT$_2$:D$_2$ ratio). Both (a) and (b) seem to contribute to the reduction in EPSE. In addition, these properties may also result in patients having fewer 'negative' symptoms when taking these drugs. The second-generation drugs differ from each other in chemical structure and in their propensities to antagonize other neurotransmitter receptors. Thus, they have individual profiles of adverse effects and cannot usefully be subclassified into various subgroups.

In the region of 30 per cent of patients with schizophrenia either show no, or very poor response, to the antipsychotic drugs described above or may have unacceptable adverse effects. Around half of these

Table 17.7   Classification of antipsychotic drugs

Drug group	Examples
First generation	
Phenothiazines	Chlorpromazine, thioridazine, trifluoperazine, fluphenazine
Thioxanthines	Flupenthixol, zuclopenthixol
Butyrophenones	Haloperidol, droperidol
Diphenylbutylpiperidines	Pimozide
Substituted benzamides	Sulpiride
Second generation	Amisulpride, olanzapine, quetiapine, risperidone, sertindole, zotepine ziprasidone (available in the USA and many European countries but not the UK)
Clozapine	Generally considered the prototype for other second generation drugs but is more non-specific in its pharmacological effects and is more effective than all other drugs for treatment-resistant patients

patients will achieve a better response with clozapine. This antipsychotic carries a 5–10 per cent risk of neutropenia and 1 per cent risk of agranulocytosis. Hence its use is restricted to patients who are treatment resistant to other antipsychotics. It is mandatory to monitor total white cell and neutrophil counts in patients on clozapine, initially weekly.

Long-term antipsychotic treatment, in patients with established schizophrenia, considerably reduces rates of relapse. For example at 1 year on placebo around 60–80 per cent will relapse compared with 20–40 per cent on active treatment. Where compliance is a problem the medication is often given in one of the slow-release depot formulations, usually administered at a frequency of every 1–6 weeks.

Pharmacokinetics

Antipsychotics are generally rapidly absorbed from the gut reaching peak serum concentrations in 2–4 hours. The elimination half-lives of most of the first-generation drugs are quite variable between individuals but are generally quite long – in the region of 20–30 hours but up to 100 hours in some individuals. Many have active metabolites, which have much longer elimination half-lives, that are usually of lower potency at the DA receptor but contribute to some of the effects of the drug. Some, such as chlorpromazine, have a number of active metabolites. This makes meaningful interpretation of serum concentrations difficult. It is almost impossible to demonstrate other than very broad relationships between serum level and clinical response. Therefore, serum level monitoring is of no value in routine clinical practice.

The second-generation drugs are also readily absorbed. Quetiapine and ziprasidone have short elimination half-lives (<10 hours) but the others have half-lives in the region of 20–30 hours. Active metabolites generally do not contribute significantly to the action of these drugs except for risperidone.

Adverse effects and toxicity

The number of different drugs and variety of adverse effects makes it impossible to comprehensively describe these. Table 17.8 lists the more important effects and the drugs most likely to give rise to them.

A rare, but potentially fatal, idiosyncratic adverse effect is neuroleptic malignant syndrome. This can occur with any antipsychotic drug. The symptoms are rigidity, hyperthermia, autonomic lability and reduced level of consciousness. Massively elevated creatine kinase is usually found. Prior to 1984 the mortality rate was around 20 per cent in unrecognized cases but improved early recognition has considerably reduced this. Management is described in Chapter 18.

Drug interactions

Pharmacokinetic

Antacids reduce absorption and enzyme-inducing drugs may decrease serum levels. The enzyme inhibitors cimetidine and propranolol both increase serum levels. There can be competition for metabolic pathways by some TCAs and SSRIs (especially fluoxetine), which may increase serum levels.

Central nervous system

Phenothiazine-type antipsychotics will potentiate the CNS depressant action of many drugs, including opiates, and will potentiate the effects of general anaesthetic agents. All antipsychotics will antagonize the effect of L-dopa in Parkinson's disease, making management of patients with psychosis and Parkinson's disease difficult.

Cardiovascular

Many antipsychotics are alpha-adrenergic receptor antagonists and may thus enhance the effect of antihypertensives, including ACE (angiotensin converting enzyme) inhibitors. In contrast, the effects of the older adrenergic neurone blocking type of antihypertensive drug may be antagonized. Drugs that may also prolong QT_c interval should be avoided if possible.

Electroconvulsive therapy

Although this is not a drug, it seems appropriate to include a brief note here. Most students will probably be aware that its use has been controversial over the years. In part this related to a public perception that it was frequently given without anaesthesia and was misused in the rather frightening manner depicted in films such as 'One Flew Over the Cuckoo's Nest'. The development of safe, short-acting anaesthetic techniques during the 1940s and 1950s consigned the rather terrifying nature of the early approach to administration to history. Good clinical observation

Table 17.8   Adverse effects of antipsychotic drugs

Adverse effect	Drugs commonly causing this
Pseudo-parkinsonism, dystonia, and tardive dyskinesia	First-generation antipsychotics
Akathisia (an unpleasant syndrome of mental and motor restlessness)	First-generation antipsychotics Clozapine
Sedation	First-generation antipsychotics
	Olanzapine, quetiapine, zotepine
	Clozapine
Anticholinergic effects (dry mouth, blurred vision, constipation, urinary retention)	First-generation antipsychotics
Weight gain	Chlorpromazine, thioridazine
	Olanzapine, zotepine, clozapine
Postural hypotension	Chlorpromazine, thioridazine
	Quetiapine, clozapine
Prolongation of QTc interval on ECG (Thought this may indicate risk of arrhythmia and sudden death)	All may cause this. Thioridazine and sertindole only available with ECG monitoring because of this
Elevated serum prolactin, galactorrhoea and altered menstrual cycle	Varying degrees with all antipsychotics except olanzapine and clozapine. Most marked with sulpiride
Sexual dysfunction	Reported least in clinical trials with olanzapine and quetiapine
Cholestatic jaundice, skin pigmentation, skin rashes, photosensitivity	Principally seen with phenothiazines and mainly chlorpromazine

and the well devised clinical trials of the 1970s and 1980s clearly defined the disorders for which ECT can be effective. It continues to be used for severe depression, usually where resistant to drug treatment, catatonia and a very small number of patients with mania and schizophrenia who do not respond to antipsychotic drugs.

The idea that induction of a seizure might be useful derived from the observation that some patients with both psychotic illness and epilepsy often showed improvement in their psychosis after having a seizure. The use of convulsions was pioneered by Meduna in 1934, when he used chemical means (IM camphor) to induce seizures. This and other chemicals were unreliable in their effects and in 1938 Cerletti and colleagues developed electrical means – electroconvulsive therapy (ECT). The lack of safe short-acting anaesthesia at that time meant this was given with only physical restraint of the patient to prevent injury. Use of general anaesthesia became routine during the 1950s. Two large clinical trials (random allocation, but not blinded) in the 1960s confirmed efficacy in depressive illness, and six placebo controlled, double-blind, random allocation studies between 1978 and 1985 further demonstrated this. The precise mode of action of ECT is not understood but it has a number of similar effects to antidepressant drugs on relevant neurotransmitter systems.

Administration of ECT

Once a clinical decision has been made that ECT may be appropriate it is important to discuss this with the patient and to make the patient aware of any potential adverse effects, the potential benefits and the risks of not having the treatment. The patient must give written consent for ECT treatment. There are only very occasional situations where a patient is extremely unwell, lacks capacity to make a decision and, at the same time, is detained under the appropriate Mental Health legislation that ECT can be given against the patient's wishes. Such a decision always requires an independent second opinion.

Before administration of the electrical stimulus the patient is anaesthetized. Standard equipment is available for administration of the stimulus and the Royal College of Psychiatrists provides guidelines and training for consultants supervising ECT. It is clear that the electrical stimulus given needs to be at least double the patient's seizure threshold and a standard formula based on age and gender is generally used to determine this. Seizures require to be at least 20 seconds in duration to be effective and usually between five and eight are required, given twice weekly. Good oxygenation of the patient immediately prior to the stimulus is important both for anaesthetic safety and to reduce the seizure threshold. Failure to have an adequate seizure should be followed, if anaesthetic conditions permit, by one restimulation with an electrical stimulus 50 per cent greater than that first used.

The prime reason for anaesthesia is to allow muscle relaxants to be used, usually suxamethonium chloride, in order to prevent injury from muscle contractions during the seizure. Benzodiazepines are avoided if possible in the patient's treatment as these will raise the seizure threshold and shorten seizures. However, if a seizure is prolonged (>60 seconds) then intravenous diazepam is used to abort the seizure.

Adverse effects

ECT is to be avoided if possible within 3 months of a myocardial infarction or a cerebrovascular accident. At least 30 per cent of patients complain of headache for a few hours post ECT. Figures for mortality reported in the 1970s suggest one death per 22 000 treatments. This is probably most often due to cardiac arrest following excessive vagal inhibition and is similar to mortality from general anaesthesia for minor surgery. There is no evidence of structural damage to the brain. Impairment of short-term memory may occur and two studies suggest this improves to normal over the 6 weeks following ECT. However, some patients do describe persistent memory difficulties that are difficult to disentangle from the effects of their depression.

Summary

At the end of this chapter you should be able to initiate appropriate psychopharmacological treatment for patients with mental illnesses. You should also understand some of the limitations of these treatments and in particular the issues relating to their adverse effects, which quite often continue to be a limiting factor. Nevertheless, progress in our understanding of the neurochemistry of severe mental disorders and in our understanding of the actions of effective treatments has led steadily towards more useful drugs and better outcomes for patients. Though effective and safe use of psychotropic drugs is very important, and is essential knowledge for doctors on mental health teams, this is usually only effective within the context of the wider range of supports and services provided. Medication will not achieve maximal effectiveness unless patients are within a structure that encourages good adherence with treatment and within which they can then develop their lives once key symptoms are suppressed or abolished.

Further reading

Anderson IM, Reid IC (2006) *Fundamentals of Clinical Psychopharmacology*, 3rd edition. London: Informa Healthcare.

King DJ (2004) *College Seminars in Clinical Psychopharmacology*, 2nd edition. London: Gaskell.

CHAPTER 18

PSYCHIATRIC EMERGENCIES

Brian Lunn and Richard Day

KEY CHAPTER FEATURES

- Deliberate self-harm
- Acute behavioural disturbance (including acute tranquillization)
- Lithium toxicity
- Acute dystonia
- Neuroleptic malignant syndrome

Introduction

There are relatively few true psychiatric emergencies. That being said there are a few important areas where prompt intervention is required. In this chapter these will be discussed with an emphasis on recognition and basic management. These are also conditions that you may come across as doctors in other specialities, which is why we have included them here. In this chapter there will be some overlap with Chapter 12 (Organic disorders) and Chapter 17 (Psychopharmacology). However, to help your learning we have cross-referenced to reduce repetition but have also included information in this chapter to enable you to consider the particular issue in the context of an emergency.

Why is this relevant to you?

This chapter is more detailed since these are situations you are likely to be faced with and have to manage in your foundation years which you must complete to become a registered doctor.

The two most common emergencies are deliberate self-harm (DSH) and acute behavioural

disturbances, principally those where extreme emotional distress, acute agitation or threatening and/or actual aggressive behaviour are involved. Such behavioural disturbances may also occur in those who have self-harmed and sometimes various aspects of behavioural disturbance may occur in the same person all together. Patients with disturbed behaviour often have to be managed in the absence of a clear diagnosis because the very existence of the behavioural problems makes it difficult to establish a diagnosis unless they are already well known to services. Acute confusional states also often present as behavioural disturbances. Another group of emergencies are the potentially life-threatening unwanted effects of psychotropic medications that require prompt intervention: dystonia, neuroleptic malignant syndrome (NMS) and lithium toxicity. The longer term, less acute adverse effects are covered in Chapter 17. A further emergency that may require urgent psychiatric input is acute delirium. This is dealt with in Chapter 12. Of specific importance are acute withdrawal from alcohol and benzodiazepines, both of which will present to newly qualified doctors on a regular basis and which it is important to recognize early. As will become evident, good nursing care is an essential part of managing any of these emergencies.

Deliberate self-harm

Before we discuss self-harm and its management, it may be useful for you to consider what comes to mind when you think of this. There is good evidence that those presenting with self-harm often receive less than optimal care. There is no doubt that when dealing with other life-threatening emergencies, being asked to assess self-harm can feel frustrating. However, it is important to remember that the patient presenting may be distressed and lack effective strategies to manage at that time. A professional approach without judgement can have enormous benefits.

It is important to recognize at the outset that DSH is a behaviour rather than a diagnosis and that the behaviour of DSH is influenced by a complex interplay of personal, psychological, health and illness, environmental and cultural factors. Greater understanding of these issues over the last 10–20 years has led to the terminology 'deliberate self-harm' to be preferred over the previous commonly used terminologies 'parasuicide' and 'attempted suicide'. The significance of any act of DSH can only really be understood once you have tried to understand and integrate these different factors.

It is important to differentiate between the antecedents of and behaviours involved in deliberate self-harm and suicide as they are often different and not part of a continuum, although there can be overlap. Some DSH is certainly an unsuccessful attempt at suicide. However, sometimes DSH unintentionally results in death, which was not an intended or anticipated outcome. It is important not to look at single demographic factors (such as gender or age) or characteristics of the attempt but to consider the picture as a whole. With suicide there generally tends to be a plan in place with the attempt having been planned. The patient anticipates that the action they take will lead to death. The attempt is made so that there is little if any chance that they will be discovered. There is often coexisting comorbidity with mental illness and/or chronic physical health problems (especially painful conditions which impact negatively on quality of life). Elderly men recently widowed are at high risk of suicide but at low risk of DSH, whereas the reverse is true for young women.

There can be many other motives for an act of DSH. The commonest are as a form of escape, or even temporary distraction (e.g. from an intolerable situation), or an appeal (to mobilize support or express distress). However, it is preferable to avoid the term 'cry for help' as that tends to bring about unhelpful responses from health professionals.

Risk factors

DSH is a common phenomenon. UK rates are between 250 and 300 per 100 000 population. It is the commonest single reason for admission to hospital for women aged less than 65 years (in men aged less than 65 it comes second only to ischaemic heart disease). It must also be remembered that many acts of DSH do not come to medical attention at all. It is a behaviour that is most prevalent in young adults and becomes less common with advancing age. In the past there has been a clear female preponderance for DSH, but over recent years in the UK there has been a significant increase in DSH among young men and the gender ratio is now almost equal. Risk factors are listed in Box 18.1. Only about 30 per cent of DSH presentations are associated with a specific mental disorder, such as depressive disorders, adjustment disorders, personality disorders, drug and alcohol dependence.

Up to half of people who present with DSH have a history of previous DSH and up to 1 in 5 will engage in further DSH over the next year. There is also a significant minority (about 1 in 7) who have a history of more than five episodes of self-harm. This group of people who engage in repetitive DSH are much more likely to have a diagnosis of personality disorder than people who only self-harm occasionally. Only a small minority of people who self-harm go on to commit suicide – about 1 per cent in the year following an episode of self-harm and 2–3 per cent over 5 years.

Box 18.1: Factors that increase the risk of deliberate self-harm

Age (effect varies with gender)

Low social class

Unemployed

Stressful life events in preceding 6 months

Relationship difficulties

Drug and alcohol misuse

Impulsivity/hostility

Physical/sexual abuse in childhood

Psychiatric disorder

Suicide

Suicide is much less common than DSH – the overall UK rate each year is about 10 per 100 000, although it has reduced by about 20 per cent between 1997 and 2006. Nevertheless, it still accounts for about 1 per cent of all deaths and, after accidents, is the second most common cause of death in young men. The demographics for completed suicide are significantly different to those of non-fatal DSH. However, the single best indicator for those at risk of suicide is a past history of DSH – 20 per cent of people who commit suicide have a history of DSH in the previous year and 50 per cent have a history of previous DSH at some point in the past. Gender is another main risk factor for suicide – 75 per cent of suicides are men (Fig. 18.2). The relationship of rates of suicide to age has varied over time. Up to around 20 years ago, rates of successful suicide increased with age. In the UK, over the last 20 years, there has been a significant rise in suicide among younger men. At present, the highest rate of death by suicide is in the 25–44 years age group (Fig. 18.1).

A diagnosis of mental disorder is a significant risk factor for suicide in that those people who are in contact with mental health services are 10 times more likely to die by suicide that the general population. Of these, about half have an affective disorder (bipolar disorder or unipolar depression), with schizophrenia, personality disorder, alcohol dependence and drug dependence being the other most common primary diagnoses.

Other risk factors for suicide are shown in Box 18.2.

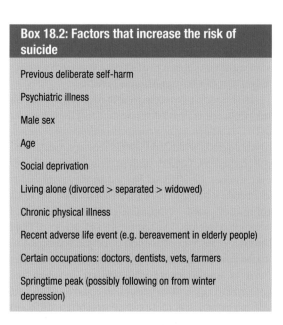

Box 18.2: Factors that increase the risk of suicide

Previous deliberate self-harm

Psychiatric illness

Male sex

Age

Social deprivation

Living alone (divorced > separated > widowed)

Chronic physical illness

Recent adverse life event (e.g. bereavement in elderly people)

Certain occupations: doctors, dentists, vets, farmers

Springtime peak (possibly following on from winter depression)

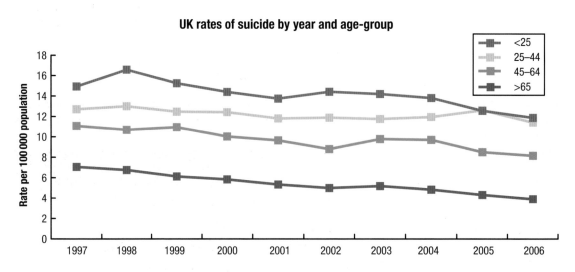

UK rates of suicide by year and age-group

Fig. 18.1   Rates of general population suicide by year and age group. (Source: National Confidential Inquiry Report, 2009.)

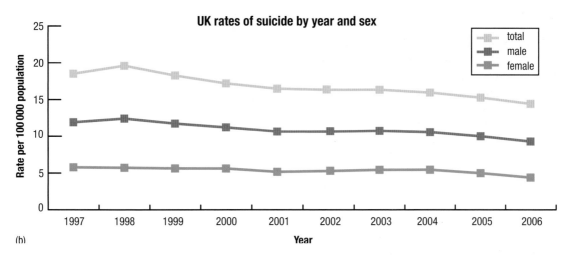

Fig. 18.2   Rates of general population suicide by year and sex. (Source: National Confidential Inquiry Report, 2009.)

Clinical presentation

There are many ways that people can self-harm. Some methods are not associated with lethality: burning the skin with a cigarette; superficial lacerations to the arms, legs or other parts of the body; picking at healing scars. Others may be more dangerous: deeper lacerations that may involve arterial damage; overdoses of over-the-counter, prescription or illicit drugs; carbon monoxide poisoning (e.g. with a car exhaust); hanging, drowning or jumping from a height. In the UK, hanging is the commonest method of suicide (40 per cent), followed by self-poisoning (25 per cent) and jumping (10 per cent). Men are more likely to use more violent methods than women, which may mean that impulsive attempts are more likely to be fatal even when there was no suicidal ideation.

The method of self-harm or suicide is influenced to some degree by availability. Thus there are now limitations on the number of paracetamol and aspirin tablets that can be sold over the counter at one time, in an attempt to make it less likely that people will have large numbers of them readily available at home. Death by firearms is common in the USA, because of availability, but very uncommon in the UK. Deaths by carbon monoxide poisoning have reduced very significantly over the past 20 years since catalytic converters became universal on new motor vehicles.

People who have self-harmed may present themselves to medical services or may be brought, more or less reluctantly, by friends or family, or even may be found coincidentally by a stranger. There may be the added complication of alcohol or drug intoxication. The disinhibition caused by alcohol may have made the self-harm behaviour more likely to occur, or the individual may have used alcohol or illicit drugs to give them 'courage' to self-harm or to increase the perceived lethality of the self-harm. Intoxication also impairs judgement and may make the person feel less hopeful, which may lead to the self-harm.

Assessment

There are a number of distinct but related aspects to consider in the assessment of DSH (Box 18.3). Box

Box 18.3: Factors to consider in the assessment of DSH

Medical safety and fitness

Circumstances of the DSH

Current suicidal ideation and mental state

Presence of mental illness

Options for immediate and future treatment

Box 18.4 Assessment of risk: typical questions in assessment of risk of harm to self

Have you ever felt that life is not worth living?

How long do those feelings last?

Do they come and go or are they there all the time?

Can you manage the feelings?

Have you thought about acting on the feelings?

Have you made any plans?

How close have you come to acting on the thoughts?

What stopped you doing anything?

Have you tried anything before?

How can I trust that you will be able to keep yourself safe?

Do you feel unsafe?

If the feelings of self-harm are pervasive and there is an urge to act on them and plans have been made the risk is high

18.4 summarizes the key features to consider when assessing the component risk in a DSH assessment.

Usually the first priority when someone is admitted with DSH is to ensure that they are medically safe and stable. Medical treatment will clearly be determined by the nature and severity of the method of self-harm. Unless the person is considered to be at high risk of a further attempt at suicide or is insisting on being discharged, assessment of the DSH itself is best left for a period of time, commonly until the following day, as admission with DSH is often in the evening or at night. This may allow what can be an unduly emotional situation to settle and facilitate a more clear assessment of the underlying mental state and level of ongoing risk. In cases of self-poisoning or intoxication, this also gives a chance for the effects of drugs or alcohol to wear off.

As discussed in Chapter 5, the various Mental Health Acts in the different parts of the UK do not allow compulsory treatment except for an individual's mental disorder. Thus, if a patient refuses a treatment for their physical health, for example, acetylcysteine after a paracetamol overdose, they cannot be forced to accept this under the terms of the Mental Health Act. It is a common misperception among other doctors

that somehow a psychiatrist can invoke legislation to permit such treatment. However, it is also important to recognize that such treatment can be given if a patient is assessed as lacking capacity to make proper decisions regarding their physical health. Assessment of capacity is something that will often require an opinion from a psychiatrist though is only rarely required in DSH.

Patients being assessed after DSH may be quite difficult to interview – the effects of self-poisoning or alcohol may make them irritable; some may be unhappy to be found alive and therefore resentful of medical attention; others may be acutely embarrassed, feel foolish and just want to forget about the episode. In any case, after an episode of self-harm the person may be experiencing a variety of distressing and conflicting emotions and so require extra care and empathy during the consultation. A patient's distress may also be exacerbated by staff who are dismissive of them or openly hostile, indicating that their time is for those who cannot 'help their illnesses'. Sometimes patients may be very reluctant to speak following DSH and may volunteer very little other than superficial information. They may in particular not wish to say much about how they are feeling, or simply respond with very limited answers such as 'fine'. It is important to combine a detailed history (including corroboration from other sources where possible) with careful mental state examination and to consider how well the history and mental state correspond. For example, a patient who denies any recent symptoms of psychiatric illness, denies intent of suicide and now says that they feel 'fine' and 'just want to go home', but who cannot make eye contact, appears agitated and distressed, is low and unreactive in affect and/or has reduced amount and volume of speech should be assessed very carefully to decide whether discharge home is the best option.

Events/circumstances leading to self-harm

The history should concentrate initially on the circumstances of the self-harm. This means obtaining information about events leading to the act of deliberate self-harm. It is helpful to know if any single incident (such as an argument with partner or parents) led to distress, which in turn led to impulsive self-harm. It is of greater concern in terms of risk if the person had thoughts of self-harm for a period of time, and cumulative factors led them then to act on these feelings.

The self-harm incident

The assessment then focuses on the means of self-harm and the effect the individual thought would result. Sometimes staff will erroneously say a serious overdose has occurred because a large number of tablets were taken, but this may have been because the patient was unaware of the potential effects of these. A patient who has taken 20 mg of diazepam but thought this might be fatal may have much greater intent. The seriousness of the attempt may not correlate with the nature of the attempt: more important is what the patient *thought* could happen. Further, if a patient has deliberately self-harmed and did not expect to be found, this may indicate a greater intent. Leaving a note may also be significant.

After the self-harm

It is also important to establish what happened after the attempt. Many patients will almost immediately regret the incident and/or be overwhelmed by guilt, panic or fear, especially if the attempt was impulsive. Some may be very distressed that the attempt has failed or that they have been found. There may be anger and hostility and it is likely that for many there is ambivalence about the situation in which they find themselves. A good risk assessment is an important part of assessment that all doctors should be able to undertake to some degree.

Management

There are two phases of management: acute and longer term. As mentioned above, the immediate aim is to ensure that the patient is medically safe and stable. Once this has been established it will be necessary to complete a full assessment. Given the risk factors discussed above, management will depend on:

- The assessed level of risk which, if high, needs to be managed through inpatient care or outreach support.
- Any comorbidity, commonly anxiety, depression or substance misuse, which will require appropriate assessment and management.

- Was this an impulsive self-harm now genuinely regretted? Such cases do not usually warrant follow up in adults and non-vulnerable groups.
- Was this part of a pattern of episodes of repeated self-harm? Such may be indicative of personality disorder. The two personality disorders most frequently associated with completed suicide are emotionally unstable personality disorder (EUPD) and dissocial personality disorder (DPD). Both can be challenging to manage and shared care arrangements between accident and emergency departments and psychiatric services may need to be in place.

Acute behavioural problems

It is not uncommon for various types of psychiatric disorder to present with an extreme abnormality of behaviour rather than what you might expect to be the typical symptoms of that disorder. In general medical settings a common reason for a patient to present with acute behavioural problems is the development of acute confusional states, characterized by concurrent disturbances of consciousness and attention, perception, thinking, memory, psychomotor behaviour, emotion and the sleep–wake schedule. The presentation can also include aggression and irritability that may put the patient and/or others at risk of harm. In settings such as A&E departments and acute psychiatric wards, acute intoxication with alcohol or illicit drugs, psychosis and agitation associated with extreme anxiety are common causes. An assessment should enable the cause to be identified and managed appropriately. (This section should be read in conjunction with Chapter 12, in which delirium was discussed.)

Management of acute behavioural problems

In managing acute behavioural disturbance the management plan needs to consider both pharmacological and non-pharmacological strategies. In psychiatric intensive care units (PICUs) it is commonly found that skilled non-pharmacological approaches can resolve the majority of behavioural disturbances. In less ideal circumstances, such as A&E departments, where staff may not possess the same skill set as PICU nurses, the chances are that strategies will need pharmacological intervention as a key component. The goals of medication in the management of acute agitation are to quickly calm the patient without excessive sedation and to ensure the safety of the patient and sometimes staff, if the patient is violent. However, there is also a need to nurse the patient appropriately so that minimal medication is used.

Non-medical interventions

Regardless of the environment in which the patient is encountered, there are several key elements to non-pharmacological interventions. These are summarized in Box 18.5. Other elements are much more environment dependent and are listed in Box 18.6.

> ### Box 18.5: The first element of any non-pharmacological approach is to try and de-escalate the situation
>
> Communication needs to be clear, consistent, firm and non-confrontational
>
> When speaking to the patient one person at a time should do the talking
>
> They need to use a slightly slower rate and lowered tone to aid clarity
>
> Lighting needs to be bright enough to allow for the patient to see clearly and not misinterpret shadows etc.

> ### Box 18.6: Environmental considerations in non-pharmacological management of acutely disturbed behaviour
>
> Remove items that confer risk for the patient or those around them. This can include cables to trip over or items that can be used as an improvised weapon
>
> The amount of stimulation should be minimized
>
> 'Time-out' away from the situation provoking or driving behaviour can have value

Rapid tranquillization

There have been a number of guidelines for rapid tranquillization (RT) published by national as well as local bodies. In England since the publication of National Institute for Health and Clinical Excellence (NICE) guidance, individual trusts should have an easy to understand algorithm in their rapid tranquillization protocols.

Two main classes of drugs tend to be used for RT. These are antipsychotic drugs and benzodiazepines. These, in the UK at least, tend to be primarily administered orally or intramuscularly. Very rarely intravenous use may be required. Only in very extreme circumstances would intravenous use be considered and then only if good resuscitation facilities were available. This would only be carried out after discussion with a consultant.

Antipsychotics

In younger patients and those who are antipsychotic drug naive (that is, have not previously taken antipsychotic medications), NICE guidance recommends that the first-line antipsychotic treatment should be a newer generation drug such as olanzapine as this decreases the risk of acute dystonia (see below). If the patient will accept an oral antipsychotic, this should be the primary method of delivery. In patients where there is a need to intervene urgently or their behavioural disturbance is of a level that requires a rapid response, then there may be no option but to give the medication intramuscularly.

When giving oral medication it is important to remember that a disturbed patient may attempt to secrete tablets. To address this, oro-dispersible forms of drugs and syrups can be used, although even with these vigilance is required to ensure medication is ingested.

When giving antipsychotic drugs it is important to remember there is a risk of significant extrapyramidal side-effects (EPSEs), particularly dystonia and akathisia, and that apart from the distress possible for the patient there is a risk of these fuelling the patient's agitated behaviour. Thus, if the antipsychotic has to be given intramuscularly, concomitant administration of an antimuscarinic medication should be considered. Where an intramuscular drug is required, haloperidol is probably the most widely used and has a good safety record as it has a relatively low propensity for sedation and hypotension compared with other intramuscular agents. However, it is more likely to cause EPSEs. Its effects will usually last for a period of between 6 and 18 hours. Chlorpromazine should never be given intramuscularly because of marked hypotensive effects. Intramuscular olanzapine and aripiprazole are alternatives to haloperidol.

In the setting of a psychiatric unit, and only for those few patients requiring repeated short-acting, intramuscular antipsychotics, intramuscular zuclopenthixol acetate, with effects lasting up to 72 hours, can be considered for patients with a known diagnosis and who are not overly sensitive to the development of adverse effects. (Do not confuse this with the depot preparation zuclopenthixol decanoate.) This should not be used in those already receiving a depot antipsychotic or as a first line in those who are neuroleptic naive. However, the long duration of action compared with the most commonly used drug, haloperidol, is a drawback in a situation where you may be uncertain of the diagnosis and potential risk factors might be masked. Depot antipsychotic drugs should never be used for RT as they do not act rapidly and are only slowly washed out.

Benzodiazepines

In some cases, particularly when the patient is already on a high dose of antipsychotics, has a previous history of serious adverse effects with antipsychotics, is antipsychotic naive or has a history of epilepsy, benzodiazepines may be given on their own. Lorazepam is the best benzodiazepine to use in this situation because of its high potency at the receptor and reasonably short elimination half-life. It is also better absorbed when given intramuscularly than other benzodiazepines. Lorazepam is said to have a similar efficacy whether given orally or intramuscularly but that is only in ideal circumstances and when the patient is compliant. Thus, it may be given orally or intramuscularly in doses of 1–2 mg and titrated against patient response.

The clear advantage of benzodiazepines when given alone is that they are anxiolytic and sedative while not having the risk of EPSEs and cardiotoxicity associated with antipsychotics.

Combining an antipsychotic with a benzodiazepine is commonly required. The combination of a benzodiazepine and a typical antipsychotic (i.e. haloperidol) has been shown to be superior to monotherapy with either agent, and may allow for decreased doses of the antipsychotic medication.

The combination can cause excessive sedation. After treatment with intramuscular agents, clinical status and vital signs should be monitored at regular intervals. Allow adequate time for clinical response between doses. A typical combination is 5–10 mg of haloperidol with 1–2 mg of lorazepam either orally or intramuscularly. In the patients mentioned above where a newer generation antipsychotic is used olanzapine 10 mg can be given intramuscularly, but concomitant use of a benzodiazepine is to be avoided due to the increased risk of oversedation and severe hypotension.

If the initial treatment fails to produce an adequate response, options include:

- giving another dose of the same medication if partially effective, or a different medication if the first medication was ineffective;
- giving a dose of lorazepam if the first medication was an antipsychotic;
- giving a combination of the same antipsychotic and lorazepam (except olanzapine).

It is also worth noting that for elderly patients lower starting and maximum doses need to be observed.

Risks

There is a significant risk associated with acute tranquillization over and above the EPSEs highlighted already, and this is why guidelines and treatment algorithms have been introduced. The potential hazards are shown in Box 18.7.

Box 18.7: Risks of acute tranquillization

Cardiac

- bradycardia
- tachycardia
- hypotension
- prolongation of QTc interval
- arrhythmias

Respiratory depression

EPSEs and acute dystonia (see below)

Local pain at injection sites

Seizures

Neuroleptic malignant syndrome (see below)

As there are significant potential problems, patients who have been medicated in this way require close monitoring of their pulse, respiration, temperature and blood pressure in the period following medication administration. In those more profoundly sedated this may include monitoring their airway. Staff need to be trained to recognize and manage these and a ward should have flumazenil and oral and intramuscular antimuscarinics available.

Lithium toxicity

The adverse effects of lithium have been covered in Chapter 17. Lithium toxicity is a more serious, potentially fatal, consequence of treating patients with lithium. Toxicity will begin to emerge if serum lithium concentration rises above 1.2 mmol/l, and worsens as plasma levels of lithium increase. At 1.6 mmol/l almost all patients would demonstrate toxicity. It is also important to remember that it is a clinical diagnosis and that in a few patients it can occur at lithium levels below 1.2 mmol/l. Further, once the clinical signs are recognized appropriate management should begin immediately without waiting for the result of a confirmatory plasma level, which must be sent along with a request for electrolytes, creatinine and estimated glomerular filtration rate (eGFR). It is important to realize that disorders in sodium pump function can shift lithium intracellularly, resulting in a more severe clinical picture than might have been expected by measured serum concentrations. Clinical signs are set out in Box 18.8.

Lithium toxicity most commonly arises from dehydration or a drug interaction. Important drugs in this respect are non-steroidal anti-inflammatory drugs (NSAIDS), angiotensin converting enzyme (ACE) inhibitors and thiazide diuretics. Accidental prescription of the wrong dose and development of renal failure are other causes. Education of patients and their families is thus essential for anyone being prescribed lithium. It is particularly important to point out the risks of dehydration and over-the-counter NSAIDs. It is also important that all doctors are aware of this potentially dangerous consequence of lithium as lithium toxicity is not infrequently seen in medical wards where either a patient has been inadvertently prescribed a drug which interacts with lithium or a patient has become dehydrated as a result of their illness but the effect of this on lithium is

---

Box 18.8: Signs of lithium toxicity

Plasma lithium concentration 1.5–2.0 mmol/l

Nausea, vomiting, diarrhoea

Coarse tremor

Apathy

Ataxia

Plasma lithium concentration >2.0 mmol/l

Dysarthria

Muscle twitching

Hyperreflexia

Cardiovascular collapse

Renal failure

Convulsions

Coma

---

forgotten about. Proper monitoring of lithium helps to reduce the risk.

The first step in management in such circumstances, if toxicity is even suspected, is to stop lithium immediately. Management should normally be on a medical ward. The underlying issue to remember in management is that the kidney excretes lithium. Unless suffering from renal failure, the patient should be kept extremely well hydrated with fluids containing a high concentration of sodium chloride to facilitate movement of lithium out of cells. In patients with impaired renal function dialysis is necessary.

If not managed promptly and assertively there is the potential for this to prove fatal. In more severe cases there is a risk of long-term neurological sequelae even following successful management of the acute toxic stage.

Acute dystonia

As covered in the Chapter 17, antipsychotic medications act on the dopaminergic system. One unwanted consequence of this can be acute dystonia. This can occur at any time following commencement of an antipsychotic but most typically occurs in the first 72 hours. It is most common in young men in the first stages of their illness. The first-generation antipsychotics, particularly the butyrophenones, are more likely to cause an acute dystonia but any of the antipsychotics can do so. The classic clinical signs of dystonia are set out in Box 18.9.

Acute treatment involves the administration of antimuscarinic drugs either orally or, in more severe instances, intramuscularly or even intravenously. This needs to be followed by review of the dose and type of antipsychotic prescribed.

Box 18.9: Acute dystonia

Involuntary sustained, painful muscular spasms affecting

- neck (spasmodic torticollis)
- jaw (trismus)
- eyes rolled upwards (oculogyric crisis)
- tongue protrusion
- trunk (opisthotonus)

Neuroleptic malignant syndrome

Neuroleptic malignant syndrome (NMS) is a rare condition but its severity, morbidity and potential mortality warrant its inclusion here. Although this disorder can occur at any stage of treatment, it occurs most commonly in the first 4–11 days, especially if there has been rapid dose escalation. The characteristic clinical features are set out in Box 18.10. There is some evidence it may more commonly occur in very hot conditions. Serotonin syndrome (see page 205) may present with some similar features and may have to be considered as a differential in patients on serotoninergic drugs.

As a first principle the patient should be treated in an environment where intensive medical support is available. The most important measures are supportive and no medication is specifically useful. The first thing to do is to stop all psychotropic medication but especially antipsychotic medication. Keeping the patient cool and well hydrated is of primary importance. It is important to monitor the patient's temperature, pulse, blood pressure and respiratory rate. In all cases a comprehensive infection screen should be performed. Diazepam may be useful and in more severe cases dantrolene has been used for muscle rigidity.

In the days before early recognition of this syndrome, up to 20 per cent of untreated cases of NMS proved fatal. It is important that following recovery any introduction of further antipsychotics is managed extremely cautiously and should only be attempted by a specialist, with careful monitoring of the patient's symptoms and vital signs.

Summary

In this chapter we have covered psychiatric emergencies and their management. DSH and acute behavioural disturbances are common and very likely to be encountered in your first few weeks of practice. Although lithium toxicity, dystonia and NMS are much less common, they carry potential for mortality if not identified and managed early. Their management is an essential skill for you to acquire.

Box 18.10: Signs of NMS

Muscle rigidity/severe extrapyramidal side-effects

Hyperthermia

Fluctuating consciousness

Autonomic disturbance (tachycardia, raised blood pressure, sweating)

Tachypnoea

Elevated white cell count

Raised creatine phosphokinase (CPK)

Further reading

Hawton K, van Heeringen K (2009) Suicide. *Lancet* 373: 1372–1381.

http://www.medicine.manchester.ac.uk/psychiatry/research/suicide/prevention/nci/inquiry reports/

NICE Guidance, 'Violence: The short-term management of disturbed/violent behaviour in psychiatric in-patient settings and emergency departments' (http://guidance.nice.org.uk/CG25/NICEGuidance/pdf/English)

CASE STUDY

A 56-year-old bank manager was admitted with acute dyspepsia and concerns that this was related to a significant gastric pathology. He was settled for the first 30 hours or so but shortly after the ward lights were dimmed he appeared to become distressed. When nursing staff approached him he appeared frightened and accused them of trying to harm him. He was sweating profusely and he appeared to be responding to auditory hallucinations.

Admission bloods were all within 'normal' limits apart from a mild RBC macrocytosis.

What might be your primary diagnosis?

What might be a useful avenue to pursue in obtaining useful information?

What might first steps in managing this man be?

The picture of sudden deterioration in mental state at darkness is characteristic of 'sundowner' syndrome, which typically is caused by an acute confusional state. Obviously the usual list of possible causes of confusion needs to be considered but with a gastric problem and a RBC macrocytosis an acute withdrawal state from alcohol would be top of your diagnostic list; in particular delirium tremens.

In all such cases corroborative histories are very useful but delay in obtaining one should not delay therapeutic intervention. See the chapter on substance misuse for details of what to look for in a drinking history.

In the first instance behavioural approaches such as turning on a brighter light and reducing unnecessary stimulation would be appropriate. Communication should be clear and use simple language. More detail is given above.

In addition to these non-pharmacological approaches he will need benzodiazepines. Hopefully he would accept them orally. High doses may need to be given and in addition to the regular medication, 'as required' medication should be available to allow the staff to titrate dosage against response. It will be important to closely monitor his basic vital signs.

Because of the risk of this man developing a Wernicke's encephalopathy parenteral thiamine should be given (see Chapter 12 for a discussion).

INDEX

Note: 'vs' indicates differential diagnosis.